Handbook of
Perinatal Clinical Psychology

The handbook examines the major issues in perinatal clinical psychology with the presence of theoretical information and operational indications, through a biopsychosocial approach.

The multiplicity of scientific information reported makes this handbook both a comprehensive overview on the major perinatal mental health disorders and illnesses, and a clinical guide. It covers perinatal clinical psychology through a journey of 15 chapters, putting the arguments on a solid theoretical basis and reporting multiple operational indications of great utility for daily clinical practice. It has well documented new evidence bases in the field of clinical psychology that have underpinned the conspicuous current global and national developments in perinatal mental health.

As such, it is an excellent resource for researchers, policy makers, and practitioners – in fact, anyone and everyone who wishes to understand and rediscover, in a single opera, the current scientific and application scenario related to psychological health during pregnancy and after childbirth.

Rosa Maria Quatraro (PhD, PgD Clinic Psy) is a psychologist, psychotherapist, and specialist in clinical psychology. For over 20 years, she has carried out clinical, research, training, and supervision duties in the field of perinatal psychology and psychopathology.

Pietro Grussu (PhD, PgD Clinic Psy) is a psychologist, psychotherapist, and specialist in clinical psychology. For over 30 years, he has carried out clinical and research duties in the field of perinatal psychology and psychopathology in the National Health Service and at Italian universities.

Handbook of Perinatal Clinical Psychology

From Theory to Practice

Edited by
Rosa Maria Quatraro and Pietro Grussu

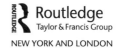

NEW YORK AND LONDON

English edition published 2020
by Routledge
52 Vanderbilt Avenue, New York, NY 10017

and by Routledge
2 Park Square, Milton Park, Abingdon, Oxon, OX14 4RN

Routledge is an imprint of the Taylor & Francis Group, an informa business

© 2020 Taylor & Francis

Original edition published 2018 by EDIZIONI CENTRO STUDI
ERICKSON S.p.A., TRENTO (ITALY)

Library of Congress Cataloging-in-Publication Data
Names: Quatraro, Rosa Maria, editor. | Grussu, Pietro, editor.
Title: Handbook of perinatal clinical psychology: from theory to practice /
edited by Rosa Maria Quatraro and Pietro Grussu.
Other titles: Psicologia clinica perinatale. English
Description: English edition. | New York, NY: Routledge, 2020. |
Originally published in Italian as Psicologia clinica perinatale.
Trento, Italy: Edizioni centro studi Erickson, S.p.A., c2018. |
Includes bibliographical references and index.
Identifiers: LCCN 2019050376 (print) | LCCN 2019050377 (ebook) |
ISBN 9780367369378 (hbk) | ISBN 9780367369385 (pbk) |
ISBN 9780429351990 (ebk)
Subjects: MESH: Pregnancy Complications—psychology |
Depression, Postpartum | Perinatal Death | Prenatal Diagnosis—psychology
Classification: LCC RG852 (print) | LCC RG852 (ebook) | NLM WQ 240 |
DDC 618.7/6—dc23
LC record available at https://lccn.loc.gov/2019050376
LC ebook record available at https://lccn.loc.gov/2019050377

ISBN: 978-0-367-36938-5 (pbk)
ISBN: 978-0-367-36937-8 (hbk)
ISBN: 978-0-429-35199-0 (ebk)

Typeset in Bembo
by codeMantra

Originally published in Italian as:
Psicologia clinica perinatale – Dalla teoria alla pratica

© 2018, BY EDIZIONI CENTRO STUDI ERICKSON S.p.A., TRENTO (ITALY)
All rights reserved

www.erickson.it
www.erickson.international

to those who have already given birth
to those who are about to give birth
to those who will give birth
to those who have been born

Contents

Contents

Authors' and Contributors' Biographies

Editors

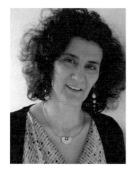

Rosa Maria Quatraro is a Psychologist, Psychotherapist, and Specialist in clinical psychology. For over 20 years, she has carried out clinical, research, training, and supervision duties in the field of perinatal psychology and psychopathology. She maintains a private practice in Padua and Vicenza (www.maternitaindifficolta.it) and works as contract psychologist at the San Bortolo Hospital, Azienda ULSS 8 Berica, Veneto Region, Italy in the Hospital Psychology Unit, Obstetrics and Gynecology Section, and at the Regional Center for Craniofacial Malformations. She is the author of over 50 national and international scientific publications on maternity psychology. Dr. Quatraro is currently Secretary of the Italian Marcé Society for Perinatal Mental Health, and a member of the International Marcé Society.

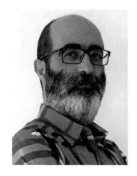

Pietro Grussu is a Psychologist, Psychotherapist, and Specialist in clinical psychology. He is the Head of the Family Service Unit and ONDa Italian Excellence Center "Integrated Services for Perinatal Depression", Padua South District, Azienda ULSS 6 Euganea, Veneto Region, Italy. He is the cofounder and current Vice President of the Italian Marcé Society for Perinatal Mental Health and the author of over 100 scientific publications. He has served as reviewer for major national and international mental health and clinical psychology journals. Dr. Grussu has taught courses in psychology, obstetrics, and educational sciences in the degree programs at the Italian Universities of Padua and Bolzano.

Authors

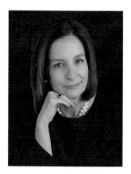

Cheryl Tatano Beck (DNSc, CNM, FAAN) is a Distinguished Professor at the University of Connecticut, School of Nursing. She also has a joint appointment at the Department of Obstetrics and Gynecology in the School of Medicine. She is a fellow in the American Academy of Nursing. Over the past 30 years, Cheryl has focused her research efforts on developing a research program on postpartum mood and anxiety disorders. She developed the Postpartum Depression Screening Scale (PDSS) which is published by Western Psychological Services. She is a prolific writer who has published over 150 journal articles and numerous award winning books such as *Nursing Research: Generating and Assessing Evidence for Nursing Practice.*

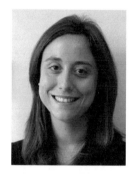

Alessandra Biaggi (PhD), is a Psychologist and a Researcher in perinatal psychiatry at the Institute of Psychiatry, Psychology & Neuroscience, King's College London. Since 2013, she has been working at the Institute on two longitudinal research projects on perinatal depression and postpartum psychosis, with a particular focus on risk factors, mother-infant relationship and infant development in the first year of life. In the past, through working with different institutions such as the University of Pavia and Fatebenefratelli Hospital in Milan and with different associations for women and parent-infant health, she has developed competence in perinatal psychiatry and in the observation and support of the parent-infant relationship.

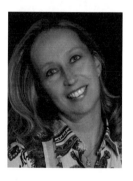

Alessandra Bramante is a Psychologist, Cognitive Psychotherapist, PhD in neuroscience. Consultant for Humanitas San Pio X Hospital, perinatal psychopathology service, Milan, and for Policentro Donna, Milan. President of the Marcé Italian regional Group for Perinatal Mental Health. She is the author of numerous scientific publications on filicide and maternal suicide and perinatal psychopathology. She is also speaker at national and international conferences.

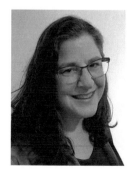

Wendy Davis (PhD) is the Executive Director of Postpartum Support International (PSI, www.postpartum.net). She also provided a counseling and consulting practice in Portland, Oregon, USA, specializing in pregnancy, birth, and postpartum mental health. She is the Founding Director of Baby Blues Connection (www.babybluesconnection.org), which is Oregon's first perinatal mental health support organization, and now serves as their volunteer training consultant. She chaired Oregon's Maternal Mental Health Workgroup convened by legislation in 2009, and the committee that wrote Oregon's Maternal Mental Health Patient and Provider Education Act in 2011. Wendy consults to community, clinical, and public health systems. She is dedicated to improving public awareness and provider capacity to increase resources for pregnant, post-loss, and postpartum families.

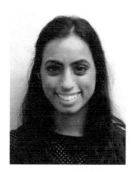

Preeya Desai (BA) is a Research Assistant at the Perinatal Pathways Lab of Columbia University Medical Center. She coordinates a randomized control trial assessing the efficacy of an intervention for postpartum depression on maternal mood and mother-infant bonding in a sample of low-income women. Her research interests are focused on the impacts of the parent-infant dyad on early child development, and interventions that may improve parent and child outcomes. She is planning to pursue a PhD in Clinical Psychology.

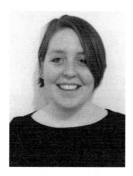

Sophie Foss (MA) is a PhD candidate in Clinical Psychology at Long Island University, Brooklyn, and a doctoral research student at the Perinatal Pathways Lab of Columbia University. Her graduate research investigates intergenerational and prenatal influences on childhood neurocognitive development. More specifically, her projects examine long-term effects of maternal childhood adversity on the prenatal environment, and how prenatal experiences influence and predict neurocognitive and behavioral development in infants and children. Her research utilizes a biopsychosocial framework, aiming to integrate biological factors and vulnerabilities with psychological experiences and social/environmental influences to understand and describe developmental processes in a comprehensive, holistic manner.

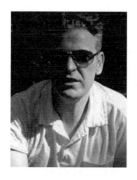

Alan W. Gemmill is Senior Research Fellow at the Parent-Infant Research Institute in Melbourne, Australia. He has conducted research on perinatal mental health for 17 years with a particular focus on randomized controlled trials of treatment and preventive intervention programs for maternal depression and anxiety. He has published widely on topics such as the neuro-developmental benefits of early stress reduction for premature infants, the major risk factors for perinatal depression and anxiety, and the predictive value of screening instruments for perinatal mood disorders. His ongoing work focuses on e-Mental Health solutions and protecting future child developmental outcomes by treating maternal mental disorders during pregnancy.

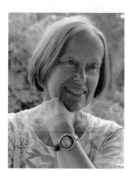

Nine M.-C. Glangeaud-Freudenthal (PhD) was trained in clinical and pathological psychology and in biochemistry. She was Research Fellow (retired) and Past-President of Marcé Society International. She hosted the international Biennial congress of this society in Paris, October 3–5, 2012. She is one of the founders and presently honorary member of the Francophone group of the Marcé society (SMF). In 1999, she initiated a national database (more than thousand inclusions). She researches on mother-baby joint inpatient admissions to mother-baby units in France and Belgium. She has also published several epidemiologic studies in collaboration with the working group UMB-SMF.

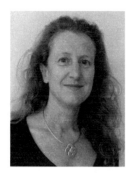

Elisabeth Glatigny (DESS, Master) is a psychologist. She did her master on mother-baby interactions under the supervision of Pr. Lebovici and was trained in attachment, CBT, and interpersonal psychotherapy (certified therapist, trainer, and supervisor by International Institute of Psychotherapy IsIPT). She contributed to a longitudinal study on postpartum depression and impact on infant development. She presently works at the "Perinatal Psychiatry Network" (inpatient mother-baby unit, liaison psychiatry) of the University Department of Adult Psychiatry in Bordeaux, France. She contributes to the networking perinatal mental health care organization in her region. She is a member of the Marcé Society and also a representative of the Francophone group.

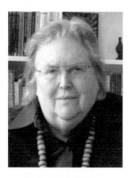

Vivette Glover is Visiting Professor of Perinatal Psychobiology at Imperial College London. Her group has shown how maternal prenatal stress, depression or anxiety increases the probability for a range of adverse neurodevelopmental outcomes for the child, together with some underlying biological mechanisms, including alterations to placental functioning. She has published over 450 papers, and has been awarded the Marcé Society Medal and the John Cox medal. She is currently an advisor to the All Party Parliamentary Group on the First 1001 Days, the Early Intervention Foundation, and the Global Alliance for Maternal Mental Health.

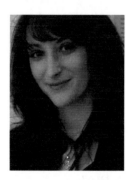

Nelly Goutaudier is Associate Professor in Psychopathology and Clinical Psychology at the University of Poitiers, France. She conducts research at the Center for Research on Cognition and Learning of the French National Center for Scientific Research (CNRS). Her main interests are perinatal psychopathology, adolescent psychopathology, and trauma- and stress-related disorders. She is the author of over 30 papers.

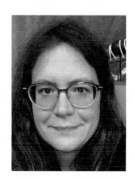

Florence Gressier (MD, PhD) is a Psychiatrist, and Head of the Perinatal Psychiatric Services including an inpatient mother-baby psychiatric unit, liaison psychiatry services, and perinatal consultations at Bicêtre University Department of Adult Psychiatry, in Le Kremlin Bicêtre, France. She is also a member of the research team at CESP, Inserm UMR1178. Since 2011, she has been involved in the Francophone Marcé Society and is presently president of the society. She has published critical reviews and studies on pharmacology and on perinatal mental health and psychiatry, in Journals such as *JAMA Pediatrics*, *J Psychiatr Res*, *Eur Neuropsychopharm*, *J Affect Disord*, *Am J Psychiatry*, and *Human Reproduction*.

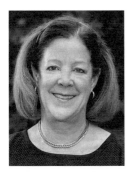

Sue L. Hall has been a Neonatologist for more than 25 years. She has a BA from Stanford University, an MSW from Boston University, and an MD from the University of Missouri-Kansas City. She was trained in Pediatrics and Neonatology at the Children's Mercy Hospital in Kansas City, Missouri, and then joined the faculty at UCLA's David Geffen School of Medicine where she was affiliated for 19 years. Now in practice at a community hospital NICU in Oxnard, California, Dr. Hall was Co-Editor of the paper "Interdisciplinary Recommendations for Psychosocial Support of NICU Parents" published in the *Journal of Perinatology* in December 2015.

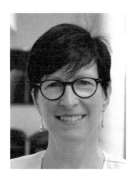

Dawn Kingston is Professor at the Faculty of Nursing in the University of Calgary.

Dr. Kingston holds the Lois Hole Hospital Cross-Provincial Chair in Perinatal Mental Health, and a national New Investigator Award from Canadian Institutes of Health Research.

Her research focuses on improving perinatal mental healthcare by developing and evaluating approaches to prevent and reduce depression and anxiety during pregnancy and beyond. She and her team are leading the field in using e-technology to build and evaluate integrated models of e-screening, e-referral, and e-therapy.

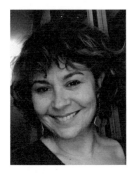

Ingrid Lacaze de Cordova has been trained as a Perinatal Psychiatric. She has a master's degree in alcohol abuse and clinical psychology. She has been working as a psychologist at the "Perinatal Psychiatry Network" in Bordeaux since 2011 and especially at the day care unit and at a neonatal unit and ambulatory care for children. She is also trained in psychoanalytic family therapy and in International Institute of Psychotherapy (IsIPT). She is presently doing supervision and training in this domain and more generally in perinatal mental health child early development. She is a member of Société Marcé Francophone (Association francophone pour l'étude des pathologies psychiatriques puerpérales et périnatales).

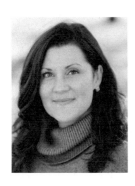

Kimberly McCue (PhD, MA) is Clinical Supervisor of the AMITA Health Perinatal Intensive Outpatient Program. Kimberly completed her PhD in clinical psychology from Illinois Institute of Technology. She earned a Master's Degree in Social Cognitive Neuroscience from the University of Chicago and a Bachelor of Science in Psychology and Biology from Northwestern University. She completed her Clinical Psychology Internship at Alexian Brothers Behavioral Health Hospital in Child & Adolescent Psychology. Kimberly has worked as a Perinatal and Infant Mental Health Specialist at Chicago's Stroger Hospital of Cook County. She also has specialized training in developmental neurophysiology and pediatric neuropsychology. Kimberly is a member of Postpartum Support International, the Association for Psychological Sciences, the Midwest Neuropsychological Society, the Society for Research in Child Development, and the American Psychological Association.

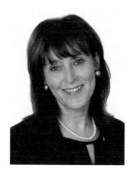

Jeannette Milgrom is Professor of Psychology at Melbourne School of Psychological Sciences, University of Melbourne and Director of the Parent-Infant Research Institute, Austin Health, Melbourne. She has supervised 9 PhD, 17 DPsych, 8 MA/Sc, and 5 BGrad Dip students. Jeannette established the Parent-Infant Research Institute (PIRI) in 2001 conducting basic and applied research (ante and postnatal depression, prematurity, developing psychological treatments – mothers, fathers, and babies), and she has been working with *beyondblue* since 2001. She is the recipient and CI of over 70 research grants and also the author of 8 books, 18 chapters, and 126 scientific articles.

Jeannette is Past President of International Marcé Society for Perinatal Mental Health.

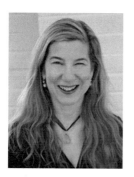

Catherine Monk is Professor of Medical Psychology in the Departments of Psychiatry and Obstetrics & Gynecology, Director of Research of the Women's Program at Columbia University Medical Center, and Research Scientist VI at the New York State Psychiatric Institute. She studies prenatal influences on children's development — and how to intervene early to improve children's health trajectories. Her research has identified maternal prenatal depression effects in fetal behavior, placental DNA methylation, and newborn brain development via imaging. She is an advisor to Zero to Three and the Seleni Institute. Her work is supported by the National Institutes of Health, the March of Dimes, the Brain Behavior Research Foundation, the Robin Hood Foundation, and Johnson & Johnson.

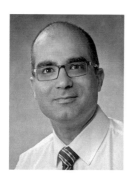

Muhammad Kashif Mughal is a Postdoctoral Fellow at the Faculty of Nursing in the University of Calgary.

His research work aims to understand the impact of early childhood adversities, including poor perinatal mental health, on child's mental and physical health and development. His current postdoctoral project involves investigating the underlying genetic, epigenetic, and biological causes of child resiliency in a large prospective pregnancy cohort of mothers and children in Canada.

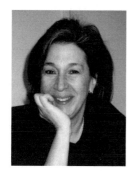

Joann Paley Galst (PhD) is a Psychologist in private practice in New York City specializing in mind-body medicine and reproductive health issues including infertility, pregnancy loss, pregnancy termination due to fetal anomaly, pregnancy and parenting after loss, infertility, third-party reproduction, and postpartum reactions. She is a past Chair of the Mental Health Professional Group of the American Society for Reproductive Medicine, Past Chair of the Mental Health Advisory Council, past Co-Director of Support Services of the Path2Parenthood (formerly the American Fertility Association), and a member of the Board of Advisors of the Pregnancy Loss Support Program of the National Council of Jewish Women-NY Section. She is a co-author of *Ethical Dilemmas in Fertility Counseling*, published by the American Psychological Association in 2010, and a co-editor and chapter author of *Prenatal and Preimplantation Diagnosis: The Burden of Choice*, published by Springer in 2015.

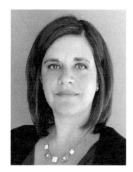

Brenda Papierniak (PsyD, LCPC, MT-BC, PMH) has 20 years of experience in the fields of mental health and medicine. She has worked in hospital, outpatient, and community mental health settings where much of her work has been with women and children with a special focus on maternal mental health of women and teens. Dr. Papierniak is a Perinatal Health Psychologist with AMITA Health/Alexian Brothers in the Pregnancy and Postpartum Mood & Anxiety Disorder Program. She also recently started a Perinatal Health Psychology Program at AMITA Health in the NICU and Antepartum units where she will be developing a training program for future psychologists. She has degrees in Music Therapy, Counseling, and a PsyD in Clinical Psychology. She has served as the Social Services Coordinator for Postpartum Support International's Illinois Chapter.

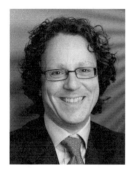

Carmine M. Pariante, (MD, FRCPsych, PhD), is Professor of Biological Psychiatry at the Institute of Psychiatry, Psychology and Neuroscience, King's College London, and Consultant Perinatal Psychiatrist at the South London and Maudsley NHS Trust. He investigates the role of stress in the pathogenesis of mental disorders and in the response to psychotropic drugs, both in clinical samples and experimental settings. His work focuses on depression and fatigue, with a particular interest in the perinatal period and in subjects with medical disorders. Professor Pariante has received numerous awards for his research, most recently the 2012 "Academic Psychiatrist of the Year" Award from the Royal College of Psychiatrists, the 2015 Anna-Monika Prize for Research on Depression, and the 2017 Andrea Leadsom Award for Outstanding Contribution to the Field of Infant Mental Health. He can be followed on Twitter @ParianteSPILab and on http://www.huffingtonpost.co.uk/carmine-pariante/.

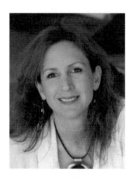

Jenny Perkel is a Clinical Psychologist working in private practice in Cape Town, South Africa. She is the author of *Babies in Mind* and a founder member of the *Babies in Mind* service. She is on the editorial board of the professional journal, *Psychoanalytic Psychotherapy in South Africa* and she is past chairperson of the *Western Cape Association for Infant Mental Health*. She works with infants, children, and their parents, as well as individual adults. She is also involved in training, supervision, and consultation with practitioners involved in child and infant mental health care. She can be reached online at www.jennyperkel.com, www.babiesinmind.co.za, and www.childreninmind.co.za; or on her e-mail at jenny@perkel.co.za.

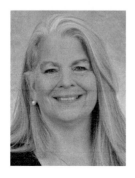

Christena Raines (RN, MSN, APRN-BC) is an Associate Professor at the University of North Carolina in Chapel Hill Perinatal Psychiatry Program within the UNC Center for Women's Mood Disorders. Chris is trained in Women's Health and is board certified in Psychiatric-Mental Health. She works as a Perinatal Psychiatric Nurse Practitioner and was a member of the planning team instrumental in opening the first in-patient Perinatal Mental Health unit in the country. She also serves on the Board of Directors of Postpartum Support International as Vice President.

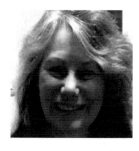

Joan Raphael-Leff is both Transcultural Psychologist and Psychoanalyst. Since qualification with the British Psychoanalytical Society in 1976, she specialized in treating reproductive and early parenting issues. As an academic, she was Professor of Psychoanalysis at the Centre for Psychoanalytic Studies at the University of Essex, UK, and Head of University College London's MSc in Psychoanalytic Developmental Psychology. She is Now retired, and leads the Anna Freud Centre Academic Faculty for Psycho-analytic Research. In 1998, she co-founded and was overall chair of COWAP, the International Psychoanalytic Association's committee on Women and Psychoanalysis. She is author or editor of 12 books and over 150 single-authored peer-reviewed professional publications. Her writings are translated into Chinese, Dutch, French, Flemish, Greek, Hebrew, Hungarian, Italian, Japanese, Polish, Portuguese, and Spanish. She continues to teach in many countries, where she is consultant to perinatal and women's projects.

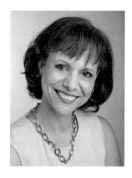

Lisa S. Segre is an Associate Professor at the College of Nursing in the University of Iowa. She is the President of the International Marcé Society. As a graduate of the Community/Clinical doctoral program at the University of Illinois, Urbana Champaign, her research focuses on the dissemination and evaluation of (1) maternal depression screening programs and (2) Listening Visits, a depression treatment delivered by non-mental health specialists. In partnership with Iowa's Department of Public Health, Dr. Segre implemented depression screening and Listening Visits in social service agencies throughout Iowa. Her recent research extends Listening Visits to mothers of hospitalized newborns.

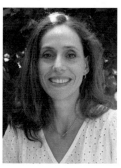

Natalène Séjourné is an Associate Professor in psychopathology at the University of Toulouse Jean-Jaurès in France. She works on perinatal psychopathology and has published several papers on miscarriage and perinatal loss.

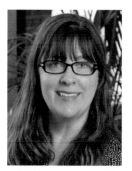

Lita Simanis (MSW, LCSW, PMH-C) is the Coordinator of the Pregnancy & Postpartum Mood & Anxiety Disorder Program at AMITA Health/Alexian Brothers. Here, she developed the first perinatal intensive outpatient program in the state of Illinois that opened its doors in August, 2015.

She is also a Perinatal Crisis Counselor for the Illinois Mom's Line, is Secretary on the Board of Directors for Postpartum Support International, and is a Board Member of the International Marcé Society for Perinatal Mental Health. She is the co-coordinator of the Postpartum Depression Illinois Alliance.

Lita started a quarterly Perinatal Mental Health Provider breakfast. She participates in the National Partnership for Women & Families and is a member of the Illinois Department of Public Health Maternal Mortality Review Committee.

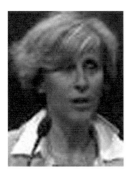

Anne-Laure Sutter-Dallay is an Adult and Child Psychiatrist, and head of the "Perinatal Psychiatry Network" (inpatient and day-care mother-baby units, liaison psychiatry) of the University Department of Adult Psychiatry in Bordeaux, France. She is a researcher at Research Center INSERM 1219 (Population Health). She is also involved in the ELFE survey (French longitudinal study since childhood) and Mother-Baby Units database analysis. Since 1993, she has been an active member of the International Marcé Society and is a founder, past president and presently scientific coordinator of the Société Marcé Francophone.

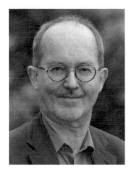

Tewes Wischmann (Ph.D. Senior Research Associate, Chair of the project team "Gynaecological Psychology") is an Associate Professor at the Institute of Medical Psychology of Heidelberg University Hospital, Heidelberg, Germany. He earned his MSc (Diploma) in psychology in 1984 and his Ph.D. (Dr. sc. hum.) in medical psychology at the Heidelberg University in 1998. In 2001, he became a trained Jungian psychoanalyst at the CG Jung Institute Stuttgart. His current work field is counseling for infertile couples, for patients with recurrent pregnancy loss, and for patients with endometriosis. He has published several books and scientific papers on the topic and is a co-author of national and international guidelines in the field. For more detail on Wischmann, visit www.dr-wischmann.com.

Acknowledgments

Handbook of Perinatal Clinical Psychology: From Theory to Practice comes from Rosa Maria's idea, from Pietro's perseverance, and from our like-mindedness and compatibility. But above all, it comes from a small project that started with a local connotation and that instead ended with a work of international standing.

In reality, all this began many years ago, thanks to the teachings of Ruggero Cerutti and Mariapia Sichel, to whom we address our special thanks.

The experience, and the clinical and research skills we gained at the Department of Obstetrics and Gynecology, University of Padua (Italy), led us to develop an extensive publishing project in perinatal psychology. This initial intent has been warmly welcomed by Dario Ianes and Riccardo Mazzeo, from the Italian publishing house Edizioni Centro Studi Erickson. They have supported the publication of numerous books and the possibility of opening a constructive scientific and cultural debate on the psychology of motherhood in Italy. After our first publication over 15 years ago, *Handbook of Perinatal Clinical Psychology* – thanks to the support of numerous collaborators and friends – is our first handbook contribution to international literature. Therefore, we are extremely grateful to Dario, Riccardo, and the Erickson group for starting this invaluable publishing experience. Thank you so much.

A special word of gratitude goes to Carmine Pariante and Lisa S. Segre for accepting our proposal to be part of the scientific committee of the series "Psychology of motherhood", also published by Erickson, and, after a careful analysis of the index and the contents of this book, for giving us useful suggestions, competent and accurate support, and all their generous and precious assistance.

Certainly, the amazing Erickson editorial team has been fundamental in building *Handbook of Perinatal Clinical Psychology*. In particular, we are grateful to Elena Martinelli, Nicoletta Rivelli, and Silvia Moretti for their help, support, and availability. We thank Tania Eccher for her painstaking work. We would also like to thank Valeria Agliuzzo for her commitment and dedication to the international diffusion of this book.

The *dream team* of international authors who agreed to be part of this publishing project honors and gratifies us: it has been a lengthy project lasting three intense years. Many thanks to Dawn and Kashif, Catherine, Sophie, Preeya and Vivette, Joan, Tewes, Joann, Natalène and Nelly, Cheryl, Lisa and Sue, Wendy, Kimberly, Brenda, Christena and Lita, Jenny, Jeannette and Alan, Alessandra and Carmine, Alessandra, Florence, Ingrid, Elisabeth, Nine and Anne-Laure, Fiona, and John.

We also thank Donna Ann Wawrykow for her important contribution relative to the linguistic form of some parts of this book, and Alessandra Biaggi and Lita Simanis for their collaboration in the correction of various drafts.

Our apologies go to Anna and Margherita, for the many hours we spent in front of the computer sending hundreds of e-mails and working late into the weekend evenings. We promise, the next weekends – and many to follow – will be devoted entirely to them.

Foreword

There have been many shocking statistics related to perinatal mental health in recent news head-lines, for example, one in four women has a mental health problem during pregnancy and a quar-ter of women who died between six weeks and one year after pregnancy in the UK died from mental health-related causes. These statistics are just some examples that can be found worldwide and they demonstrate the breadth and severity of the psychological problems women may face around the time of birth. Much can and needs to be done to support these women and their fam-ilies. It is also important to be mindful of the many women who will have a relatively uneventful, healthy pregnancy and adjust well to parenting. For these women, a greater focus on psychological well-being in the perinatal period can *optimize* health around the time of birth and have a signif-icant impact on their longer term health and well-being. This handbook provides clear examples of how we can make a difference to the health and well-being of all women, and their families, as they manage perinatal decisions and events.

Mental health care continues to languish in the shadow of physical health care. On reading this book you quickly become aware of the folly of mind-body dualism as a too simplistic solution to a complex problem. If, like me, you work in the field of reproductive health, you will recognize your own biases toward identifying and treating the physical outcomes of infertility, miscarriage, and complications in pregnancy, during and after birth. This book helps you to delve into the complex relationship between physical and mental health when considering these unique events. Each chapter is a testament to the international work that has been done to date to try and disen-tangle the unique features of psychological health in the perinatal period – exploring contexts and factors that can mask psychological problems, and highlighting the psychological challenges that parents face in their decision making and when complications arise.

This handbook provides a wealth of information, from research and practice, from experts in the field covering an array of psychological issues: the experience of perinatal stress; psychological issues during pregnancy, delivery, and the postnatal period; and the risk of psychopathology and prevention. It is striking that on many occasions research findings suggest there should be simple solutions to psychological problems that arise at this time. For example, the importance of social support in the perinatal period to maintain psychological well-being seems common sense and yet we often fail to offer support to those women who need it. Conversely, giving birth can feel like an increasing complex event and this book also offers us support in understanding much of the complexity that new technology and scientific progress brings, for example, in the fields of reproducible biotechnology, prenatal diagnosis, and neonatal care. In addition to understanding the reproductive impact on women and their families, the book highlights the main social and ethical issues these new developments bring to us all.

Many topics covered are challenging for parents, health professionals, and society alike and this book provides a balanced and sensitive approach. The chapter on prenatal screening for congenital anomalies highlights the decisions that parents have to make and provides guidance on how to sup-port parents through the range of potential outcomes. Examples are given of a psychotherapeutic intervention for women who have chosen to terminate a pregnancy with fetal anomaly as well as how to offer psychological support for those who chose to continue a pregnancy with either a viable or nonviable fetal anomaly.

The *Handbook of Perinatal Clinical Psychology: From Theory to Practice* is an excellent resource for researchers, policy makers, and practitioners – in fact, anyone who wants to understand something of the importance of perinatal psychology. It also provides us with challenges – a challenge to change how we think about perinatal health and perinatal clinical psychology and a challenge to truly work to an integrated psychological and physical health model.

Professor Fiona Alderdice
National Perinatal Epidemiology Unit
University of Oxford
United Kingdom

Introduction

Rosa Maria Quatraro and Pietro Grussu

The ever-increasing attention being given to perinatal psychological and psychiatric disorders has led to the continuing exponential growth in the number of research studies on the topic and, consequently, an increase in our knowledge of perinatal clinical psychology and psychiatry. In the United Kingdom, in a document concerning the economic burden of the problems of perinatal mental health, Bauer and colleagues (2014) point out that the long-term costs of perinatal depression, anxiety and postpartum psychoses equal £8.1 million yearly – in other words, £10,000 for each newborn, the largest part of which is committed to the adverse effects on the baby. Different parts of this book illustrate elements like this, and make it clear that perinatal mental health cannot and should not be a luxury of the few. This is not a discussion about the well-being of a single individual, but of the whole family and, above all, of future generations. In this context, perinatal clinical psychology can and must give maximum attention not only to women and their families, but also to the training of the healthcare providers who work in the perinatal field.

In a document published in 2016 on the role of perinatal clinical psychology in the English perinatal services, the British Psychological Society maintains that a clinical psychologist should be included in maternity wards and neonatal intensive care units of hospitals with more than 3,000 deliveries annually, as well as within integrated perinatal mental health service departments of both local health units and their hospital counterparts. The scope of the clinical psychologist's involvement is not just the care of the patient, but also the supervision and training of the personnel and the multidisciplinary teams that deal with perinatal mental health. It is important to remember that women who are emotionally ill during the perinatal period have a clear preference for psychological support rather than for psychotropic drugs (Buist, O'Mahen and Rooney, 2015) which are, in certain situations, the first line of treatment, but, in others, may not be considered necessary if there is an alternate means of arriving at a correct diagnosis and effective treatment. This reality makes the need for perinatal clinical psychology even more important so that efficient and effective interventions can be structured for both the prevention and the treatment of perinatal emotional disorders. From this perspective, the projects and strategies for reducing the suffering and the stress which may be associated with pregnancy and the postpartum period are of significant importance. In other words, the clinical psychologist cannot and should not be concerned exclusively with perinatal psychopathology, but must be available to intervene – before as well as after the birth of the child – when events that can cause stress and emotional hardship arise.

In the last 20 years, increasing attention has been focused on depressive, anxiety and psychotic disorders of the perinatal period. Recently, attention to subclinical disorders has become such a health necessity that the National Institute of Health and Care Excellence (2018) places particular emphasis on the advisability of detecting and treating the anxious and depressive symptoms that arise in the perinatal period. The idea is to enhance the emotional health and well-being of all women who face the delicate transition to motherhood (Alderdice, McNeill and Lynn, 2013). Alongside this, we must consider that recently, with the advances of biotechnologies and with the progress of perinatal medicine, it is increasingly critical to devote the proper attention to all of those conditions of serious physical and emotional stress that can arise when one is trying to become pregnant or to carry a pregnancy to term, during labor and delivery, and immediately after the birth of the child.

From a preventive perspective and with a view to reducing emotional suffering that sometimes takes the form of real pathology, it is important, then, to offer support and appropriate psychological interventions to women and couples who face assisted fertilization, cope with a prenatal diagnosis, deal with pregnancy-related grief (repeated miscarriages, repeated and/or late spontaneous abortions, fetal or neonatal endo-uterine deaths), experience premature births with the related admission to Neonatal Intensive Care, face high-risk pregnancies and/or traumatic deliveries, go through emotional difficulties typical of the postpartum period, have concerns about nurturing and caring for their baby, or struggle with breastfeeding.

Perinatal clinical psychology is called upon to intervene in all of these areas with effective and appropriate methods that limit the consequences of these perinatal events on the health of the mother, of the couple and, above all, on the health of the child. It is an investment in future generations – a chance to intervene while the child's mind is still developing and being shaped by the attitudes and perspectives of the mother and the parental couple. It is precisely by intervening with supportive and therapeutic strategies on the mental and emotional functioning of the mother and the parental couple that we can have the maximum results in terms of interrupting the transgenerational transmission of trauma and stress to the offspring, thus reducing the risk of psychopathology in the children.

This handbook originates from our "field experience" as clinical psychologists who have been dealing with most of the issues covered in this text for many years. We wanted to put forward an idea that goes beyond the mind-body dualism. In this spirit, it seems important to open wide the field of perinatal mental health and its clinical conditions to attract the attention and concern of governments and health policy makers, as well as clinicians in the social context, be they psychologists, obstetricians, pediatric nurses, perinatal healthcare providers or numerous specialists who take care of women and children during the perinatal period (psychiatrists, child neuropsychiatrists, pediatricians, general practitioners).

The specific objective of this collection is to explore all the situations that, in the period preceding and following childbirth, can cause emotional distress to the woman, the couple and the family, including the children to come. Each part deals with one aspect of perinatal clinical psychology and in each part, different authors – everyone an expert in a specific field of the clinical psychology of pregnancy and the postnatal period – develop their subject matter to offer an updated configuration of the literature and, subsequently, to discuss the principal intervention techniques that can be implemented by the clinical psychologist.

The first part, comprised of the two opening chapters, provides an in-depth knowledge of the literature on stress and its effects on the mother and the child during pregnancy and after delivery. This very important topical issue is addressed by two of the foremost research groups engaged for many years in the study of perinatal stress: the team of Dawn Kingston and Muhammad Kashif Mughal from the University of Calgary; and that of Catherine Monk and Vivette Glover, assisted by their associates Sophie Foss and Preeya Desai. In their contributions, the authors describe the effects of stress on future generations and the related transmission mechanisms on which research is steadily moving forward with increasingly interesting findings. In addition, there is a focus on stress reduction programs and on screening methods for women who experience situations of intense perinatal distress.

The second part, which covers procreation, pregnancy and delivery, focuses instead on the adverse events that can lead to risk factors for perinatal emotional disorders, whether simultaneously with an established or interrupted pregnancy or during subsequent pregnancies and postpartum periods. The chapters of this second part unfold from a starting point of the clinical reality of those who work with women daily and who find themselves dealing with ever more complex maternity situations. Increased maternal and paternal age, environmental pollutants and stress have led to a reduction in fertility which is increasingly being overcome by homologous- and heterologous-assisted fertilization, as well as by biotechnology. All of this, though, has personal and social costs that can only be partially foreseen and that give us cause to reflect, as put forward by Joan Raphael-Leff. The costs, however, are also emotional. These women and couples are in fact often bearers of intense suffering that is little expressed and shared, and which needs to be seen, accepted and listened to by society, by doctors and by healthcare workers so that the women and the couples themselves can take charge of it. This option, as Tewes Wischmann explains in Chapter 4, also has a preventive value with respect to perinatal emotional health and to the parent-child relationship.

Progress has also brought with it the increasingly sophisticated possibility of carrying out prenatal diagnoses, permitting practitioners to detect the health of the fetus and the presence of eventual genetic and/or functional anomalies. This prospect, with the associated choice of how to intervene, opens up an ethical and human dilemma that couples rarely face with indifference, and this topic is explored in depth by Joann Paley Galst. The decision that presents itself – therapeutic abortion or continuation of the pregnancy despite fetal deformities or health problems – requires specific interventions that reduce the adverse impacts of these actions not only on the woman and the couple, but also on any other children, current or future.

Another situation with comparable repercussions and additional unique aspects is the grief related to pregnancy in which it is important to include not only fetal endo-uterine deaths and neonatal deaths, but also spontaneous abortions and recurrent spontaneous abortions. All of these events, discussed extensively and comprehensively by Natalène Séjourmé and Nelly Goutaudier, can give rise to reactions of emotional suffering and, in some cases, to real psychopathologies such as post-traumatic stress disorder or a grief disorder. Clinical situations like these, until a few years ago, were barely taken into account by health professionals, and were experienced only within the intimacy of the affected couple. Today, more and more events such as these are becoming moments to be shared and to be acted upon by perinatal practitioners, with both preventive and remedial interventions.

Another issue that is also currently receiving a great deal of attention in the clinical setting is traumatic births and their negative psychological impact not only on the woman/couple but also on the healthcare practitioners who assist the new mothers. The topic is masterfully developed in all its facets by Cheryl Tatano Beck. Her innovative interpretation of each actor's role in the birth scene calls for the clinical psychologist to intervene (directly or indirectly) using suitable means to limit a negative ripple effect.

The third part is dedicated to the postpartum period, a time of transition and of physical, psychological, social and relational changes. A woman must carry out or satisfy multiple demands, and now that the baby is a real living being, the mother experiences a period of physical and psychological adjustment, as well as a time of adaptation to her new role. This transition and its challenges are described in Chapter 8 by Rosa Maria Quatraro and Pietro Grussu. Particular attention is focused on the experiences, the emotional sensitivity and the stress reactions that characterize the first postpartum weeks. Our contribution also confronts the thorny issue of assistance – during the hospital stay and after the return home – and the health needs exhibited by women. The chapter gives a number of practical clinical hints and describes the support interventions that are of greatest efficacy when seeking to prevent stress from leading to psychopathology.

The birth of a child is not always a joyous event. Premature births, or newborns with physical problems requiring hospitalization in Neonatal Intensive Care are, in fact, a continually growing reality. Parents who must face this delicate and difficult situation can experience emotional distress and practical difficulties of various kinds. In Chapter 9 by Lisa S. Segre and Sue L. Hall, following their complete and exhaustive review of the literature on the topic, the authors introduce diverse methodologies for psychological efforts and psychosocial support to assist these "special" parents of "special" children.

The importance of social support – be it emotional or practical – to help women who are suffering emotionally during the perinatal period is comprehensively discussed in Chapter 10 written by an outstanding team from the American group Postpartum Support International (Wendy Davis, Kimberly McCue, Brenda Papierniak, Christena Raines and Lita Simanis). Starting from a review of the most current research on the role of social support in maternal well-being and in the treatment of perinatal emotional disorders, the chapter provides a complete overview of different types of support – both institutional and informal – and provides useful operational guidelines for relatives and healthcare providers. In our opinion, of special interest is the attention given to the support directed toward populations with specific needs, such as adolescent mothers, homosexual couples and families who come from other cultures or who have specific religious beliefs.

A subject that is particularly dear to mothers and healthcare providers – and that is also the object of important international initiatives by UNICEF and the World Health Organization, not to mention various national governments – is breastfeeding. In this book, the breastfeeding theme has been developed as an issue regarding the mother-child relationship, which from birth is mediated by nutrition. The psychological factors related to breastfeeding and weaning are exhaustively developed by Jenny Perkel, who underscores how conflicts, hopes and fears are focused on this subject. Often for mothers, and unfortunately sometimes even for healthcare providers, breastfeeding becomes the litmus test of how much a woman knows about being a good mother, and how good of a mother she feels herself to be for her child. This has important psychological repercussions for both mother and child. The difficulties of breastfeeding and weaning can, however, also be an opportunity for growth. The author in fact invites the reader to reconsider these stalemates in breastfeeding and weaning, and to view them as an opportunity to explore deeper emotional problems potentially linked to the mental state of the mother and/or the newborn and their relationship.

Finally, in the fourth and final part, we thought it necessary to also make room for perinatal psychopathology to which clinical psychology is devoted in its own right alongside perinatal psychiatry, not only in the screening and primary prevention phases, but also in the treatment phase by means of psychotherapeutic interventions focused on the woman, and on the mother-child relationship.

The contribution from Jeannette Milgrom and Alan W. Gemmill in Chapter 12 places different forms of emotional suffering not only within the new DSM-5 criteria, but also in terms of a sub-threshold disorder that does not permit a classical psychiatric diagnosis. As it unfolds, the chapter takes into account maternal illness and considers the most up-to-date research on the outcomes of cognitive-behavioral psychotherapy. The authors also explore the possible consequences of maternal psychological distress on the mother-child relationship, and offer their own working model.

The following two chapters cover two very important topics regarding the prevention of perinatal emotional disorders: the risk factors, and screening programs for early detection of women who are suffering.

Alessandra Biaggi and Carmine M. Pariante in Chapter 13 give us an overview, based on the most current data, of the principal psychosocial, environmental and gynecological risk factors which can lead to an onset of prenatal and postnatal depression and anxiety. The authors point out that an accurate risk assessment, carried out through multidimensional screening during the perinatal period, could enable the timely application of preventive interventions focused on modifiable risk factors. Subsequently, in Chapter 14 on screening and detection of women at risk of perinatal psychopathology, Alessandra Bramante helps us to understand not only why the implementation of screening procedures is desirable and what is the state of the art at an international level, but also what is the best action to take after identifying women who are at risk or who are already emotionally suffering. Additional issues under discussion include the tools to use, the practitioners to involve in screening procedures, how and when to activate the procedures and the recommendations endorsed by the principal international agencies dealing with the mental health of pregnant and postpartum women, including the International Guidelines on Perinatal Psychopathology.

The handbook closes with a chapter on psychotic conditions and bipolar disorders during the perinatal period which, although rare, require an in-depth investigation not only by psychiatrists, but by all clinicians. Being familiar with acute psychopathology is necessary in order to distinguish minor from ostensibly major psychopathology.

The clinical psychologist is, in fact, also called upon to work in these specific contexts both as therapist and as supervisor of a psychosocial team engaged in individual situations that have an immense impact on the health not only of the woman, but also of the child and the family. Early recognition of the onset of perinatal psychosis and its prodromal symptoms can not only save the life of a mother and her child, but also permit timely therapeutic intervention.

The distinction between psychoses, depression and bipolar disorder is well defined by a team from the French Marcé group (Florence Gressier, Ingrid Lacaze de Cordova, Elisabeth Glatigny, Nine Glangeaud-Freudenthal and Anne-Laure Sutter-Dallay). In those situations referred to above, according to the authors of this chapter, it is of primary importance to be able to prescribe suitable pharmacological treatments and psychological therapies integrated within a remedial broad-spectrum therapeutic strategy that is aimed at the mother, but also at the mother-child-father relationship, such as the therapies offered by the mother-baby units in many countries of the world.

Today, in many parts of the world, the assistance given to mothers with psychotic perinatal disorders is unquestionably inadequate. These women are admitted to hospital in the psychiatric wards without the possibility of having their child nearby, causing a profound negative impact on their lived experience as a mother, and on the mother-baby relationship.

In the face of all this, *Handbook of Perinatal Clinical Psychology: From Theory to Practice* was conceived and written to offer a far-reaching overview of this broad area of application and research.

The content developed within this work – greatly needed and painstakingly realized – is directed not only toward those who are showing their first interest in clinical psychology in the perinatal field, but also toward those who have been working in the field for years and sense the need to keep up to date by delving into a high-level narrative on the subject.

In this handbook, students, interns, researchers and professionals of various disciplines will find updated knowledge as well as encouragement and motivation to take an integrated and multidisciplinary approach to safeguard and sustain perinatal health. Moreover, there are suggestions of how and when to intervene in an appropriate way when the situation requires it.

Being aware of all that is available in the scientific literature thanks to the enormous body of work carried out and disseminated by researchers all over the world must not, in our opinion, be the privilege or the duty of a few. Knowledge in the perinatal field is in continual evolution, but what we know today must dutifully and responsibly be made known to the widest possible audience of professionals.

If we have an in-depth knowledge of all that the scientific literature makes available to us, we are in possession of an initial wealth of skills. Thanks to these fundamentals, we can structure effective and efficient prevention interventions at various levels.

It is also our belief that investing in this project of dissemination and instruction worldwide will stimulate future generations of colleagues, and will enrich the training and knowledge of health professionals. It is their contribution that is of primary importance so that the experience of motherhood and parenthood can be a time of growth and development for the individual, the couple and the family, and not a hardship or, in some cases, even a disease.

We believe it.
Buona lettura.

Padova (Italy), May 26, 2019

References

Alderdice, F., McNeill, J., & Lynn, F. (2013). A systematic review of systematic reviews of interventions to improve maternal mental health and well-being. *Midwifery*, *29*(4), 389–399.

Bauer, A., Parsonage, M., Knapp, M., Iemmi, V., & Adelaja, B. (2014). *The Costs of Perinatal Mental Health Problems*. London, UK: Centre for Mental Health and London School of Economics.

British Psychological Society (2016). Perinatal psychology provision in specialist perinatal community mental health services. Position paper.

Buist, A., O'Mahen, H., Rooney, R. (2015). Acceptability, attitudes, and overcoming stigma. In Milgrom, J., & A. Gemmill (Eds.), *Identifying Perinatal Depression and Anxiety: Evidence-based Practice in Screening, Psychosocial Assessment and Management* (pp. 51–62). John Wiley & Sons, Ltd: New York.

National Institute for Health and Care Excellence NICE (2018). Antenatal and postnatal mental health. Clinical management and service guidance. Updated edition. National Clinical Guideline Number 192. Published by The British Psychological Society and The Royal College of Psychiatrists.

Part I

Stress

1

Overview of Perinatal Maternal Stress

Dawn Kingston and Muhammad Kashif Mughal

The Concept of Perinatal Maternal Stress

The "definition" of stress has been hotly debated for decades – a reflection of its conceptual, behavioral, and physiological complexity. At the heart of the stress process is the body's adaptive response to a threatening environmental stress by instigating the sympathetic nervous system and the hypothalamic-pituitary-adrenal (HPA) axis. The resultant release of glucocorticoids – the endpoint of the stress response – leads to a cascade of events in the brain that contributes to epigenetic changes, remodeling of neurons and synapses, neurogenesis, neuroinflammation, and circuitry remapping (McEwen, Bowles, et al., 2015; Sapolsky, 2015). While intended as an acute, adaptive response to promote safety and survival in a threatening situation, the persistent activation of the stress response that characterizes modern social stress can lead to physiological (e.g., over-activation of the HPA axis, over-secretion of glucocorticoids) and experiential (e.g., physical and emotional exhaustion, a feeling of not being in control, low self-esteem) overload over months and years (McEwen et al., 2015).

Some of the key aspects of stress that have emerged with the resurgence of stress research over the past few decades are:

- The stress response can be activated solely by psychological states and thoughts, especially those of loss of control and unpredictability, the experience of low social support (Sapolsky, 2015), and the perception of whether stress is a negative (i.e., damaging) or positive (i.e., growth-producing) force (Crum, Akinola, Martin, & Fath, 2017; Crum, Salovey, & Achor, 2013).
- The experience of stress and its outcomes vary dramatically across individuals (Sapolsky, 2015). Indeed, Sapolsky argues that the stressor itself is of less consequence than the individual's perception as they manage life's challenges (Sapolsky, 2015).
- Prenatal stress can have deleterious physical and emotional effects not only for the immediate offspring, but also across generations through epigenetic mechanisms (Babenko, Kovalchuk, & Metz, 2015; Metz, Ng, Kovalchuk, & Olson, 2015).
- Most physiologic endpoints, structural outcomes (e.g., synaptic plasticity in the hippocampus), and behavior show an inverted-U pattern in response to a stressor and the concomitant stress response. In other words, at ranges of very low and high stress, an individual's outcomes are worse than at a level of mild to moderate stress, which acts to optimize outcomes (Sapolsky, 2015).

- The notion that early life stress can result in adverse neurobiological outcomes that can persist across the life course needs to be balanced by the advantage of neuroplasticity, a process that is also active through adulthood (Sapolsky, 2015).

Prenatal maternal stress is of particular concern, given its dual impact on the mother-child dyad. Much research has focused on the life-long influence of prenatal stress on the offspring's physical, psychological, behavioral, and developmental outcomes – a body of evidence collectively brought under the "fetal programming" paradigm of the developmental origins of disease (Lewis, Austin, Knapp, Vaiano, & Galbally, 2015; Moisiadis & Matthews, 2014).

However, at times this research shows inconsistent results that are likely the reflection of the lack of a distinct conceptualization of stress in general (Peters, McEwen, & Friston, 2017), and in particular prenatal maternal stress. Several primary studies and reviews of "prenatal stress" operationalize stress as stress, depression, and/or anxiety, which only serves to cloud our ability to understand the unique contribution of prenatal stress. However, the correlations between stress, depression, and anxiety are low to moderate at best (Liou, Wang, & Cheng, 2014). In addition, recent research demonstrates that the relationships between stress, depression, and anxiety and child outcomes differ, as do the associations between various operationalizations of stress (e.g., as objective or subjective stress) and child outcomes. Different factors also predict subjective and objective stress (Kingston, Heaman, Fell, Dzakpasu, & Chalmers, 2012). Taken together, these findings suggest that stress is a form of distress that is distinct from depression and anxiety. Future research would benefit from distinguishing stress from depression and anxiety when studying the influence of maternal psychological distress on child outcomes, and when exploring the patterns (severity, duration) of maternal stress and its role in the risk, comorbidity, and treatment of depression and anxiety.

In addition, it is important to highlight recent studies' results of the clear, differential relationship between various forms of objective and subjective stress (e.g., objective life event stress, cognitive appraisal of a stressor, perceived impact of life events) and child outcomes when simultaneously assessed within the same study (see discussion in Stress Effects On Child Development). While life event assessments (the most common approach to measuring stress) represent objective measures of stress, they cannot account for the contribution of individual variability that occurs through stress perception – the individual appraisal of whether a stressor is threatening, controllable, predictable – and therefore manageable – or threatening and unpredictable – with the concomitant cascade of stress hormones. Indeed, stress expert, Robert Sapolsky, has highlighted the need to understand the modulating effect of perception on stress-related outcomes as critical in the future of stress research:

> Individual differences in stress biology were once mostly an experimental irritant: oh no, because of variability we need a bigger sample size. However, individual variability as to whether something is perceived as stressful, and in resilience and vulnerability to stress-related disease, should be viewed as the most important topic in the field … To best appreciate the importance of individual differences in stress responsiveness, it is worth focusing on the single most important concept in the field.
>
> *(Sapolsky, 2015) (p.1346)*

Perinatal Stress and Women's Psychological Health

Prevalence Rates

Rates of subjective psychological stress in the perinatal period are not well reported. In a Canadian population-based study of 6,421 new mothers, 12% reported high levels of perceived stress in the 12 months preceding the infant's birth, with 17.1% reporting three or more stressful life events during the same period (Kingston, Heaman, et al., 2012). In a second Canadian study ($N = 441$), a similar prevalence of perceived stress was found with 12.3% of pregnant women reporting the past year as extremely or very stressful and 31.8% as moderately stressful (Kingston, Sword, Krueger, Hanna, & Markle-Reid, 2012). Using data from a Canadian pregnancy cohort to conduct latent class analysis, Mughal et al. reported three trajectories of stress generated from measures of perceived stress at five time points from the second trimester of pregnancy to three years postpartum: low stress symptoms ($n = 762$, 38.4%), moderate stress symptoms (the second and largest trajectory of $n = 969$, 48.9%), and persistent high stress symptoms ($n = 251$, 12.7%) (Mughal et al., 2017, under review).

The majority of studies of stress in the perinatal period conceptualize stress as objective life event stress and thus prevalence rates of life event stress are more common than those of perceived stress. Giallo et al. (2014) reported that 36% of women with minimum depression symptoms experienced "some to many" stressful life events, whereas this prevalence was almost double in women with persistently high depression symptoms (70.6%) (Giallo, Cooklin, & Nicholson, 2014). Using data from the US Pregnancy Risk Assessment Monitoring System ($N = 115,704$), Mukherjee et al. reported that 35% of pregnant women experienced multiple stressors or illness-/death-related stressors, with 70% of participants reporting at least one stressful life event in the year prior to delivery (Mukherjee, Coxe, Fennie, Madhivanan, & Trepka, 2017b). This is consistent with research by Whitehead et al. (Whitehead, Hill, Brogan, & Blackmore-Prince, 2002), who have also identified that 65–70% of pregnant women report having one stressful life event in the year before birth. Mukherjee also reported the most common stressful life events during pregnancy as moving to a new address (33.1%), arguing with the partner more than usual (24.0%), and having a sick close family member (22.5%) (Mukherjee et al., 2017b).

Predictors of Stress

Studies demonstrate that different psychological, demographic, behavioral, and health variables are associated with different forms of stress. For instance, using data from the population-based Canadian Maternity Experiences Survey, Kingston et al. reported that demographic factors were associated only with life stress, while psychological factors contributed to both life event and perceived stress (Kingston, Heaman, et al., 2012). The factor most strongly associated with perceived stress was having three or more stressful life events in the year prior to delivery (AOR 3.18, 95% CI 2.65–3.82). Other significant factors included being unhappy or ambivalent about being pregnant – having a diagnosis of depression or been prescribed antidepressants before becoming pregnant; having none, little, or some support available during pregnancy; having a previous miscarriage; having a medical condition before or during pregnancy, not attending prenatal classes; and having three or more ultrasounds (a proxy for pregnancy-related complications). Having three or more stressful life events was most strongly associated with demographic factors (single marital status, AOR 3.14, 95% CI 2.48–3.98; income below the low-income cut-off level, AOR 2.32, 95% CI 1.95–2.77) and having a diagnosis of depression or being prescribed antidepressants pre-pregnancy (AOR 2.19, 95% CI 1.81–2.65). Other significant risk factors included demographic variables such as young age and being Aboriginal (recent immigrant status was protective), and psychological/health factors such as being unhappy or ambivalent about the pregnancy, wanting to become pregnant later or not at all, having no, little, or some social support during pregnancy, having a previous miscarriage or abortion, and developing a new medical condition during pregnancy (Kingston, Heaman, et al., 2012). Another Canadian study of pregnant women ($N = 441$) used structural equation modeling to demonstrate that prenatal stress is an interplay of perceived and life stress in childhood and adult stressors and perceived stress, with retrospectively reported childhood stress (combined life event and perceived stress) having a significant impact on prenatal stress (Std β = .54, p <.001) after controlling for adult factors, including perceived stress, family cohesion, social support, and socioeconomic position (Kingston, Sword, et al., 2012).

Stress as a Predictor of Depression and Anxiety

Parker et al. have reported that psychological stress is a preceding factor in 85% of cases of depression (Parker, Schatzberg, & Lyons, 2003). Other studies have shown causal commonalities between stress and depression, in that the dysregulation seen in the HPA axis in psychological stress has also been observed in depressed patients, including elevated cortisol. Indeed, dysregulation of the HPA axis is the most prominent endocrine change observed in depression (Brummelte & Galea, 2010). In the Longitudinal Study of Australian Children (N = 4,879), women reporting "some to many" stressful life events at three months postpartum had over three times the odds of having persistently elevated depression from three months to seven years post-delivery compared with women who reported "none or few," after adjusting for relevant confounders (AOR 3.06, 95% CI 2.29–4.11) (Giallo et al., 2014). In a sample of 230 ethnically diverse women, perceived stress (but not stressful life events) was associated with depression symptoms at 14 weeks' gestation (AOR 1.18, 95% CI 1.04–1.34) (Kinser et al., 2017).

Several studies highlight the significant impact of prenatal stress as a risk for postpartum depression. In an Australian cohort of 7,797 pregnant women, having minimal daily hassles reduced the odds of postpartum depression at six weeks postpartum by over 20% compared to having high or moderate level (AOR 0.79, 95% CI 0.64–0.97) (Milgrom et al., 2008). Using 2009–2011 Pregnant Risk Assessment Monitoring System data (N = 91,253), women who experienced all four types of stressful life events (e.g., partner-related, traumatic, emotional, financial) had the highest odds of experiencing postpartum depression (AOR 5.43, 95% CI 5.36–5.51) (Mukherjee, Coxe, Fennie, Madhivanan, & Trepka, 2017a). In exploring the impact of single stressful life events, this study noted that partner-related stressors (arguments with partner) contributed the most to postpartum depression (AOR 2.21, 95% CI 2.18–2.25), a finding that was replicated using data from Georgia's Pregnancy Risk Assessment System (2004–2011) (Salm Ward, Kanu, & Robb, 2017). A national Swedish study recruiting women during the first antenatal visit (N = 2,430) also found that those with two or more stressful life events in the past year were three times as likely to have an elevated Edinburgh Postnatal Depression Scale (EPDS) score compared with women with one or no event (Rubertsson, Wickberg, Gustavsson, & Radestad, 2005). Importantly, this study also reported a dose–response relationship between the number of stressful life events in the year before pregnancy and the mean EPDS score.

Two recent systematic reviews also highlighted prenatal stress, especially negative life events, as a significant predictor of antenatal anxiety and depression (Biaggi, Conroy, Pawlby, & Pariante, 2016; Lancaster et al., 2010), with a moderate effect size found for the association with antenatal depression (Lancaster et al., 2010). A third recent systematic review of 203 studies also identified prenatal stressful life events as a predictor of postpartum depression in both developed and developing countries (Norhayati, Hazlina, Asrenee, & Emilin, 2015). Taken together, prenatal stress is consistently noted as one of the strongest predictors of postpartum depression and anxiety.

Psychological stress has also been used to characterize clinical depression sub-types and to define predictors of recovery. For example, in a small study exploring psychosocial characteristics of women with postpartum depression who had recovered and those with sustained depression (N = 154), the mean number of stressful life events was lower in the group experiencing recovery (M 2.7, SD 2) than that with sustained depression (M 4.6, SD 3), although this difference was non-significant (p = .057) (Putnam et al., 2017). In another study of non-pregnant, middle-aged inpatients admitted to hospital for depression (N = 270), participants experiencing their first episode of depression perceived that the severity of acute stressors in the 12 months prior to symptom onset was greater than those experiencing depression relapse. While 75% of all participants reported at least one major stressor in the year before symptom onset, more than 60% identified this stressor as chronic or enduring (Mitchell, Parker, Gladstone, Wilhelm, & Austin, 2003). Few studies have explored patterns of stress across pregnancy or comorbidity patterns. While some studies have reported increasing trends in stress across gestation, others have identified decreasing levels. In a prospective study of 16–36 weeks' gestation (N = 215), Rallis et al. found that higher stress levels during early pregnancy predicted higher stress levels throughout, and that higher depression scores during early pregnancy also predicted higher stress scores in later gestation (Rallis, Skouteris, McCabe, & Milgrom, 2014). In terms of comorbidity, we have identified that high stress is *always* a component of severe depression and anxiety (unpublished).

Moderators and Mediators of Stress

Social support is the most common mediator and moderator of psychosocial stress to be explored. In a community-based sample of over 2,000 pregnant women, Glazier et al. found that the effect of second trimester stress (measured as partner conflict and life events) on symptoms of depression and anxiety was mediated by high social support (Glazier, Elgar, Goel, & Holzapfel, 2004). In a sample of women who were pregnant at the time of the 2008 Iowa state flood, Kroska et al. found that social support moderated the relationship between prenatal maternal stress and child BMI at 30 months of age (Kroska et al., 2017). In other words, women who perceived that the flood had significant, negative personal consequences were more likely to have children with greater BMIs at 30 months (with higher birth weight as a mediator), but only if they had also reported low social support (or less satisfaction with their support) during pregnancy. This relationship did not exist for women who reported that they received adequate social support (and were satisfied with this support) during pregnancy, suggesting that support influenced women's subjective perception of stress and buffered its impact on child outcomes 2.5 years later (Kroska et al., 2017). The buffering effects of prenatal partner support on the relationship between prenatal stress and cortisol reactivity in six-week-old infants were also reported in another study of low-income Mexican-American families (N = 220) (Luecken et al., 2013).

It Is Not Just the Absence of Distress That Counts

While lower perceived stress and fewer stressful life events have been found to be protective of future adverse maternal and child outcomes (Milgrom et al., 2008), Phua et al. have proposed that positive mental health during pregnancy is itself distinctly associated with optimal child outcomes (Phua et al., 2017). Using data from the prospective birth cohort study, Growing Up in Singapore Towards Healthy Outcomes Study (N = 1,066), investigators evaluated the relationships between the positive items of the EPDS, the State-Trait Anxiety Inventory (STAI), and the Beck Depression Inventory (BDI) administered at 26 week's gestation and child developmental outcomes at 12, 18, and 24 months of age. Examples of positive items from these scales included: *In the past seven days, I have been able to laugh and see the funny side of things, I feel self-confident at this moment, I feel satisfied at this moment, I feel secure,* and *I make decisions easily.* Following bifactor analyses, Phua et al. found that positive maternal mental health during pregnancy was uniquely associated with improved cognitive, language, socio-emotional, and motor development (Phua et al., 2017). These emergent findings suggest that identifying positive aspects of mental health may be beneficial clinically as a component of prenatal psychosocial assessment and in research in understanding the effect of positive maternal mental health on maternal and child outcomes.

Assessment of Stress

The concluding remarks of the majority of studies reporting the substantial prevalence of prenatal stress and linking prenatal to poor maternal and child outcomes highlight the need to conduct prenatal psychosocial assessment with inquiry about stressful life events women have experienced in the previous year as well as their perception of the personal and familial impact of those events. As Graignic-Philippe et al. note:

> It appears necessary to assess individual stress reactivity prospectively and separately at each trimester of pregnancy, to discriminate chronic from acute stress, and to take into consideration moderator variables such as past life events, sociocultural factors, predictability, social support and coping strategies.
>
> (Graignic-Philippe, Dayan, Chokron, Jacquet, & Tordjman, 2014)

A limitation in evaluating perceived stress is its inherently subjective nature, individual differences to recognize circumstances as stressful, and relying on self-reported measures of stress in the majority of studies.

Another major challenge in implementing stress assessment as a component of prenatal care is the lack of tools that are appropriate for clinical use. For example, although the Perceived Stress Scale has been widely used in and outside of the perinatal field, standardized cut-off points are not available to support clinical judgment. The Antenatal Risk Questionnaire (ANRQ) (Austin, Colton, Priest, Reilly, & Hadzi-Pavlovic, 2013), a validated antenatal psychosocial risk assessment questionnaire, includes two items that inquire about the presence and impact of stressful life events in the previous year:

Box 1.1 Stressful Life Event Items of the ANRQ

Have you had any major stresses, changes or losses in the last 12 mo†nths? (*Yes, No*)

How distressed were you by these major stresses, changes or losses? (*Not at all, a little, somewhat, quite a lot, very much*)

The scores from these two items are incorporated in an overall psychosocial assessment score that is linked to recommendations for referral and care.

The Depression, Anxiety and Stress Scale (DASS-21) also offers normed data and standardized cut-offs for the seven-item stress subscale: normal (0–14), mild stress (15–18), moderate stress (19–25), severe stress (26–33), and extremely severe stress (34+) (Lovibond, 1995) (Table 1.1).

Effects of Prenatal Maternal Stress on Child Development

Cross-sectional and longitudinal birth cohort studies demonstrate a moderate association between prenatal stress (conceptualized variably as objective stress, subjective stress, CRH, and cortisol) and adverse child outcomes (Dunkel Schetter & Tanner, 2012; Glover, 2011, 2014, 2015; Kingston, McDonald, Austin, & Tough, 2015; Kingston & Tough, 2014). Such outcomes include mental health problems (Entringer, Buss, & Wadhwa, 2015; Glover, 2014, 2015; Kingsbury et al., 2016), physical health problems, such as asthma and diabetes (Entringer et al., 2015; Fatima, Srivastav, & Mondal, 2017), and sub-optimal neurobehavioral development (Glover, 2014, 2015; Graignic-Philippe et al., 2014; Grizenko, Fortier, Gaudreau-Simard, Jolicoeur, & Joober, 2015).

Table 1.1 DASS-21 Scale

Over the past week...	0 = Did not apply to me at all	1 = Applied to me to some degree, or some of the time	2 = Applied to me a considerable degree or a good part of time	3 = Applied to me very much or most of the time
I found it hard to wind down.				
I tended to over-react to situations.				
I felt that I was using a lot of nervous energy.				
I found myself getting agitated.				
I found it difficult to relax.				
I was intolerant of anything that kept me from getting on with what I was doing.				
I felt that I was rather touchy.				

(Lovibond e Lovibond, 1995).

Other studies exploring the biological underpinnings of these associations have found that high glucocorticoid (GC) exposure during pregnancy contributes to life-long cardiovascular, metabolic, reproductive, and neurological diseases through dysregulation of the HPA axis (Moisiadis & Matthews, 2014). For this reason, GC programming of the HPA axis has been identified "as a pivotal link between early life experience and the development of chronic disease later in life" (Moisiadis & Matthews, 2014, p. 392).

Across this body of work, some observations that form the foundation of our understanding of the role of prenatal stress in child outcomes – and challenge us as we move forward in this field – are:

• Although associations between prenatal stress and offspring outcomes are evident in both animal and human studies, the mechanisms for transmission of prenatal stress to offspring and subsequent generations are less clear (but likely largely due to epigenetic mechanisms) (Babenko et al., 2015; Cao-Lei et al., 2017).
• Animal studies show a transgenerational effect of prenatal stress that can be extended (and worsen) through third and fourth generations (Babenko et al., 2015; Metz et al., 2015).
• Exposure to prenatal stress can generate positive outcomes for the offspring, demonstrating an adaptive role of prenatal stress (Glover, 2011).
• Child outcomes definitely vary by the type and timing of stress exposure (King & Laplante, 2015).
• Acute and chronic prenatal stress (Karatsoreos & McEwen, 2013a), and perceived/subjective and objective stress (Cao-Lei, Veru, et al., 2016; Moss et al., 2017; Simcock et al., 2017) have differential effects on child outcomes.

In this section, we review the associations between child outcomes and prenatal stress by the type of stress: objective/life event, subjective/perceived, disaster-related, and biological (e.g., cortisol). It is not a comprehensive review, but rather a review of exemplars that highlights findings that form the foundation for advancing perinatal stress research.

Perceived/Subjective Stress

Perceived stress captures an individual's appraisal of their ability to manage day-to-day problems, and is largely influenced by how predictable and controllable these problems are (Sapolsky, 2015). Studies evaluating the impact of perceived/subjective stress are less common than those operationalizing stress as objective, life event stress. In addition, the findings are less consistent, the magnitude of effect is more variable than life event stress studies, and there are few studies that distinguish between acute and chronic subjective stress. In a recent study exploring trajectories of stress from pregnancy to three years post-delivery (N = 1,983), persistent moderate (n = 878, 48.4%) and high stress (n = 228, 12.5%) symptoms throughout this period were associated with sub-optimal global child development in bivariate analyses (moderate: OR 1.40, 95% CI 1.01–1.95; high: OR 1.92, 95% CI 1.23–2.99). However, neither association was significant in multivariate models that controlled for anxiety trajectories, socioeconomic variables, and child sex (Mughal et al., 2017, under review).

Using 15 years of data from the Australian-based pregnancy cohort, the Mater University Study of Pregnancy (N = 3,925 mother-child dyads), Betts et al. conducted a similar analysis to assess the long-term trajectories of anxiety, depression, and stress on internalizing and externalizing problems in young adolescents (Betts, Williams, Najman, & Alati, 2014). To model the comorbidity that frequently occurs among depression, anxiety, and stress, these investigators combined all three disorders in the trajectory analysis. Stress – measured at seven time points from pregnancy to five years postpartum – was conceptualized as self-perceived daily strain resulting from personal or social situations (e.g., daily hassles) using the Reeder Stress Inventory. When controlled for relevant confounders, the only trajectory that was significantly associated with internalizing behavior at age 14 was high stress/anxiety/depression during pregnancy (AOR 2.36, 95% CI 1.22–3.51); no trajectories were associated with externalizing behavior. In their discussion, the authors note the value of not isolating stress, depression, and anxiety in exploring the effects of psychological distress on child outcomes (Betts et al., 2014). In the same cohort, young adults (age 21) whose mothers experienced ongoing high perceived stress during pregnancy had a greater tendency of experiencing internalizing (B = 2.76, 1.33–4.17) and externalizing problems (B = 1.45, CI 0.28–2.62) as well as depressive symptoms (OR 1.87, 95% CI 1.27–2.73) (N = 3,099); no other trajectories showed an association (Betts, Williams, Najman, & Alati, 2015). Davis et al. found that maternal perceived stress assessed at five time points across the second and third trimesters was associated with infant stress regulation (N = 116) (Davis, Glynn, Waffarn, & Sandman, 2011). Following a heel-stick procedure at 24 hours of age, term infants of mothers who experienced psychological stress throughout their second and third trimesters demonstrated a slower rate of recovery from the stressor, after adjustment for relevant confounders.

In this study, Davis et al. also explored the association between maternal cortisol (also collected at five time points during pregnancy) on the same infant outcome, and concluded that while perceived stress can have a programming effect on infant stress regulation, it is likely not mediated by cortisol (Davis et al., 2011). Recent research by Cao-Lei and colleagues has shed more light on the mechanisms underlying the effect of perceived stress. Using data from the pregnant cohort of women who experienced the 1998 Quebec ice storm, Cao-Lei et al. evaluated whether objective stress and subjective stress were associated with DNA methylation in 13-year-old offspring (N = 34) (Cao-Lei et al., 2015). They found that the children of mothers who reported negative appraisals in which they perceived the natural disaster to have significant negative consequences were more likely to show widespread DNA methylation across the genome. This study is one of the first to demonstrate that perceived stress during pregnancy may play a role in child outcomes several years later through widespread epigenetic changes. Cao-Lei et al. reported a similar finding in the same cohort in which negative cognitive appraisal was associated with lower BMI and central adiposity in 13-year-old offspring, mediated by DNA methylation of genes in the pathway for diabetes type I and II (Cao-Lei, Dancause, et al., 2016). In this case, DNA methylation mediated a protective effect between prenatal stress and child BMI, demonstrating an adaptive influence of prenatal cognitive appraisal of stress on the offspring's health.

Studies from other cohorts show differential outcomes of perceived stress by timing of exposure and sex (Herbison, Allen, Robinson, Newnham, & Pennell, 2017). The Western Australian Pregnancy Cohort (Raine) Study collected stress data (DASS-21) during pregnancy and at eight time points from age 1 to 17 years. In a recent study examining the association between trajectories of life course stress and depression and anxiety in early adulthood, Herbison et al. reported clear differences in the adult offsprings' mental health by timing, level, and sex. In the whole cohort, high prenatal stress early during pregnancy (0–18 weeks) was associated with significantly higher stress, depression, and anxiety in the adult offspring, whereas this relationship did not remain significant when the exposure to prenatal stress occurred in later pregnancy (18–34 weeks). Looking at sex-specific difference, among females, medium to high chronic stress exposure across the life course was associated with depression and anxiety symptoms. In males, however, high stress early during pregnancy was related to depression and anxiety symptoms in adulthood. Of interest, among the five trajectories of stress experienced by the adult children, only 7.8% of the cohort were members of the descending trajectory, in which stress was highest in childhood and declined throughout the life course. In the remaining trajectories, offspring experienced stable low (16.7%), stable medium (30.7%), or stable high (17.2%) stress, or increasing stress from childhood through the life course (27.5%). This study also examined the relative contributions of prenatal and postnatal stress, reporting that while prenatal stress had a significant influence on adult depression and anxiety in males, postnatal stress had a greater influence in females.

There is also growing interest in the overall influence of prenatal stress on offspring microbiota. A recent study by Zijlmans and colleagues (Zijlmans, Korpela, Riksen-Walraven, de Vos, & de Weerth, 2015) demonstrated that prenatal appraisal of daily hassles (e.g., whether the situation felt like a hassle or an uplift) influenced infant microbiota at three months of age, after controlling for postnatal perceived stress and other relevant confounders ($N = 25$). Infants of mothers who experienced greater stress had more prevalent diarrhea, gastroenteritis, and allergic reactions (43%) as a result of having a colonization pattern characterized by an increased abundance of Proteobacteria (e.g., Escherichia and Enterobacter) and a decreased abundance of lactic acid bacteria and Actinobacteria, compared with infants of mothers with low/no stress (0%) (Zijlmans, Korpela, et al., 2015).

Much of the research examining the effects of prenatal perceived stress extended from animal studies of its influence on gestational age to human studies of preterm birth. The relationship between prenatal stress/glucocorticoids and preterm birth remains a significant issue, particularly the mechanisms driving this association. In a recent systematic review, Staneva et al. (Staneva, Bogossian, Pritchard, & Wittkowski, 2015) reported that four of five studies of perceived stress showed a small to moderate significant effect on preterm birth, with relative risks ranging from 1.75 (95% CI 1.20–2.54) to 2.32 (95% CI 1.18–4.60).

Stressful Life Events

Stressful life events remain the most common approach to assessing stress clinically and in research, and are based on the notion that cumulative stress can result from several major life changes (Graignic-Philippe et al., 2014). Research exploring the effect of stressful life events (using a variety of tools) shows consistent associations with adverse child outcomes. For example, using data from the Avon Longitudinal Study of Parents and Children (ALSPAC; $N = 10,569$), high numbers of stressful life events during pregnancy have been linked to adolescent depression (AOR 1.03,

95% CI 1.01–1.06) (Kingsbury et al., 2016). Using latent class growth analysis, this study also found that adolescents of mothers with stressful life events during pregnancy were more likely to experience stable, high levels of depression from age 10/11 to 18/19 (OR 1.72, 95% CI 1.09–2.71). Kingsbury and colleagues concluded that these results show support for a fetal programming hypothesis and highlighted the need for prenatal stress management. Also using the ALSPAC cohort for trajectory analyses, MacKinnon et al. examined the association between prenatal life event stress at 18 weeks' gestation and trajectories of externalizing symptoms from age 6 to 16 years using the Strengths and Difficulties Questionnaire (N = 7,699) (MacKinnon, Kingsbury, Mahedy, Evans, & Colman, 2018). Children in the high externalizing symptom trajectory were more likely to have mothers who were members of the highest quartile of stressful life events. Notably, this study also found a dose-response relationship between prenatal stress and externalizing symptoms.

Disaster Exposure

As another type of stressor, Moss et al. have noted that it is beneficial to study disaster exposure in that 17–20% of individuals will experience psychological morbidity following a natural disaster (Moss et al., 2017). A series of studies were conducted following the 2008 Iowa flood, recruiting women <20 weeks' gestation from University of Iowa hospitals and maternity clinics. Life event stress was assessed at recruitment and 30 months following recruitment, along with subjective measures of distress (e.g., psychological reaction to the flood, perceived stress). During simultaneously examining the impact of both objective and subjective prenatal stress on toddler cognitive functioning, Laplante et al. found that high subjective stress early during pregnancy was associated with lower cognitive functioning and language scores in 30-month–old toddlers (Laplante, Hart, O'Hara, Brunet, & King, 2017). The effect of objective stress was moderated by child sex, demonstrating the complexity of prenatal stress effects. Specifically, sex differences were not apparent at low degrees of maternal hardship; however, at moderate or high levels, boys had higher vocabulary scores. Laplante et al. note, "it appears that maternal flood-related objective hardship eliminated the usual superiority of girls in early language development by accelerating language acquisition in boys" (Laplante et al., 2017, p. 89). Consistent with findings reported using data from pregnant women exposed to the 1998 Quebec ice storm (Laplante et al., 2004), both studies found that exposure during early pregnancy had the most dramatic effects on cognitive and language development. As such, these studies demonstrate the differential effects of subjective and objective stress, the unique sex-specific effects that prenatal stress can exhibit on some child outcomes, and the influence of timing of exposure on outcomes.

Studies of the Queensland flood in 2011 provided additional opportunity to study the influence of type and timing of stress exposure on child development. In a cohort of 16-month-old children whose mothers were exposed to the flood during pregnancy (N = 145) (Moss et al., 2017), objective hardship related to flood exposure was associated with poorer cognitive development while negative cognitive appraisal was related to motor development. Further analyses revealed that these relationships were moderated by timing of exposure. In particular, cognitive performance was better if a child's mother experienced severe hardship as a result of the flood during the first month of pregnancy, but worse if she experienced it after 30 weeks' gestation. In another study using data from the Queensland flood, Simcock et al. reported (Simcock et al., 2016) that children of mothers who were exposed to the flood later during pregnancy (after 22 weeks) and who had a negative cognitive appraisal of the personal impact of the flood experienced poorer gross motor development. However, children of mothers who were exposed to the flood early during pregnancy (before 17 days) and who had a positive appraisal of the flood effects had better motor development at 6 and 16 months of age. This study provides important empiric evidence that cognitive appraisal can buffer the effects of stress exposure on child development.

Biological Measures: Cortisol

Early studies exploring the underlying mechanisms of prenatal stress on child outcomes focused on chemical hormones, such as cortisol. However, most evidence for cortisol as a mediator between prenatal stress and child development is weak and inconsistent (Davis et al., 2011). Indeed, a recent systematic review of studies exploring the relationship between maternal prenatal cortisol and child outcomes shows few significant associations (Zijlmans, Riksen-Walraven, & de Weerth, 2015). Zijlmans et al. note that when the association is significant, higher cortisol is generally linked to a more adverse/negative developmental outcome. However, the variability across studies suggests that maternal cortisol may not be the sole or main underlying mechanism linking prenatal stress to child outcomes (Zijlmans, Riksen-Walraven, et al., 2015). Indeed, the low or absent correlations that are consistently reported between self-report measures of prenatal stress and cortisol levels support this position (Baibazarova et al., 2013; Glover, Bergman, Sarkar, & O'Connor, 2009). Finally, Graignic-Philippe et al.'s review provides evidence of the complex interplay between the sympathetic nervous system and the HPA axis overall, and especially during pregnancy, with the caveat that cortisol measures are limited as indicators of acute stress during pregnancy (Graignic-Philippe et al., 2014).

Prenatal Stress: An Adaptive Perspective

A common assumption underlying the study of the influence of prenatal stress on child outcomes is that prenatal stress only acts adversely on child development and health. However, in a classic and widely cited paper, Gluckman and Hanson describe the advantage that programmed changes in the fetus, instigated by an adverse intrauterine environment, have for preparing the child to survive in a similar adverse extrauterine environment (Gluckman & Hanson, 2004). Indeed, the Project Ice Storm study discussed previously demonstrates that prenatal stress early in gestation can advance language outcomes in boys, preparing them to function better and earlier in a challenging world (Laplante et al., 2017). However, a mismatch can (the "mismatch hypothesis") occur when this programming does not fit the requirements of the extrauterine environment, and programs the child for disease instead (Gluckman & Hanson, 2006). Glover proposes several adaptive programmed changes that the child may experience as a result of exposure to prenatal stress (Glover, 2011). For example, she suggests that ADHD and hyperactivity may optimize attention and support greater vigilance. The aggressive behavior that characterizes externalizing behavior may enable the offspring to meet needs in a resource-deprived environment. Changes in cognitive function may enable the offspring to generate new solutions and strategies to unpredictable, novel situations. Adopting an adaptive perspective may contribute to better interpretation of findings of prenatal stress–child outcome studies.

Transmission of Prenatal Stress to Offspring

There is substantial evidence that the transmission of prenatal stress to the offspring in the form of adverse developmental outcomes, poor physical and mental health, or programming of the HPA axis for enhanced vulnerability to stress and affective disorders occurs through epigenetic mechanisms. In brief, epigenetic changes are those alternations to the chromatin that do not involve changes in DNA sequencing. Research over the past decade highlights three types of stress-induced epigenetic mechanism: chromatin remodeling, DNA modification, and micro-RNA (Babenko et al., 2015; Cao-Lei et al., 2017; Metz et al., 2015).

Stress-induced chromatin remodeling occurs when the N-terminal tails of histones (protein around which DNA coils itself and condenses during cell division) are chemically modified through the addition of acetyl, methyl, or phosphate groups (Constantinof, Moisiadis, & Matthews, 2016). This opens up the DNA structure, making it more available for transcription (and subsequent gene expression) (Constantinof et al., 2016).

DNA methylation occurs with the addition of a methyl group to the DNA molecule (Constantinof et al., 2016). The methyl group suppresses gene expression by preventing transcription factors from binding so that the DNA is less available for transcription (Kundakovic & Jaric, 2017). With respect to prenatal stress, most DNA methylation occurs in genes within the HPA-related glucocorticoid pathway (Cao-Lei et al., 2017).

Three genes in particular have been implicated in the epigenetic transmission of maternal prenatal stress to offspring. First, NR3C1, the gene responsible for encoding the glucocorticoid receptor, in its methylated state has been linked to increase HPA activity. In a study of 82 pregnant women, methylation of NR3C1 was significantly higher in leukocytes in cord blood of infants whose mothers experienced prenatal stress compared with those who did not (Oberlander et al., 2008). In follow-up, NR3C1 methylation was found to be linked to increased salivary cortisol in three-month-old infants (Oberlander et al., 2008). Conradt et al. also found that greater placental DNA methylation of NR3C1 in psychologically distressed women was associated with poorer self-regulation, hypotonia, and greater lethargy in newly delivered infants, compared with women with little psychological distress during pregnancy (Conradt, Lester, Appleton, Armstrong, & Marsit, 2013). In the cohort of pregnant women exposed to the Quebec ice storm in 1998, Cao-Lei et al. (2016) found correlations between objective prenatal stress and cytokine production in 13-year-old children, mediated by DNA methylation (Cao-Lei, Veru, et al., 2016).

Second, FK506 Binding Protein 5 (FKBP5), the gene responsible for encoding an immunophilin protein, is responsible for regulating the immune system and glucocorticoid receptors (Cao-Lei et al., 2017). In a study of 61 pregnant women in their second and third trimesters, DNA methylation of this gene was correlated with perceived prenatal stress, and further associated with reduced fetal coupling (i.e., the relationship between fetal movement and heart rate) – a precursor to poor neurodevelopmental outcomes (Monk et al., 2016).

Third, 11β-HSD2 is the gene responsible for cortisol regulation in the placenta. It codes for production of the enzyme, 11-β-hydroxysteroid dehydrogenase, which metabolizes active cortisol into inactive cortisone. Methylation of this gene has been associated with sub-optimal neurobehavioral outcomes and increased cortisol in infants (Cao-Lei et al., 2017). Another study showed that infants of women who were psychologically distressed during pregnancy had greater 11β-HSD2 methylation than infants of mothers who were not distressed, and this was associated with infant hypotonia (Conradt et al., 2013).

Micro-RNAs are also emerging as key players in epigenetic transmission. They tend to reduce gene expression by inhibiting transcription (Babenko et al., 2015) and are involved in brain development (Sun, Crabtree, & Yoo, 2013). Animal studies have shown that altered micro-RNA profiles are associated with neurodegenerative disease and abnormal psychological behaviors (Zucchi et al., 2013), as well as altered stress responses (Gapp et al., 2014).

Transgenerational Programming

Transgenerational programming – the transmission of early life influences on multigenerational outcomes – is gaining attention as a mechanism for transmission of prenatal stress across generations (Babenko et al., 2015; Metz et al., 2015). Strong evidence from animal studies exists for the heritability of prenatal stress to the second and third generations of offspring through epigenetic mechanisms (Constantinof et al., 2016). For example, in guinea pig models, administration of synthetic glucocorticoid (to F0) pregnant guinea pigs, who were then mated with control mates, resulted in F2 offspring showing reduced HPA-axis responses to stress through altered glucocorticoid negative feedback sensitivity, decreased secretion of pituitary ACTH, and decreased CRH mRNA (Iqbal, Moisiadis, Kostaki, & Matthews, 2012). Altered m-RNAs have also been implicated in transgenerational transmission. For example, Yao et al. exposed pregnant dams to stress and then divided their pregnant daughters (F1) and granddaughters (F2) into stressed and non-stressed groups. They found that gestational age became shorter, maternal weight gain became less, and behavior became more dysfunctional with each generation, with the most dramatic effects apparent in the F3 generation. Compared with non-stressed rats, micro-RNAs regulating brain plasticity and parturition were altered significantly, with the most dramatic influences on preterm birth occurring in the F3 generation (Yao et al., 2014). Understanding the implications of these findings in human pregnancy will likely dominate research in the next decades (Metz et al., 2015).

Resilience

While resilience is often defined as the ability to respond positively from challenging situations, McEwen expands this by noting that resilience involves not only the ability to recover from stress-related damage, but also the capacity to flexibly adapt to changes in the environment toward the end goal of "achieving a positive outcome in the face of adversity" (McEwen et al., 2015, p. 1). McEwen's idiom of "bending and not breaking" is particularly apt within the context of the importance of early life experiences that contribute to the development of healthy brain architecture. Indeed, McEwen notes that healthy brain development underlies the establishment of flexible cognition, high self-esteem, a sense of internal control and mastery, and effective self-regulation – major determinants of our appraisal of challenging situations as threatening or controllable and our overall experience of stress as positive, tolerable, or toxic (McEwen et al., 2015). As such, resilience involves responses both at the level of the brain and in our behavior. For instance, a resilient brain responds to both acute and chronic stress with structural remodeling, especially in the hippocampus, amygdala, and prefrontal cortex. In this case, when the stressor is over, the remodeled neurons and synapses tend to recover, although not always to the optimal level of the pre-stress state. Animal and human studies show that the deficits that remain post-stress exposure can include cognitive impairment, over-reactivity to future stressors, and mood disorders, although there are clear sex-specific differences in these stress-related outcomes.

Early maternal care is critical to the development of a resilient brain and flexible, adaptive responses to adversity (Gunnar & Donzella, 2002; Karatsoreos & McEwen, 2013b; McEwen et al., 2015). For instance, a small but promising study by Sharp et al. ($N = 243$) demonstrated that the association between prenatal depression and physiological and emotional reactivity of seven-month-old infants was modulated by maternal holding and stroking (Sharp et al., 2012). In other words, in this sample of prenatally depressed women, infants whose mothers held and stroked them more during the first two months postpartum did not experience the adverse effects of prenatal depression compared to infants with less maternal care experienced. A second study by this team followed up the infants at 2.5 years, and found that infants whose mothers with prenatal depression had stroked them more in the early postpartum period did not experience increased risk for internalizing behavior, whereas the association between prenatal stress and internalizing behavior was significant for mothers who stroked their infants less (Sharp, Hill, Hellier, & Pickles, 2015). Other studies comparing children in the two-year period of being adopted following orphanage institutionalization or fostering with children remaining with their birth families show changes in cortisol responses (blunting) in institutionalized/fostered children, indicative of HPA programming (Koss, Hostinar, Donzella, & Gunnar, 2014) – changes that also mediated increased behavioral problems at school entry (Koss, Mliner, Donzella, & Gunnar, 2016). Studies using animal models also demonstrate that epigenetic changes in the form of DNA methylation of genes in the stress regulation pathway can transmit the positive influences of maternal care across generations (Meaney & Szyf, 2005). On a clinical level, these studies provide a basis for encouragement for pregnant women struggling with anxiety or depression. The emerging evidence that stroking an infant can moderate the effect of prenatal depression on child outcomes is a hopeful message of a powerful, doable maternal intervention. Given the lack of long-term child-related follow-up that limits most trials of antenatal mental health intervention (Kingston et al., 2014), future research exploring other means of mitigating the potentially adverse effects of prenatal depression, anxiety, and stress on child outcomes is warranted.

References

Austin, M. P., Colton, J., Priest, S., Reilly, N., & Hadzi-Pavlovic, D. (2013). The antenatal risk questionnaire (ANRQ): Acceptability and use for psychosocial risk assessment in the maternity setting. *Women Birth, 26*(1), 17–25. doi:10.1016/j.wombi.2011.06.002

Babenko, O., Kovalchuk, I., & Metz, G. A. (2015). Stress-induced perinatal and transgenerational epigenetic programming of brain development and mental health. *Neuroscience Biobehavioral Reviews, 48*, 70–91. doi:10.1016/j.neubiorev.2014.11.013

Baibazarova, E., van de Beek, C., Cohen-Kettenis, P. T., Buitelaar, J., Shelton, K. H., & van Goozen, S. H. (2013). Influence of prenatal maternal stress, maternal plasma cortisol and cortisol in the amniotic fluid on birth outcomes and child temperament at 3 months. *Psychoneuroendocrinology, 38*(6), 907–915. doi:10.1016/j.psyneuen.2012.09.015

Betts, K. S., Williams, G. M., Najman, J. M., & Alati, R. (2014). Maternal depressive, anxious, and stress symptoms during pregnancy predict internalizing problems in adolescence. *Depression and Anxiety, 31*(1), 9–18. doi:10.1002/da.22210

Betts, K. S., Williams, G. M., Najman, J. M., & Alati, R. (2015). The relationship between maternal depressive, anxious, and stress symptoms during pregnancy and adult offspring behavioral and emotional problems. *Depression and Anxiety, 32*(2), 82–90. doi:10.1002/da.22272

Biaggi, A., Conroy, S., Pawlby, S., & Pariante, C. M. (2016). Identifying the women at risk of antenatal anxiety and depression: A systematic review. *Journal of Affective Disorders, 191*, 62–77. doi:10.1016/j.jad.2015.11.014

Brummelte, S., & Galea, L. A. (2010). Depression during pregnancy and postpartum: Contribution of stress and ovarian hormones. *Progress in Neuro-Psychopharmacology and Biological Psychiatry, 34*(5), 766–776. doi:10.1016/j.pnpbp.2009.09.006

Cao-Lei, L., Dancause, K. N., Elgbeili, G., Laplante, D. P., Szyf, M., & King, S. (2016). Pregnant women's cognitive appraisal of a natural disaster affects their children's BMI and central adiposity via DNA methylation: Project Ice Storm. *Early Human Development, 103*, 189–192. doi:10.1016/j.earlhumdev.2016.09.013

Cao-Lei, L., de Rooij, S. R., King, S., Matthews, S. G., Metz, G. A. S., Roseboom, T. J., & Szyf, M. (2017). Prenatal stress and epigenetics. *Neuroscience Biobehavioral Reviews.* doi:10.1016/j.neubiorev.2017.05.016

Cao-Lei, L., Elgbeili, G., Massart, R., Laplante, D. P., Szyf, M., & King, S. (2015). Pregnant women's cognitive appraisal of a natural disaster affects DNA methylation in their children 13 years later: Project Ice Storm. *Translational Psychiatry, 5*, e515. doi:10.1038/tp.2015.13

Cao-Lei, L., Veru, F., Elgbeili, G., Szyf, M., Laplante, D. P., & King, S. (2016). DNA methylation mediates the effect of exposure to prenatal maternal stress on cytokine production in children at age 13(1/2) years: Project Ice Storm. *Clinical Epigenetics, 8*, 54. doi:10.1186/s13148-016-0219-0

Conradt, E., Lester, B. M., Appleton, A. A., Armstrong, D. A., & Marsit, C. J. (2013). The roles of DNA methylation of NR3C1 and 11beta-HSD2 and exposure to maternal mood disorder in utero on newborn neurobehavior. *Epigenetics, 8*(12), 1321–1329. doi:10.4161/epi.26634

Constantinof, A., Moisiadis, V. G., & Matthews, S. G. (2016). Programming of stress pathways: A transgenerational perspective. *Journal of Steroid Biochemistry and Molecular Biology, 160*, 175–180. doi:10.1016/j.jsbmb.2015.10.008

Crum, A. J., Akinola, M., Martin, A., & Fath, S. (2017). The role of stress mindset in shaping cognitive, emotional, and physiological responses to challenging and threatening stress. *Anxiety, Stress and Coping, 30*(4), 379–395. doi:10.1080/10615806.2016.1275585

Crum, A. J., Salovey, P., & Achor, S. (2013). Rethinking stress: The role of mindsets in determining the stress response. *Journal of Personality and Social Psychology, 104*(4), 716–733. doi:10.1037/a0031201

Davis, E. P., Glynn, L. M., Waffarn, F., & Sandman, C. A. (2011). Prenatal maternal stress programs infant stress regulation. *Journal of Child Psychology and Psychiatry, 52*(2), 119–129. doi:10.1111/j.1469-7610.2010.02314.x

Dunkel Schetter, C., & Tanner, L. (2012). Anxiety, depression and stress in pregnancy: Implications for mothers, children, research, and practice. *Current Opinion in Psychiatry, 25*(2), 141–148. doi:10.1097/YCO.0b013e3283503680

Entringer, S., Buss, C., & Wadhwa, P. D. (2015). Prenatal stress, development, health and disease risk: A psychobiological perspective-2015 Curt Richter Award Paper. *Psychoneuroendocrinology, 62*, 366–375. doi:10.1016/j.psyneuen.2015.08.019

Fatima, M., Srivastav, S., & Mondal, A. C. (2017). Prenatal stress and depression associated neuronal development in neonates. *International Journal of Developmental Neuroscience, 60*, 1–7. doi:10.1016/j.ijdevneu.2017.04.001

Gapp, K., Jawaid, A., Sarkies, P., Bohacek, J., Pelczar, P., Prados, J., ... Mansuy, I. M. (2014). Implication of sperm RNAs in transgenerational inheritance of the effects of early trauma in mice. *Nature Neuroscience, 17*(5), 667–669. doi:10.1038/nn.3695

Giallo, R., Cooklin, A., & Nicholson, J. M. (2014). Risk factors associated with trajectories of mothers' depressive symptoms across the early parenting period: An Australian population-based longitudinal study. *Archives of Women's Mental Health, 17*(2), 115–125. doi:10.1007/s00737-014-0411-1

Glazier, R. H., Elgar, F. J., Goel, V., & Holzapfel, S. (2004). Stress, social support, and emotional distress in a community sample of pregnant women. *Journal of Psychosomatic Obstetrics and Gynecology, 25*(3–4), 247–255. doi:10.1080/01674820400024406

Glover, V. (2011). Annual research review: Prenatal stress and the origins of psychopathology: An evolutionary perspective. *Journal of Child Psychology and Psychiatry, 52*(4), 356–367. doi:10.1111/j.1469-7610.2011.02371.x

Glover, V. (2014). Maternal depression, anxiety and stress during pregnancy and child outcome; what needs to be done. *Best Practice & Research: Clinical Obstetrics & Gynaecology, 28*(1), 25–35. doi:10.1016/j.bpobgyn.2013.08.017

Glover, V. (2015). Prenatal stress and its effects on the fetus and the child: Possible underlying biological mechanisms. *Advanced Neurobiology, 10*, 269–283. doi:10.1007/978-1-4939-1372-5_13

Glover, V., Bergman, K., Sarkar, P., & O'Connor, T. G. (2009). Association between maternal and amniotic fluid cortisol is moderated by maternal anxiety. *Psychoneuroendocrinology, 34*(3), 430–435. doi:10.1016/j.psyneuen.2008.10.005

Gluckman, P. D., & Hanson, M. A. (2004). Developmental origins of disease paradigm: A mechanistic and evolutionary perspective. *Pediatric Research, 56*(3), 311–317. doi:10.1203/01.PDR.0000135998.08025.FB

Gluckman, P. D., & Hanson, M. A. (2006). The consequences of being born small – An adaptive perspective. *Hormonal Research, 65 Suppl 3*, 5–14. doi:10.1159/000091500

Graignic-Philippe, R., Dayan, J., Chokron, S., Jacquet, A. Y., & Tordjman, S. (2014). Effects of prenatal stress on fetal and child development: A critical literature review. *Neuroscience Biobehavioral Reviews, 43*, 137–162. doi:10.1016/j.neubiorev.2014.03.022

Grizenko, N., Fortier, M. E., Gaudreau-Simard, M., Jolicoeur, C., & Joober, R. (2015). The effect of maternal stress during pregnancy on IQ and ADHD symptomatology. *Journal of the Canadian Academy of Child and Adolescent Psychiatry, 24*(2), 92–99.

Gunnar, M. R., & Donzella, B. (2002). Social regulation of the cortisol levels in early human development. *Psychoneuroendocrinology, 27*(1–2), 199–220.

Herbison, C. E., Allen, K., Robinson, M., Newnham, J., & Pennell, C. (2017). The impact of life stress on adult depression and anxiety is dependent on gender and timing of exposure. *Development and Psychopathology, 29*(4), 1443–1454. doi:10.1017/S0954579417000372

Iqbal, M., Moisiadis, V. G., Kostaki, A., & Matthews, S. G. (2012). Transgenerational effects of prenatal synthetic glucocorticoids on hypothalamic-pituitary-adrenal function. *Endocrinology, 153*(7), 3295–3307. doi:10.1210/en.2012-1054

Karatsoreos, I. N., & McEwen, B. S. (2013a). Annual research review: The neurobiology and physiology of resilience and adaptation across the life course. *Journal of Child Psychology and Psychiatry, 54*(4), 337–347. doi:10.1111/jcpp.12054

Karatsoreos, I. N., & McEwen, B. S. (2013b). Resilience and vulnerability: A neurobiological perspective. *F1000Prime Reports, 5*, 13. doi:10.12703/P5-13

King, S., & Laplante, D. P. (2015). Using natural disasters to study prenatal maternal stress in humans. *Advanced Neurobiology, 10*, 285–313. doi:10.1007/978-1-4939-1372-5_14

Kingsbury, M., Weeks, M., MacKinnon, N., Evans, J., Mahedy, L., Dykxhoorn, J., & Colman, I. (2016). Stressful life events during pregnancy and offspring depression: Evidence from a prospective cohort study. *Journal of the American Academy of Child and Adolescent Psychiatry, 55*(8), 709–716.e702. doi:10.1016/j.jaac.2016.05.014

Kingston, D., Austin, M. P., Hegadoren, K., McDonald, S., Lasiuk, G., McDonald, S., … van Zanten, S. V. (2014). Study protocol for a randomized, controlled, superiority trial comparing the clinical and cost-effectiveness of integrated online mental health assessment-referral-care in pregnancy to usual prenatal care on prenatal and postnatal mental health and infant health and development: The Integrated Maternal Psychosocial Assessment to Care Trial (IMPACT). *Trials, 15*, 72. doi:10.1186/1745-6215-15-72

Kingston, D., Heaman, M., Fell, D., Dzakpasu, S., & Chalmers, B. (2012). Factors associated with perceived stress and stressful life events in pregnant women: Findings from the Canadian maternity experiences survey. *Maternal and Child Health Journal, 16*(1), 158–168. doi:10.1007/s10995-010-0732-2

Kingston, D., McDonald, S., Austin, M. P., & Tough, S. (2015). Association between prenatal and postnatal psychological distress and toddler cognitive development: A systematic review. *PLoS One, 10*(5), e0126929. doi:10.1371/journal.pone.0126929

Kingston, D., Sword, W., Krueger, P., Hanna, S., & Markle-Reid, M. (2012). Life course pathways to prenatal maternal stress. *Journal of Obstetric, Gynecologic & Neonatal Nursing, 41*(5), 609–626. doi:10.1111/j.1552-6909.2012.01381.x

Kingston, D., & Tough, S. (2014). Prenatal and postnatal maternal mental health and school-age child development: A systematic review. *Maternal and Child Health Journal, 18*(7), 1728–1741. doi:10.1007/s10995-013-1418-3

Kinser, P. A., Thacker, L. R., Lapato, D., Wagner, S., Roberson-Nay, R., Jobe-Shields, L., … York, T. P. (2017). Depressive symptom prevalence and predictors in the first half of pregnancy. *Journal of Women's Health (Larchmt)*. doi:10.1089/jwh.2017.6426

Koss, K. J., Hostinar, C. E., Donzella, B., & Gunnar, M. R. (2014). Social deprivation and the HPA axis in early development. *Psychoneuroendocrinology, 50*, 1–13. doi:10.1016/j.psyneuen.2014.07.028

Koss, K. J., Mliner, S. B., Donzella, B., & Gunnar, M. R. (2016). Early adversity, hypocortisolism, and behavior problems at school entry: A study of internationally adopted children. *Psychoneuroendocrinology, 66*, 31–38. doi:10.1016/j.psyneuen.2015.12.018

Kroska, E. B., O'Hara, M. W., Elgbeili, G., Hart, K. J., Laplante, D. P., Dancause, K. N., & King, S. (2017). The impact of maternal flood-related stress and social support on offspring weight in early childhood. *Archives of Women's Mental Health*. doi:10.1007/s00737-017-0786-x

Kundakovic, M., & Jaric, I. (2017). The epigenetic link between prenatal adverse environments and neurodevelopmental disorders. *Genes (Basel), 8*(3). doi:10.3390/genes8030104

Lancaster, C. A., Gold, K. J., Flynn, H. A., Yoo, H., Marcus, S. M., & Davis, M. M. (2010). Risk factors for depressive symptoms during pregnancy: A systematic review. *American Journal of Obstetrics and Gynecology, 202*(1), 5–14. doi:10.1016/j.ajog.2009.09.007

Laplante, D. P., Barr, R. G., Brunet, A., Galbaud du Fort, G., Meaney, M. L., Saucier, J. F., … King, S. (2004). Stress during pregnancy affects general intellectual and language functioning in human toddlers. *Pediatric Research, 56*(3), 400–410. doi:10.1203/01.PDR.0000136281.34035.44

Laplante, D. P., Hart, K. J., O'Hara, M. W., Brunet, A., & King, S. (2017). Prenatal maternal stress is associated with toddler cognitive functioning: The Iowa Flood Study. *Early Human Development, 116*, 84–92. doi:10.1016/j.earlhumdev.2017.11.012

Lewis, A. J., Austin, E., Knapp, R., Vaiano, T., & Galbally, M. (2015). Perinatal maternal mental health, fetal programming and child development. *Healthcare (Basel), 3*(4), 1212–1227. doi:10.3390/healthcare3041212

Liou, S. R., Wang, P., & Cheng, C. Y. (2014). Longitudinal study of perinatal maternal stress, depressive symptoms and anxiety. *Midwifery, 30*(6), 795–801. doi:10.1016/j.midw.2013.11.007

Lovibond, S. H., & Lovibond, P. F. (1995). *Manual for the Depression, Anxiety and Stress Scales* (2nd ed.). Sydney: Psychology Foundation.

Luecken, L. J., Lin, B., Coburn, S. S., MacKinnon, D. P., Gonzales, N. A., & Crnic, K. A. (2013). Prenatal stress, partner support, and infant cortisol reactivity in low-income Mexican American families. *Psychoneuroendocrinology, 38*(12), 3092–3101. doi:10.1016/j.psyneuen.2013.09.006

MacKinnon, N., Kingsbury, M., Mahedy, L., Evans, J., & Colman, I. (2018). The association between prenatal stress and externalizing symptoms in childhood: Evidence from the Avon longitudinal study of parents and children. *Biological Psychiatry, 83*(2), 100–108. doi:10.1016/j.biopsych.2017.07.010

McEwen, B. S., Bowles, N. P., Gray, J. D., Hill, M. N., Hunter, R. G., Karatsoreos, I. N., & Nasca, C. (2015). Mechanisms of stress in the brain. *Nature Neuroscience, 18*(10), 1353–1363. doi:10.1038/nn.4086

McEwen, B. S., Gray, J., & Nasca, C. (2015). Recognizing resilience: Learning from the effects of stress on the brain. *Neurobiology of Stress, 1*, 1–11. doi:10.1016/j.ynstr.2014.09.001

Meaney, M. J., & Szyf, M. (2005). Environmental programming of stress responses through DNA methylation: Life at the interface between a dynamic environment and a fixed genome. *Dialogues in Clinical Neuroscience, 7*(2), 103–123.

Metz, G. A., Ng, J. W., Kovalchuk, I., & Olson, D. M. (2015). Ancestral experience as a game changer in stress vulnerability and disease outcomes. *Bioessays, 37*(6), 602–611. doi:10.1002/bies.201400217

Milgrom, J., Gemmill, A. W., Bilszta, J. L., Hayes, B., Barnett, B., Brooks, J., … Buist, A. (2008). Antenatal risk factors for postnatal depression: A large prospective study. *Journal of Affective Disorders, 108*(1–2), 147–157. doi:10.1016/j.jad.2007.10.014

Mitchell, P. B., Parker, G. B., Gladstone, G. L., Wilhelm, K., & Austin, M. P. (2003). Severity of stressful life events in first and subsequent episodes of depression: The relevance of depressive subtype. *Journal of Affective Disorders, 73*(3), 245–252.

Moisiadis, V. G., & Matthews, S. G. (2014). Glucocorticoids and fetal programming part 1: Outcomes. *Nature Reviews Endocrinology, 10*(7), 391–402. doi:10.1038/nrendo.2014.73

Monk, C., Feng, T., Lee, S., Krupska, I., Champagne, F. A., & Tycko, B. (2016). Distress during pregnancy: Epigenetic regulation of placenta glucocorticoid-related genes and fetal neurobehavior. *American Journal of Psychiatry, 173*(7), 705–713. doi:10.1176/appi.ajp.2015.15091171

Moss, K. M., Simcock, G., Cobham, V., Kildea, S., Elgbeili, G., Laplante, D. P., & King, S. (2017). A potential psychological mechanism linking disaster-related prenatal maternal stress with child cognitive and motor development at 16 months: The QF2011 Queensland Flood Study. *Developmental Psychology, 53*(4), 629–641. doi:10.1037/dev0000272

Mukherjee, S., Coxe, S., Fennie, K., Madhivanan, P., & Trepka, M. J. (2017a). Antenatal stressful life events and postpartum depressive symptoms in the United States: The role of women's socioeconomic status indices at the state level. *Journal of Women's Health (Larchmt), 26*(3), 276–285. doi:10.1089/jwh.2016.5872

Mukherjee, S., Coxe, S., Fennie, K., Madhivanan, P., & Trepka, M. J. (2017b). Stressful life event experiences of pregnant women in the United States: A latent class analysis. *Women's Health Issues, 27*(1), 83–92. doi:10.1016/j.whi.2016.09.007

Norhayati, M. N., Hazlina, N. H., Asrenee, A. R., & Emilin, W. M. (2015). Magnitude and risk factors for postpartum symptoms: A literature review. *Journal of Affective Disorders, 175*, 34–52. doi:10.1016/j.jad.2014.12.041

Oberlander, T. F., Weinberg, J., Papsdorf, M., Grunau, R., Misri, S., & Devlin, A. M. (2008). Prenatal exposure to maternal depression, neonatal methylation of human glucocorticoid receptor gene (NR3C1) and infant cortisol stress responses. *Epigenetics, 3*(2), 97–106.

Parker, K. J., Schatzberg, A. F., & Lyons, D. M. (2003). Neuroendocrine aspects of hypercortisolism in major depression. *Hormones and Behavior, 43*(1), 60–66.

Peters, A., McEwen, B. S., & Friston, K. (2017). Uncertainty and stress: Why it causes diseases and how it is mastered by the brain. *Progress in Neurobiology, 156*, 164–188. doi:10.1016/j.pneurobio.2017.05.004

Phua, D. Y., Kee, Mkzl, Koh, D. X. P., Rifkin-Graboi, A., Daniels, M., Chen, H., … Growing Up In Singapore Towards Healthy Outcomes Study Group. (2017). Positive maternal mental health during pregnancy associated with specific forms of adaptive development in early childhood: Evidence from a longitudinal study. *Development and Psychopathology, 29*(5), 1573–1587. doi:10.1017/S0954579417001249

Putnam, K. T., Wilcox, M., Robertson-Blackmore, E., Sharkey, K., Bergink, V., Munk-Olsen, T., … Treatment, Consortium. (2017). Clinical phenotypes of perinatal depression and time of symptom onset: Analysis of data from an international consortium. *Lancet Psychiatry, 4*(6), 477–485. doi:10.1016/S2215-0366(17)30136-0

Rallis, S., Skouteris, H., McCabe, M., & Milgrom, J. (2014). A prospective examination of depression, anxiety and stress throughout pregnancy. *Women and Birth, 27*(4), e36–42. doi:10.1016/j.wombi.2014.08.002

Rubertsson, C., Wickberg, B., Gustavsson, P., & Radestad, I. (2005). Depressive symptoms in early pregnancy, two months and one year postpartum-prevalence and psychosocial risk factors in a national Swedish sample. *Archives of Women's Mental Health, 8*(2), 97–104. doi:10.1007/s00737-005-0078-8

Salm Ward, T., Kanu, F. A., & Robb, S. W. (2017). Prevalence of stressful life events during pregnancy and its association with postpartum depressive symptoms. *Archives of Women's Mental Health, 20*(1), 161–171. doi:10.1007/s00737-016-0689-2

Sapolsky, R. M. (2015). Stress and the brain: Individual variability and the inverted-U. *Nature Neuroscience, 18*(10), 1344–1346. doi:10.1038/nn.4109

Sharp, H., Hill, J., Hellier, J., & Pickles, A. (2015). Maternal antenatal anxiety, postnatal stroking and emotional problems in children: Outcomes predicted from pre- and postnatal programming hypotheses. *Psychological Medicine, 45*(2), 269–283. doi:10.1017/s0033291714001342

Sharp, H., Pickles, A., Meaney, M., Marshall, K., Tibu, F., & Hill, J. (2012). Frequency of infant stroking reported by mothers moderates the effect of prenatal depression on infant behavioural and physiological outcomes. *PLoS One, 7*(10), e45446. doi:10.1371/journal.pone.0045446

Simcock, G., Elgbeili, G., Laplante, D. P., Kildea, S., Cobham, V., Stapleton, H., … King, S. (2017). The effects of prenatal maternal stress on early temperament: The 2011 Queensland flood study. *Journal of Developmental and Behavioral Pediatrics, 38*(5), 310–321. doi:10.1097/dbp.0000000000000444

Simcock, G., Kildea, S., Elgbeili, G., Laplante, D. P., Stapleton, H., Cobham, V., & King, S. (2016). Age-related changes in the effects of stress in pregnancy on infant motor development by maternal report: The Queensland flood study. *Developmental Psychobiology, 58*(5), 640–659. doi:10.1002/dev.21407

Staneva, A., Bogossian, F., Pritchard, M., & Wittkowski, A. (2015). The effects of maternal depression, anxiety, and perceived stress during pregnancy on preterm birth: A systematic review. *Women and Birth, 28*(3), 179–193. doi:10.1016/j.wombi.2015.02.003

Sun, A. X., Crabtree, G. R., & Yoo, A. S. (2013). MicroRNAs: Regulators of neuronal fate. *Current Opinion in Cell Biology, 25*(2), 215–221. doi:10.1016/j.ceb.2012.12.007

Whitehead, N., Hill, H. A., Brogan, D. J., & Blackmore-Prince, C. (2002). Exploration of threshold analysis in the relation between stressful life events and preterm delivery. *American Journal of Epidemiology, 155*(2), 117–124.

Yao, Y., Robinson, A. M., Zucchi, F. C., Robbins, J. C., Babenko, O., Kovalchuk, O., … Metz, G. A. (2014). Ancestral exposure to stress epigenetically programs preterm birth risk and adverse maternal and newborn outcomes. *BMC Medicine, 12*, 121. doi:10.1186/s12916-014-0121-6

Zijlmans, M. A., Korpela, K., Riksen-Walraven, J. M., de Vos, W. M., & de Weerth, C. (2015). Maternal prenatal stress is associated with the infant intestinal microbiota. *Psychoneuroendocrinology, 53*, 233–245. doi:10.1016/j.psyneuen.2015.01.006

Zijlmans, M. A., Riksen-Walraven, J. M., & de Weerth, C. (2015). Associations between maternal prenatal cortisol concentrations and child outcomes: A systematic review. *Neuroscience & Biobehavioral Reviews, 53*, 1–24. doi:10.1016/j.neubiorev.2015.02.015

Zucchi, F. C., Yao, Y., Ward, I. D., Ilnytskyy, Y., Olson, D. M., Benzies, K., … Metz, G. A. (2013). Maternal stress induces epigenetic signatures of psychiatric and neurological diseases in the offspring. *PLoS One, 8*(2), e56967. doi:10.1371/journal.pone.0056967

2

Fetal Exposure to Mother's Distress

New Frontiers in Research and Useful Knowledge for Daily Clinical Practice

Catherine Monk, Sophie Foss, Preeya Desai, and Vivette Glover

Introduction

Research over the last 20 years has shown the importance of the mother's emotional state during pregnancy, for the neurodevelopment of her fetus and future child. It is clear that it is not only extreme or toxic stress or a diagnosed mental illness that can affect fetal development but a wide range of stresses that can have effects. These include symptoms of prenatal anxiety and depression (O'Connor et al., 2002), stressful life events (Bergman et al., 2007), daily hassles (Huizink et al., 2002), exposure to a natural disaster such as an ice storm in Canada (King & Laplante, 2005), or human made disaster such as Chernobyl (Huizink et al., 2007) in Russia. It is not clear yet whether different types of stress have differential effects on outcome, or whether, for example, symptoms of prenatal anxiety have a different effect from symptoms of prenatal depression. One study found that symptoms of prenatal anxiety, but not depression, had a significant effect on child academic achievement at 16 years (Pearson et al., 2016). The mother's own early experiences of trauma may also have an effect on the development of her fetus, independently of her current emotional state, as is discussed further below.

Some women feel very anxious about their pregnancy, about the labor, or whether the child will be normal at birth. Several studies have found that such pregnancy-specific anxiety is especially associated with altered child outcome, e.g., in telomere length (Entringer et al., 2013) and in the epigenetic pattern of the glucocorticoid receptor (Hompes et al., 2013) in the newborn. However, it remains to be determined whether assessments focused on pregnancy-specific anxiety are accessing a unique form of anxiety particularly relevant to fetal development — that theoretically would diminish once the baby is born healthy – or whether these assessment approaches are simply better suited to measure anxiety during the prenatal period because women typically high on anxiety focus their concerns on their pregnancy and the birth outcomes — which would imply the likelihood of continued anxiety after birth.

If the mother is stressed, anxious, or depressed while pregnant, she may drink alcohol or smoke, and she may pass on vulnerability genes to her offspring. These factors can all affect child outcome. There is a likelihood that she will be similarly affected postnatally and this may affect her interaction with her baby, the quality of her child's attachment to her, and her later parenting. There is much evidence that if the mother is depressed postnatally, this can also increase the risk of later psychopathology and compromised cognitive ability in her child. It is thus important to determine how much of any association between maternal prenatal mood and child outcome is indeed causal, and not due to these associated factors. Several large community studies have found that even after allowing for all of these factors there remains an association between prenatal mood and later child outcome, suggesting a direct association. These large community studies include the Generation R study in the Netherlands (Kooijman et al., 2016), the Finnish FinnBrain study (Nolvi et al., 2016), the Finnish PREDO study (Lahti et al., 2017), and the RAINE study in Australia (Robinson et al., 2008), as well as ALSPAC in the United Kingdom (O'Donnell et al., 2014). Some studies have found that associations with later child psychopathology are much stronger with prenatal maternal mood, than with paternal mood (Pearson et al., 2013, Glover et al., 2015), showing that these associations are not solely genetic and support the role of the prenatal maternal environment which plays a unique role in children's outcomes. O'Donnell et al. (2014) have demonstrated with the ALSPAC data set that if the mother was in the top 15% for symptoms of anxiety or depression while pregnant, her child at age of 13 years had a risk of 13% of a probable mental disorder, compared to a risk of 7% for the children of the other 85% (O'Donnell et al., 2013). This was after allowing for a wide range of possible confounders, including postnatal maternal mood, parenting, paternal mood, maternal alcohol consumption, maternal education, and socioeconomic status. Thus, in the O'Donnell study the risk of a mental disorder in the child was approximately doubled, and clinically significant, although nearly 90% of the children were not affected.

Another approach to ruling out confounds in prenatal programming research is to assess the offspring at the time of exposure to maternal distress, that is, as a fetus, or right after birth, as a newborn. Clearly, each of these methods removes the potential confounding influence of factors in the postnatal environment, though so far they do not also provide predictive developmental outcomes relating fetal-newborn observations to future child psychopathology – though sometimes to alterations in infant development. In some of the earliest studies, DiPietro et al. showed greater maternal stress during pregnancy; in addition, poverty status was associated with variation in fetal autonomic nervous system (ANS) regulation (DiPietro et al., 1996; Pressman et al., 1998). Others have related anxiety and depression to greater fetal movement (Groome et al., 1995; Dieter et al., 2001) and variation in fetal reactivity to various stimuli (Sandman et al., 2003; Monk et al., 2000, 2004, 2010). In particular, Monk et al. have found that fetuses of depressed or anxious mothers show greater heart rate reactivity to stimuli independent of maternal ANS and cortisol activity (Monk et al., 2000, 2004, 2010) and that greater fetal heart rate reactivity predicts more reactive temperament evidenced in motor responses to novelty at four months of age (Werner et al., 2007). In another study, sleeping, non-sedated newborns underwent magnetic resonance imaging (MRI) and showed that prenatal maternal depression is associated with alterations in the microstructure of the amygdala, a region of the brain undergirding emotion experiences, particularly fear responses (Gold et al., 1988). In related work, Posner found that prenatal maternal depression was associated with increased resting state connectivity between the dorsal lateral prefrontal cortex and the amygdala in neonates of women depressed during pregnancy (Posner et al., 2016). Interestingly, greater fetal heart rate reactivity predicted this increased functional connectivity near birth, suggesting that the identification of greater fetal responses is potentially a marker of brain development consistent with increased responses to novel or fear-inducing challenges (Posner et al., 2016).

Across a range of methodologies and time frames (clinical to epidemiologic, prospective follow-up and proximal fetal-newborn assessment), data strongly suggest that women's mental health during pregnancy has an impact on children's future neurobehavioral development.

Types of Child Outcome Affected

Prenatal stress can increase the risk for a range of different emotional and behavioral problems in the infant, child, or adolescent, as well as a range of physical outcomes (Glover, 2014; van den Bergh et al., 2017). Several studies have shown an increased probability for a difficult temperament in the infant, with more dysregulated sleeping and feeding, more crying, and being harder to soothe (e.g. Werner et al., 2013; Laplante et al., 2016; Nolvi et al., 2016). Other research has found increased risk for both internalizing and externalizing symptoms (Robinson et al., 2008; Lahti et al., 2017). Many studies have shown an increased probability for symptoms of anxiety and depression among children (O'Connor et al., 2002; Van den Bergh et al., 2008; Maxwell et al., 2017), symptoms of ADHD (O'Connor et al., 2002; Van den Bergh & Marcoen, 2004), and symptoms of conduct disorder (O'Connor et al., 2002; O'Connor et al., 2003). Other studies have shown an increased chance of autism (Kinney et al., 2008) or severity of symptoms on the autistic spectrum (Varcin et al., 2017). The increased risk for both depression (Pearson et al., 2013) and anxiety (Capron et al., 2015) has been shown to persist into early adulthood. Several studies have shown an increased likelihood of lower cognitive performance (Laplante et al., 2004; Bergman et al., 2007; Maxwell et al., 2017), and worse later school achievement (Pearson et al., 2016). Research on infants has found that effects can be different with boys and girls (Glover & Hill, 2012; Tibu et al., 2014; Braithwaite et al., 2017).

Very severe stress in the first trimester (weeks 0–12), such as the death of an older child, increases the risk of later schizophrenia (van Os & Selten, 1998; Khashan et al., 2008). Neuronal migration peaks between gestational weeks 12–20, and is largely complete by weeks 26–29 (Tau & Peterson, 2010). It is known that this pattern of migration is disturbed in schizophrenia. Most of the studies referred to above, with other outcomes, have found associations with stress later during pregnancy, in both second and third trimesters. Lahti et al. (2017), who assessed women biweekly, from week 12 to 38 during pregnancy, found an increase in child internalizing and externalizing symptoms associated with maternal depressive symptoms at all of these times. More research is needed to understand the most sensitive gestational ages for different outcomes and different exposures.

Many physical outcomes have been found to be altered by exposure to prenatal stress, including an increased risk of early delivery, preterm birth, and lower birth weight for gestational age (Glover, 2015). However, the effect sizes are somewhat inconsistent and generally smaller than those associated with altered neurodevelopment. There is an increased risk of asthma (Cookson et al., 2009; Khashan et al., 2012), allergic diseases (Suh et al., 2017), reduced telomere length (Entringer et al., 2013), which may be associated with reduced lifetime longevity, altered finger print pattern (King et al., 2009), and mixed handedness (Glover et al., 2004; Rodriguez & Waldenstrom, 2008). It does not seem that in general the effects on later psychopathology are mediated by effects of fetal physical growth (O'Donnell & Meaney, 2017).

With all these outcomes, maternal prenatal stress, anxiety, and depression only *increase risk*; they do not definitely predict poor outcomes. It is one of many exposures shaping children's future lives, e.g., maternal prenatal nutrition, environmental pollution. Most children are not affected, and those who are, are affected in different ways. Some of the differences in outcomes may lie in differences in postnatal care. The effects of postnatal depression can be additive with those of prenatal (O'Donnell et al., 2014) or ameliorative: secure mother-infant attachment can buffer against some of the prenatal effects (Bergman et al., 2010), while insecure attachment can exacerbate others (Bergman et al., 2008).

Early Life Trauma

There is currently interest in the early life causes of maternal prenatal symptoms of anxiety and depression, and also how early trauma may be related to her physiology during pregnancy and thus the development of her fetus. Early life exposure to adverse childhood experiences (ACEs) predicts later anxiety and depression as well as other mental and physical health outcomes (Lee et al., 2017). Plant et al. (2017) have shown, using the ALSPAC cohort, that a maternal history of child maltreatment is significantly associated with offspring internalizing and externalizing difficulties. Maternal antenatal depression, postnatal depression, and offspring child maltreatment all independently significantly mediated this association.

Moog et al. (2016) have shown that childhood trauma in the mother is associated with raised CRH during pregnancy, thus linking her early experience with placental-fetal stress physiology. The same group (Moog et al., 2017) have also found that early childhood trauma was associated with altered brain structure in the newborn, predominantly reduced global cortical gray matter, independently of the mother's prenatal mood. The effect was also independent of other potential confounding variables, including maternal socioeconomic status, obstetric complications, obesity, recent interpersonal violence, gestational age at birth, infant sex, and postnatal age at the MRI scan. This interesting finding suggests that early trauma can alter the mother's biochemistry in a way that in turn alters the development of the brain of her fetus.

Possible mediating factors are chemicals associated with the immune system and inflammation. Blackmore et al. (2011) found that a history of trauma, although not current symptoms of prenatal anxiety or depression, was associated with significantly elevated levels of the pro-inflammatory cytokine, TNF-alpha, after controlling for psychosocial and obstetric covariates. Similarly, in a sample of pregnant adolescents at risk for both high ACE scores and current distress, Walsh et al. found that in young women with more severe abuse histories, those with current depression versus not had higher levels of another pro-inflammatory cytokine, interleukin-6 (IL-6) (Walsh et al., 2016), another biological indicator of inflammation. Graham et al. (2017) have shown that higher than average maternal IL-6 during pregnancy was associated with brain changes in the newborn including a larger right amygdala volume. These changes were in turn associated with lower impulse control at 24 months of age in the infant. Intriguingly, a recent study showed that maternal childhood abuse was associated with variation in fetal ANS regulation independent of current psychiatric symptoms (Gustafsson et al., 2017).

The effects of trauma may even last until the grandchild generation. Serpeloni et al. (2017) have shown that if the grandmother suffered from interpersonal violence during her pregnancy, there was an altered epigenetic profile in her grandchildren.

Underlying Biological Mechanisms

Beyond the specific topic of maternal childhood trauma, the role of the hypothalamic-pituitary-adrenal (HPA) axis and cortisol has been most studied as a potential mediator of the effects of prenatal stress on the fetus and the child. There is good evidence that fetal exposure to higher levels of cortisol can alter fetal brain development. Maternal exposure to synthetic glucocorticoids during pregnancy is associated with worse mental health in childhood and adolescence (Khalife et al., 2013). Davis and colleagues have shown that babies exposed to synthetic glucocorticoids *in utero* have altered brain structure, including a thinner cortex, as shown by MRI scans (Davis et al., 2013). Also, the children of mothers who had consumed high levels of licorice during pregnancy were more likely to have ADHD symptoms, as well as lower IQ and earlier puberty (Raikkonen et al., 2017). Licorice contains a natural inhibitor of the enzyme 11-β-hydroxysteroid dehydrogenase type II (11β-HSD2), which converts cortisol to its inactive form cortisone in the placenta, and these fetuses were thus exposed to higher levels of cortisol *in utero*. In addition, Bergman et al. (2010) showed that higher levels of cortisol in amniotic fluid were negatively correlated with cognitive scores in the Bayley's Mental Developmental Index when the infant was 18 months old (Bergman et al., 2010).

However, it is not likely that prenatal stress is altering fetal neurodevelopment primarily via raised maternal cortisol levels. The maternal HPA axis becomes gradually less responsive to stressors as pregnancy progresses, and there is only a weak, if any, association between maternal mood and cortisol level, especially later during pregnancy (Sarkar et al., 2006; Evans et al., 2008; O'Donnell et al., 2009). Bleker et al. (2017), with a large cohort of pregnant Dutch women, have shown that the variables that were associated with higher cortisol levels were lower maternal age, being nulliparous, lower pre-pregnancy body mass index, higher C-reactive protein, carrying a female fetus, non-smoking, and being unemployed (Bleker et al., 2017). A total of 32% of all variance in cortisol was explained by these variables. None of the psychosocial stressors they examined were significantly associated with maternal serum cortisol levels.

It is likely that fetal programming, caused by prenatal stress, may be partly mediated by raised fetal exposure to cortisol without increases in maternal levels. Stress or anxiety may cause increased trans-placental transfer of maternal cortisol to the fetal compartment without a rise in maternal levels. The placenta clearly plays a crucial role in moderating fetal exposure to maternal factors. Thus, another mechanism by which the fetus could become overexposed to glucocorticoids is through changes in placental function, especially in a down-regulation of the barrier enzyme 11β-HSD2, which converts cortisol to the inactive cortisone. If there is less of this barrier enzyme in the placenta, then the fetus will be exposed to more maternal cortisol, independently of any change in the maternal cortisol level. If the mother has higher basal levels of cortisol, then the amount of fetal exposure will also be higher, as there is a strong correlation between maternal and fetal cortisol levels (Gitau et al., 1998). Glover et al. (2009) showed that the correlation between maternal plasma and amniotic fluid cortisol was significantly increased with greater symptoms of maternal anxiety, suggesting that with more anxiety the placenta becomes more permeable to cortisol, with potentially increased fetal exposure (Glover et al., 2009).

Several studies have examined aspects of prenatal maternal mood and the expression of HPA-related genes in the placenta. O'Donnell et al. have shown that both the expression and activity of placental 11-βHSD2 are down-regulated with higher levels of maternal anxiety (O'Donnell et al., 2012). Togher et al. (2017) have found a down-regulation of 11-βHSD2 associated with a composite measure of prenatal stress (Togher et al., 2017). Monk et al. (2016), using the Perceived Stress Scale, found an association with increased methylation of 11-βHSD2 in the placenta, which also suggests a down regulation of expression (Monk et al., 2016). This in turn was associated with reduced fetal movement and heart rate coupling, an index of fetal central nervous system (CNS) development. Coupling reliably increases over gestation, reflecting the coordination of the autonomic and somatic systems, and is positively associated with more mature neural integration at birth.

Maternal prenatal depression has been associated with an increase in the expression of the cortisol receptor (NR3C1) in the placenta in several studies (Conradt et al., 2013; Reynolds et al., 2015). Togher et al. (2017) found an upregulation associated with their composite prenatal stress measure.

Several studies have shown an association between placental HPA axis genes and infant neurobehavior, providing some evidence that the alteration in the placental expression of these genes associated with prenatal maternal mood or stress may have a direct mediating role in fetal neurodevelopment (Appleton et al., 2015; Paquette et al., 2015). Raikkonen et al. (2015) found that higher placental NR3C1 mRNA partly mediated the association between maternal depressive symptoms during pregnancy and infant regulatory behaviors (Raikkonen et al., 2015). Although HPA axis genes have been most studied in the placenta, it is likely that other systems are involved as well, including serotonin (Muller et al., 2017).

We currently do not know what biological changes in the mother are involved in fetal programming induced by prenatal stress, anxiety, or depression. As discussed above, there must be other maternal factors in addition to cortisol. Pro-inflammatory cytokines are promising candidates. Similar to findings with trauma, there is increasing evidence relating depression in general with altered function of the immune system, including raised levels of pro-inflammatory cytokines (Cattaneo et al., 2015). Exposure to early life stressful events may act through the modulation of inflammatory responses over the entire life span. As indicated, a history of exposure to trauma, specifically intimate partner violence, has been associated with raised levels of the cytokine TNF-α during pregnancy (Blackmore et al., 2011). Several studies now have related symptoms of depression or anxiety or a history of abuse to altered cytokine patterns during pregnancy (Walsh et al., 2016; Chang et al., 2017; Karlsson et al., 2017). However, we do not yet know how, if at all, this affects the function of the placenta or the development of the fetus.

Epigenetic changes are being studied in other tissues besides the placenta, underlying the long-term effects of prenatal stress on the development of the fetus and the child (Cao-Lei et al., 2017; Nemoda & Szyf, 2017). Epigenetic alterations to the DNA control the degree to which a gene is expressed or repressed, turned on or off. Epigenetic changes can last throughout the lifetime, but in some cases they can also be reversed.

Epigenetic changes in the fetus and the child after prenatal stress have been found both in animal models (Jensen Pena et al., 2012) and in humans. Several studies have looked at alterations in the methylation of specific genes, and especially in the promoter region of the glucocorticoid receptor (NR3C1) that binds cortisol. Hompes et al. (2013) have shown epigenetic changes in this region using cord blood (reflecting fetal tissue) from mothers who suffered from pregnancy-related anxiety (Hompes et al., 2013). Oberlander et al. (2008) have shown altered NR3C1 promoter methylation in cord blood from neonates born to mothers with prenatal depression.

Epigenetic changes have also been found in older children whose mothers experienced stress during pregnancy. For example, maternal prenatal stress, caused by intimate partner violence, has been shown to be associated with increased methylation of the NR3C1 promoter in the blood of their adolescent children (Radtke et al., 2011). While this finding is interesting and suggestive of intergenerational effects of domestic violence, these results, like most of the epigenetic studies in this field, should be treated with some caution. Although epigenetics remains a promising mechanism for the mediation of prenatal stress effects on the developing brain of the fetus and future child, evidence for it is still quite limited.

There is increasing interest in the influence of the microbiome on mental health, and alterations in its composition as one pathway for the effects of maternal prenatal stress on later psychopathology of the child (O'Mahony et al., 2017; Rakers et al., 2017). Gut bacteria strongly influence our metabolic, endocrine, immune, and both peripheral and central nervous systems (CNS). Thus, disruption of the microbiome in early life has the potential to influence neurodevelopment and mental health outcomes in the long term, particularly through its interaction with the immune system and the gut-brain axis. Zijlmans et al. (2015) have shown that maternal prenatal stress was strongly and persistently associated with the infants' microbiota composition.

Genes of Risk

Some of the transmission of risk, and likely some of the differences in outcome are due to differences in different genetic vulnerabilities of the children themselves. Qiu et al. (2017) have shown that the effects of both prenatal maternal depressive symptoms, and the effect of socioeconomic status, on neonatal brain development, are modulated by genetic risk. They conclude that their findings suggest gene-environment interdependence in the fetal development of brain regions implicated in cognitive-emotional function, and that candidate biological mechanisms involve a range of brain region-specific signaling pathways that converge on common processes of synaptic development.

Others have examined gene-environment interactions looking at specific genes. Chen et al. (2015) have shown that a genetic variant in BDNF affects the degree of association between maternal prenatal anxiety and neonatal DNA methylation, as well as neonatal brain structure.

O'Donnell et al. (2014), using the ALSPAC cohort, showed an interaction between prenatal anxiety and different genetic variants of *BDNF* and later child internalizing symptoms from age 4 to 15 years. O'Donnell et al. (2017) showed that there was also a significant interaction between child *COMT* genotype and symptoms of both ADHD and working memory in the child. There was no interaction between *BDNF* and working memory or ADHD, or between *COMT* and internalizing symptoms. The interactions in both the O'Donnell studies explained only a small part of the variance, and there are probably very many genes involved in the predisposition to the many types of outcomes affected by maternal prenatal distress.

Screening for Prenatal Mood Symptoms

Research in the latter part of the 20th century began to establish the association between women's mental health during pregnancy and their children's neurobehavioral development. While the mechanisms for these effects still warrant extensive investigation, the correspondence of the data from a variety of sources, and the effect sizes (e.g., a doubling of the risk for psychopathology in the ALSPAC data set) support intervention and prevention to offset this early risk exposure. Indeed, we routinely provide treatment prior to completely understanding the pathophysiology of disease etiology (e.g., cancer) and depression, stress, and anxiety are typically modifiable when there is access to decent behavioral health services. As with all clinical work, the first step is reliable screening.

Many leading professional and government bodies now call for routine screening for mental health issues during the perinatal period (Committee on Obstetric, 2015). In 2015, the American College of Obstetricians and Gynecologists formally announced the new standard to screen all pregnant women at least once for depression and anxiety using validated tools (Gynecologists, 2015). In 2016, the US Preventive Services Task Force specifically recommended screening for depression during pregnancy and the postpartum period (Siu et al., 2016). Findings from a systematic review published in *JAMA* supported the USPSTF recommendation that screening for depression in the prenatal/postpartum period reduced the prevalence of depression and increased remission or treatment response (O'Connor et al., 2016). Eight scales are typically used to screen for depression during pregnancy, and the one with the strongest sensitivity and specificity data, the Edinburgh Postnatal Depression Scale (EPDS), also includes anxiety questions as depression in the prenatal period often is comorbid with significant anxiety symptoms (Gynecologists, 2015). Each of the scales is self-report except for the Hamilton Rating Scale for Depression (HRSD) (Hamilton, 1960). In addition to the EPDS and the HRSD, six other assessment tools for depression are included: the Postpartum Depression (PPD) Screening Scale (Beck & Gable, 2001), the Patient Health Questionnaire-9 (Kroenke et al., 2001), the Beck Depression Inventory (Beck et al., 1961), the Beck Depression Inventory II (Beck et al., 1996), the Center for Epidemiologic Studies Depression Scale (Radloff, 1977), the Zung Self-Rating Depression Scale (Zung, 1965).

The Edinburgh Postnatal Depression Scale consists of ten self-reported items, is quite brief, has been translated into 12 languages, requires a low reading level, and is easy to score. As indicated, it includes anxiety symptoms and minimizes the inclusion of somatic symptoms of depression, such as changes in sleeping patterns that are common during pregnancy independent of depression. The inclusion of these constitutional symptoms in other screening instruments, such as the Patient Health Questionnaire 9, the Beck Depression Inventory, and the Center for Epidemiologic Studies Depression Scale, reduces their specificity for perinatal depression. With the exception of the Patient Health Questionnaire 9 and the Edinburgh Postnatal Depression Scale, other instruments have at least 20 questions and, thus, take more time to complete and score (Ji et al., 2011; Gynecologists, 2015).

Despite evidence that depression during pregnancy includes anxiety symptoms and that often there is a comorbid anxiety disorder (Dindo et al., 2017), as well as the demonstration of maternal anxiety having consequences for children's development, assessment of anxiety during pregnancy receives far less attention. Much of the fetal programming research focused on maternal anxiety uses research as opposed to clinical scales, e.g., Spielberger's State Trait Anxiety Scale (Spielberger & Gorsuch, 1983) or the Crown Crisp (Crown & Crisp, 1966). One scale with strong sensitivity and specificity data that is designed for use with peripartum patients and is used in research as well as in clinical settings is the Hamilton Rating Scale for Anxiety (Hamilton, 1959). As indicated, there are questionnaires focused specifically on pregnancy-related stress and anxiety (e.g., Huizink et al., 2004), though the following two are typically used in research studies: Pregnancy Experience Scale (DiPietro et al., 2004) and the Prenatal Distress Questionnaire (Yali & Lobel, 1999).

With respect to assessing past trauma, as indicated above, the standard, ten-question, ACE questionnaire has been used in fetal programming research and is a highly validated instrument in clinical settings (Glowa et al., 2016); it is suitable for clinical screening with pregnant women.

There are almost no risks in screening for mood symptoms during pregnancy, as a false positive would likely be identified by the treating clinician prior to initiating treatment, assuming they have some behavioral health expertise. In addition, an elevated score, particularly in the context of an acutely stressful event, or when screening occurs shortly after birth and the associated mood lability, likely will resolve and also be identified as a change by the professional. One caution is the false negative: lack of endorsement of symptoms could override professional judgment and is a concern, especially as stigma associated with mental health issues during the peripartum period can be an impediment to full disclosure (see below) and the current time constraints on healthcare professionals can undermine careful patient examination.

Treatment for Prenatal Mood Symptoms

Standard cognitive behavior therapy (CBT) and pharmacology have been shown to be effective for prenatal mood symptoms (O'Connor et al., 2016) — 10% of pregnant women in the USA currently are prescribed psychotropic medication, with antidepressants being the most common; 1.6% of pregnant women use drugs from two or more different categories, typically combining an antidepressant and an anxiolytic (Ayad & Costantine, 2015). Yet there can be significant disinclination to taking medications while breastfeeding or pregnant (Dennis & Chung-Lee, 2006; Goodman, 2009; Battle et al., 2013), underscoring the need for other effective treatment options during the prenatal period.

One intervention with strong outcome data for prenatal depression is interpersonal psychotherapy (IPT), first adapted by Spinelli et al. for use with this population (Spinelli, 1997; Spinelli & Endicott, 2003). IPT is a brief intervention (12–16 sessions) that assigns the patient the sick role, thereby aiming to reduce self-blame and guilt, and identifies a core current interpersonal problem related to their depression, for example grief and role transition, as well as strengthens social support. In a randomized control trial (RCT) comparing IPT to a parenting education program, 60% of the women treated with IPT reached remission, and mood improvement was correlated with improved mother-infant interaction (Spinelli & Endicott, 2003). More recently, Grote et al. developed an enhanced IPT designed to be culturally relevant to socioeconomically disadvantaged women in the USA. An intention to treat analyses showed women in enhanced IPT compared to those in usual care with added attention showing significant reductions in depression diagnoses and symptoms before childbirth and six months postpartum (Grote et al., 2009).

Other current treatment approaches include mindfulness, yoga, and stress-reduction techniques as either stand-alone interventions or add-ons to established therapies. For example, a pilot RCT testing Mindful Awareness Practices (MAPs) classes for six weeks with home practice compared to a reading control condition showed that the MAPs group had larger decreases in pregnancy-specific anxiety and pregnancy-related anxiety, though these results were not sustained six weeks post intervention (Guardino et al., 2014). In another pilot study testing a new intervention, Mindfulness-Based Childbirth and Parenting (MBCP), an eight-week therapy group, women reported a decline in depression, anxiety, and stress, with these results continuing into the postpartum period (Dunn et al., 2012). A pilot study of mindfulness-based yoga practiced over seven weeks in a group setting, which combined Iyengar yoga and mindfulness-based stress-reduction techniques, demonstrated reductions in physical pain and perceived stress and anxiety from the second to the third trimester (Beddoe et al., 2009). Finally, in an RCT leveraging mindfulness approaches to prepare for childbirth based on MBCP compared to those in a standard childbirth preparation course showed lower post-course depression scores that were maintained through postpartum follow-up (Duncan et al., 2017). A study utilizing standard stress-reduction instructions during pregnancy showed lower levels of stress, depression, and negative affect as well as morning cortisol levels (Urizar, 2004), though a recent study failed to replicate those findings (Urizar & Munoz, 2001).

Despite effective treatments, including ones specifically tailored to the prenatal period, prenatal mood symptoms are significantly undertreated similar to PPD (Dennis & Chung-Lee, 2006; Smith et al., 2009; Grote et al., 2015). One study provided nursing support for referrals and monitored treatment engagement for women with post-partum depression — an attempt to provide a referral that was 'warm', only 12% received psychotherapy and even fewer received pharmacology (Horowitz & Cousins, 2006). Barriers to treatment include shame in endorsing distress in the context of childbearing (Dennis & Chung-Lee, 2006), stigma associated with receiving mental health services (Dennis & Chung-Lee, 2006; Goodman, 2009), logistical challenges to attending added healthcare appointments typically uncoordinated with OB care and at another location (Dennis & Chung-Lee, 2006; Goodman, 2009; Byatt et al., 2012), and, as indicated, a preference not to take medications while pregnant or breastfeeding (Dennis & Chung-Lee, 2006; Goodman, 2009; Battle et al., 2013). However, the prenatal period is potentially an optimal time for engaging women in behavioral healthcare services for two reasons: (1) studies have shown that they are motivated to improve their health during this time (DiPietro et al., 2004) and (2) they have dramatically increased contact with healthcare providers due to ongoing prenatal care. Two novel treatment approaches have aimed to target some of the reasons for the low uptake rates of mental health services during the prenatal period while also taking advantage of the increased contact with healthcare personnel.

Building on the success of IPT for prenatal depression, as well as collaborative care models that embed a Depression Care Specialist (DCS) into primary care settings and coordinate care across disciplines, Grote et al. have shown significant results with their program MOMCare treating depressed pregnant women who are socioeconomically disadvantaged. Specifically, from birth through 18 months postpartum and compared to usual maternity support services, they found MOMCare patients had lower levels of depression severity, higher rates of remission, and a higher rate of receiving mental healthcare visits (Grote et al., 2017). Importantly, in a follow-up work, a MOMCare study identified 65% of its sample as having probable comorbid post-traumatic stress disorder (PTSD) and showed that it benefited more from depression reduction associated with MOMCare treatment than their non-PTSD counterparts (Grote et al., 2016).

The Massachusetts Child Psychiatry Access Program for Moms (MCPAP for Moms), directed by psychiatrist Nancy Byatt and obstetrician Tiffany Moore-Simas (www.mcpapformoms.org/), brings behavioral health services to healthcare personnel serving pregnant and postpartum women by providing: (1) trainings and toolkits on evidence-based guidelines for screening, assessment, and treatment of perinatal mental health and substance use disorders; (2) access to real-time telephonic psychiatric consultation; and (3) care coordination. Since its launch in July 2014, MCPAP for Moms has enrolled 134 Ob/Gyn practices accounting for >80% of deliveries in the state, provided over 3,800 care coordination activities, and provided 2,000 phone consultations, serving 3,000 perinatal women.

These integrated care models, bringing mental health expertise to OB patients and personnel, can serve as roadmaps for future approaches to scalable treatment of prenatal mood symptoms and disorders.

Prevention

A recent review (Werner et al., 2015) identified 37 psychological and psychosocial prevention-oriented RCTs for PPD. Of the 17 studies with effective strategies, 13 were conducted with at-risk populations, suggesting the importance of utilizing known PPD risk factors as inclusion criteria for PDD preventive treatment. Universal interventions to prevent PPD have not produced promising results (Pearlstein et al., 2009). The majority of preventive interventions target two of the most common predictors of PPD, prenatal depression or distress, which are clearly so relevant to fetal programming. This review (Werner et al., 2015) and others (Whitton et al., 1996; Boath et al., 2004; v Ballestrem et al., 2005) highlight reasons that some prevention programs have poor outcomes. Many of these factors overlap with identified barriers to successful treatment of PPD and mood disturbance during pregnancy: (1) use of pharmacology (Whitton et al., 1996; Boath et al., 2004) and (2) high attrition rates (McIntosh, 1993; Dennis & Chung-Lee, 2006; Werner et al., 2015) which may result from (a) lack of accessible treatment (v Ballestrem, 2005), (b) stigma related to mental health care (Dennis & Chung-Lee, 2006), and (c) a sole focus on the mother. This narrow focus overlooks childbearing women's child-centered orientation commencing during the prenatal period (Alhusen et al., 2013).

Here, we review three prevention interventions with promising preliminary data. An RCT of rational-emotive behavior therapy (REBT) versus community group care with pregnant women showed a greater drop in depression, anxiety, and negative emotionality for the REBT group and the results were maintained for all three mood states postpartum (Anton & David, 2015). Dimidjian et al. showed that mindfulness-based cognitive therapy versus treatment as usual had acceptable rates of compliance, including with at-home assignments, and reduced rates of depressive relapse/reoccurrence and lower symptom severity through six months postpartum (Dimidjian et al., 2015). Monk et al. (2000) and Werner et al. (2015) developed a novel intervention based on the conceptualization of maternal depression as a potential disorder of the mother-infant dyad, and one that can be approached through psychological and behavioral changes in the mother — commencing before birth — that affect her and the child. PREPP (Practical Resources for Effective Postpartum Parenting) enrolls distressed pregnant women at risk for PPD, spans late pregnancy to the six-week postpartum check-up, comprises four in-person 'coaching' sessions adjunctive to obstetrical prenatal and postnatal appointments, one phone session, and imparts (a) mindfulness and self-reflection skills, (b) parenting skills, and (c) psycho-education. Recently published results from a preliminary RCT showed that PREPP, compared to enhanced treatment as usual (providing added support for finding treatment), is associated with high attendance rates, reduced maternal depression symptoms, and less infant fuss/cry behavior six weeks postpartum. Viewing PPD as *a potential disorder of the dyad* informed PREPP treatment development by making mother-infant behavioral interactions, infant regulation, and parenting competence as central components in improving maternal mood.

Prenatal mood symptoms are modifiable by established treatments; newer approaches are emerging that are specially designed for pregnant women, and that include prevention strategies. What is not yet known is whether these therapies, if successful in treating maternal mood, will also have positive effects on the future child. In an elegantly designed study, Davis and colleagues are considering this question in a new NIH RCT study entitled 'Reducing Fetal Exposure to Maternal Depression to Improve Infant Risk Mechanisms' in which they will use IPT versus treatment as usual to treat prenatal depression and examine children's development through 14 months old. Data from this study will provide evidence for fetal programming that has experimental control (more than is typical in observational studies) in that the exposure to maternal depressed will be 'turned on or off' potentially providing cause-effect evidence of maternal depression effects on child development. It will also show the potential for treatment of prenatal mood symptoms to affect two patients, the mother and her future child.

Conclusion

The division of physical and mental illnesses is rampant in our general and professional cultures. Maternal and fetal physical health traditionally have been viewed as intertwined yet an awareness of women's mental health during pregnancy, and its possible influence on children's future neurobehavioral development has not been acknowledged. Kendler labels this a still-existing Cartesian mind-body dualism (Kendler, 2005). In this antiquated model, mental and behavioral problems, such as stress experiences and depression, are in the mind, without physical instantiation; they hold less legitimacy in terms of garnering public health attention and resources. Fetal programming research is part of modern science showing that experiences 'get under the skin' to become part of the women's biochemistry and physiology as well as part of the developing organisms. What the woman experiences is in her mind and her brain and body, which amounts to the environment shaping the fetus' future development. The life she lives – including what behavioral health treatment she receives – affects her, and – at least in terms of depression, stress, anxiety, and past trauma – her future child.

References

Alhusen, J. L., Hayat, M. J. & Gross, D. A longitudinal study of maternal attachment and infant developmental outcomes. *Archives of Women's Mental Health* **16**, 521–529, doi:10.1007/s00737-013-0357-8 (2013).

Anton, R. & David, D. A randomized clinical trial of a new preventive rational emotive and behavioral therapeutical program of prepartum and postpartum emotional distress. *Journal of Evidence-Based Psychotherapies* **15**, 3–15 (2015).

Appleton, A. A., Lester, B. M., Armstrong, D. A., Lesseur, C. & Marsit, C. J. Examining the joint contribution of placental NR3C1 and HSD11B2 methylation for infant neurobehavior. *Psychoneuroendocrinology* **52**, 32–42, doi:10.1016/j.psyneuen.2014.11.004 (2015).

Ayad, M. & Costantine, M. M. Epidemiology of medications use in pregnancy. *Seminars in Perinatology* **39**, 508–511, doi:10.1053/j.semperi.2015.08.002 (2015).

Battle, C. L., Salisbury, A. L., Schofield, C. A. & Ortiz-Hernandez, S. Perinatal antidepressant use: Understanding women's preferences and concerns. *Journal of Psychiatric Practice* **19**, 443–453, doi:10.1097/01.pra.0000438183.74359.46 (2013).

Beck, A. T., Steer, R. A. & Brown, G. K. *Beck Depression Inventory-Second Edition (BDI-II)*. (The Psychological Corporation, 1996).

Beck, A. T., Ward, C. H., Mendelson, M., Mock, J. & Erbaugh, J. An inventory for measuring depression. *The Archives of General Psychiatry* **4**, 561–571 (1961).

Beck, C. T. & Gable, R. K. Further validation of the postpartum depression screening scale. *Nursing Research* **50**, 155–164 (2001).

Beddoe, A. E., Paul Yang, C. P., Kennedy, H. P., Weiss, S. J., & Lee, K. A. The effects of mindfulness-based yoga during pregnancy on maternal psychological and physical distress. *Journal of Obstetric, Gynecologic, & Neonatal Nursing* **38**(3), 310–319 (2009).

Bergman, K., Sarkar, P., Glover, V. & O'Connor, T. G. Quality of child-parent attachment moderates the impact of antenatal stress on child fearfulness. *Journal of Child Psychology and Psychiatry* **49**, 1089–1098 (2008).

Bergman, K., Sarkar, P., Glover, V. & O'Connor, T. G. Maternal prenatal cortisol and infant cognitive development: Moderation by infant-mother attachment. *Biological Psychiatry* **67**, 1026–1032, doi:S0006-3223(10)00013-2 [pii] 10.1016/j.biopsych.2010.01.002 (2010).

Bergman, K., Sarkar, P., O'Connor, T. G., Modi, N. & Glover, V. Maternal stress during pregnancy predicts cognitive ability and fearfulness in infancy. *Journal of the American Academy of Child and Adolescent Psychiatry* **46**, 1454–1463 (2007).

Blackmore, E. R. et al. Psychiatric symptoms and proinflammatory cytokines in pregnancy. *Psychosomatic Medicine* **73**, 656–663, doi:PSY.0b013e31822fc277 [pii] 10.1097/PSY.0b013e31822fc277 (2011).

Bleker, L. S., Roseboom, T. J., Vrijkotte, T. G., Reynolds, R. M. & de Rooij, S. R. Determinants of cortisol during pregnancy – The ABCD cohort. *Psychoneuroendocrinology* **83**, 172–181, doi:10.1016/j.psyneuen.2017.05.026 (2017).

Boath, E., Bradley, E. & Henshaw, C. Women's views of antidepressants in the treatment of postnatal depression. *Journal of Psychosomatic Obstetrics & Gynecology* **25**, 221–233 (2004).

Braithwaite, E. C. et al. Maternal prenatal cortisol predicts infant negative emotionality in a sex-dependent manner. *Physiology & Behavior* **175**, 31–36, doi:10.1016/j.physbeh.2017.03.017 (2017).

Byatt, N., Simas, T. A., Lundquist, R. S., Johnson, J. V. & Ziedonis, D. M. Strategies for improving perinatal depression treatment in North American outpatient obstetric settings. *Journal of Psychosomatic Obstetrics & Gynecology* **33**, 143–161, doi:10.3109/0167482X.2012.728649 (2012).

Cao-Lei, L. et al. Prenatal stress and epigenetics. *Neuroscience and Biobehavioral Reviews*, doi:10.1016/j.neubiorev.2017.05.016 (2017).

Capron, L. E. et al. Associations of maternal and paternal antenatal mood with offspring anxiety disorder at age 18 years. *Journal of Affective Disorders* **187**, 20–26, doi:10.1016/j.jad.2015.08.012 (2015).

Cattaneo, A. et al. Inflammation and neuronal plasticity: A link between childhood trauma and depression pathogenesis. *Frontiers in Cellular Neuroscience* **9**, 40, doi:10.3389/fncel.2015.00040 (2015).

Chang, J. P. et al. Polyunsaturated fatty acids and inflammatory markers in major depressive episodes during pregnancy. *Progress in Neuro-Psychopharmacology & Biological Psychiatry*, doi:10.1016/j.pnpbp.2017.05.008 (2017).

Chen, L. et al. Brain-derived neurotrophic factor (BDNF) Val66Met polymorphism influences the association of the methylome with maternal anxiety and neonatal brain volumes. *Development Psychopathology* **27**, 137–150, doi:10.1017/S0954579414001357 (2015).

Committee on Obstetric, P. The American college of obstetricians and gynecologists committee opinion no. 630. Screening for perinatal depression. *Obstetrics & Gynecology* **125**, 1268–1271, doi:10.1097/01.AOG.0000465192.34779.dc (2015).

Conradt, E., Lester, B. M., Appleton, A. A., Armstrong, D. A. & Marsit, C. J. The role of DNA methylation of NR3C1 and 11beta-HSD2 and exposure to maternal mood disorder in utero on newborn neurobehavior. *Epigenetics: Official Journal of the DNA Methylation Society* **8**, 1321–1329 (2013).

Cookson, H., Granell, R., Joinson, C., Ben-Shlomo, Y. & Henderson, A. J. Mothers' anxiety during pregnancy is associated with asthma in their children. *The Journal of Allergy and Clinical Immunology* **123**, 847–853 e811, doi:S0091-6749(09)00158-4 [pii] 10.1016/j.jaci.2009.01.042 (2009).

Crown, S. & Crisp, A. H. A short clinical diagnostic self-rating scale for psychoneurotic patients. The Middlesex Hospital Questionnaire (M.H.Q.). *British Journal of Psychiatry* **112**, 917–923 (1966).

Davis, E. P., Sandman, C. A., Buss, C., Wing, D. A. & Head, K. Fetal glucocorticoid exposure is associated with preadolescent brain development. *Biological Psychiatry* **74**, 647–655, doi:10.1016/j.biopsych.2013.03.009 (2013).

Dennis, C. L. & Chung-Lee, L. Postpartum depression help-seeking barriers and maternal treatment preferences: A qualitative systematic review. *Birth* **33**, 323–331 (2006).

Dieter, J. N. I. et al. Maternal depression and increased fetal activity. *Journal of Obstetrics and Gynaecology* **21**, 468–473 (2001).

Dimidjian, S. et al. An open trial of mindfulness-based cognitive therapy for the prevention of perinatal depressive relapse/recurrence. *Archives of Women's Mental Health* **18**, 85–94, doi:10.1007/s00737-014-0468-x (2015).

Dindo, L., Elmore, A., O'Hara, M. & Stuart, S. The comorbidity of Axis I disorders in depressed pregnant women. *Archives of Women's Mental Health*, doi:10.1007/s00737-017-0769-y (2017).

DiPietro, J. A., Hodgson, D. M., Costigan, K. A. & Hilton, S. C. Fetal neurobehavioral development. *Child Development* **67**, 2553–2567 (1996).

DiPietro, J. A., Ghera, M. M., Costigan, K. & Hawkins, M. Measuring the ups and downs of pregnancy stress. *Journal of Psychosomatic Obstetrics & Gynecology* **25**, 189–201 (2004).

Duncan, L. G. et al. Benefits of preparing for childbirth with mindfulness training: A randomized controlled trial with active comparison. *BMC Pregnancy and Childbirth* **17**, 140, doi:10.1186/s12884-017-1319-3 (2017).

Dunn, C., Hanieh, E., Roberts, R. & Powrie, R. Mindful pregnancy and childbirth: Effects of a mindfulness-based intervention on women's psychological distress and well-being in the perinatal period. *Archives of Women's Mental Health* **15**, 139–143, doi:10.1007/s00737-012-0264-4 (2012).

Entringer, S. et al. Maternal psychosocial stress during pregnancy is associated with newborn leukocyte telo-mere length. *American Journal of Obstetrics and Gynecology* **208**, 134, e131–137, doi:S0002-9378(12)02088-1 [pii] 10.1016/j.ajog.2012.11.033 (2013).

Evans, L. M., Myers, M. M. & Monk, C. Pregnant women's cortisol is elevated with anxiety and depression – but only when comorbid. *Archives of Women's Mental Health* **11**, 239–248, doi:10.1007/s00737-008-0019-4 (2008).

Gitau, R., Cameron, A., Fisk, N. M. & Glover, V. Fetal exposure to maternal cortisol. *The Lancet* **352**, 707–708 (1998).

Glover, V. Maternal depression, anxiety and stress during pregnancy and child outcome; what needs to be done. *Best Practice & Research. Clinical Obstetrics & Gynaecology* **28**, 25–35, doi:10.1016/j.bpobgyn.2013.08.017 (2014).

Glover, V. Prenatal stress and its effects on the fetus and the child: Possible underlying biological mecha-nisms. *Advances in Neurobiology* **10**, 269–283, doi:10.1007/978-1-4939-1372-5_13 (2015).

Glover, V. & Hill, J. Sex differences in the programming effects of prenatal stress on psychopathology and stress responses: An evolutionary perspective. *Physiology & Behavior* **106**, 736–740, doi:10.1016/j.physbeh.2012.02.011 (2012).

Glover, V., O'Connor, T. G. & O'Donnell, K. Prenatal stress and the programming of the HPA axis. *Neuroscience and Biobehavioral Reviews* (2009).

Glover, V., O'Connor, T. G., Heron, J., Golding, J. & team, A. S. Antenatal maternal anxiety is linked with atypical handedness in the child. *Early Human Development* **79**, 107–118, doi:10.1016/j.earlhumdev.2004.04.012 (2004).

Glover, V., O'Donnell, K., O'Connor, T. G., Ramchandani, P. & Capron, L. Prenatal anxiety and de-pression, fetal programming and placental function. *Psychoneuroendocrinology* **61**, 3–4, doi:10.1016/j.psyneuen.2015.07.395 (2015).

Glowa, P. T., Olson, A. L. & Johnson, D. J. Screening for adverse childhood experiences in a family med-icine setting: A feasibility study. *Journal of the American Board of Family Medicine: JABFM* **29**, 303–307, doi:10.3122/jabfm.2016.03.150310 (2016).

Goodman, J. H. Women's attitudes, preferences, and perceived barriers to treatment for perinatal depression. *Birth* **36**, 60–69, doi:10.1111/j.1523-536X.2008.00296.x (2009).

Gold, P., Goodwin, F. & Chrousos, G. Clinical and biochemical manifestations of depression. Relation to the neurobiology of stress. *The New England Journal of Medicine* **319**, 413–420 (1988).

Graham, A. M. et al. Maternal systemic interleukin-6 during pregnancy is associated with newborn amygdala phenotypes and subsequent behavior at 2 years of age. *Biological Psychiatry*, doi:10.1016/j.biopsych.2017.05.027 (2017).

Groome, L. J., Swiber, M. J., Bentz, L. S., Holland, S. B. & Atterbury, J. L. Maternal anxiety during preg-nancy: Effect on fetal behavior at 38 to 40 weeks of gestation. *Developmental and Behavioral Pediatrics* **16**, 391–396 (1995).

Grote, N. K. et al. A randomized controlled trial of culturally relevant, brief interpersonal psychotherapy for perinatal depression. *Psychiatric Services* **60**, 313–321 (2009).

Grote, N. K. et al. Collaborative care for perinatal depression in socioeconomically disadvantaged women: A randomized trial. *Depression and Anxiety* **32**, 821–834, doi:10.1002/da.22405 (2015).

Grote, N. K. et al. A randomized trial of collaborative care for perinatal depression in socioeconomically disadvantaged women: The impact of comorbid posttraumatic stress disorder. *Journal of Clinical Psychiatry* **77**, 1527–1537 (2016).

Guardino, C. M., Dunkel Schetter, C., Bower, J. E., Lu, M. C. & Smalley, S. L. Randomised controlled pilot trial of mindfulness training for stress reduction during pregnancy. *Psychology & Health* **29**, 334–349, doi:10.1080/08870446.2013.852670 (2014).

Gustafsson, H., Doyle, C., Gilchrist, M., Werner, E. & Monk, C. Maternal abuse history and reduced fetal heart rate variability: Abuse-related sleep disturbance is a mediator. *Development and Psychopathology* **29**, 1023–1034, doi:10.1017/S0954579416000997 (2017).

Gynecologists, A. C. o. O. a. (2015).

Hamilton, M. The assessment of anxiety states by rating. *The British Journal of Medical Psychology* **32**, 50–55 (1959).

Hamilton, M. A rating scale for depression. *Journal of Neurology, Neurosurgery, and Psychiatry* **23**, 56–62 (1960).

Hompes, T. et al. Investigating the influence of maternal cortisol and emotional state during pregnancy on the DNA methylation status of the glucocorticoid receptor gene (NR3C1) promoter region in cord blood. *Journal of Psychiatric Research* **47**, 880–891, doi:10.1016/j.jpsychires.2013.03.009 (2013).

Horowitz, J. A. & Cousins, A. Postpartum depression treatment rates for at-risk women. *Nursing Research* **55**, S23–27 (2006).

Huizink, A. C., Mulder, E. J., Robles de Medina, P. G., Visser, G. H. & Buitelaar, J. K. Is pregnancy anxiety a distinctive syndrome? *Early Human Development* **79**, 81–91, doi:10.1016/j.earlhumdev.2004.04.014 (2004).

Huizink, A. C., Robles de Medina, P. G., Mulder, E. J., Visser, G. H. & Buitelaar, J. K. Psychological measures of prenatal stress as a predictor of infant temperament. *Journal of the American Academy of Child Psychiatry* **41**, 1078–1085 (2002).

Huizink, A. C. et al. Chernobyl exposure as stressor during pregnancy and behaviour in adolescent offspring. *Acta Psychiatrica Scandinavica* **116**, 438–446, doi:10.1111/j.1600-0447.2007.01050.x (2007).

Jensen Pena, C., Monk, C. & Champagne, F. A. Epigenetic effects of prenatal stress on 11beta-hydroxysteroid dehydrogenase-2 in the placenta and fetal brain. *PLoS One* **7**, e39791, doi:10.1371/journal.pone.0039791PONE-D-12-04077 [pii] (2012).

Ji, S. et al. Validity of depression rating scales during pregnancy and the postpartum period: Impact of trimester and parity. *Journal of Psychiatric Research* **45**, 213–219, doi:S0022-3956(10)00177-9 [pii] 10.1016/j.jpsychires.2010.05.017 (2011).

Karlsson, L. et al. Cytokine profile and maternal depression and anxiety symptoms in mid-pregnancy-the FinnBrain Birth Cohort Study. *Archives of Women's Mental Health* **20**, 39–48, doi:10.1007/s00737-016-0672-y (2017).

Kendler, K. S. Toward a philosophical structure for psychiatry. *The American Journal of Psychiatry* **162**, 433–440 (2005).

Khalife, N. et al. Prenatal glucocorticoid treatment and later mental health in children and adolescents. *PLoS One* **8**, e81394, doi:10.1371/journal.pone.0081394 (2013).

Khashan, A. S. et al. Higher risk of offspring schizophrenia following antenatal maternal exposure to severe adverse life events. *Archives of General Psychiatry* **65**, 146–152 (2008).

Khashan, A. S. et al. Prenatal stress and risk of asthma hospitalization in the offspring: A Swedish population-based study. *Psychosomatic Medicine* **74**, 635–641, doi:10.1097/PSY.0b013e31825ac5e7 (2012).

King, S. et al. Prenatal maternal stress from a natural disaster predicts dermatoglyphic asymmetry in humans. *Development Psychopathology* **21**, 343–353, doi:10.1017/S0954579409000364 (2009).

King, S. & Laplante, D. P. The effects of prenatal maternal stress on children's cognitive development: Project Ice Storm. *Stress* **8**, 35–45, doi:UP61488770455R12 [pii] 10.1080/10253890500108391 (2005).

Kinney, D. K., Miller, A. M., Crowley, D. J., Huang, E. & Gerber, E. Autism prevalence following prenatal exposure to hurricanes and tropical storms in Louisiana. *Journal of Autism and Developmental Disorders* **38**, 481–488, doi:10.1007/s10803-007-0414-0 (2008).

Kooijman, M. N. et al. Influence of fetal blood flow redistribution on fetal and childhood growth and fat distribution: The Generation R Study. *BJOG* **123**, 2104–2112, doi:10.1111/1471-0528.13933 (2016).

Kroenke, K., Spitzer, R. L. & Williams, J. B. The PHQ-9: Validity of a brief depression severity measure. *Journal of General Internal Medicine* **16**, 606–613 (2001).

Lahti, M. et al. Maternal depressive symptoms during and after pregnancy and psychiatric problems in children. *Journal of the American Academy of Child and Adolescent Psychiatry* **56**, 30–39, e37, doi:10.1016/j.jaac.2016.10.007 (2017).

Laplante, D. P., Brunet, A. & King, S. The effects of maternal stress and illness during pregnancy on infant temperament: Project Ice Storm. *Pediatric Research* **79**, 107–113, doi:10.1038/pr.2015.177 (2016).

Laplante, D. P. et al. Stress during pregnancy affects general intellectual and language functioning in human toddlers. *Pediatric Research* **56**, 400–410 (2004).

Lee, J. Y. et al. Prenatal exposure to dexamethasone in the mouse induces sex-specific differences in placental gene expression. *Development Growth Differ*, doi:10.1111/dgd.12376 (2017).

Maxwell, S. D., Fineberg, A. M., Drabick, D. A., Murphy, S. K. & Ellman, L. M. Maternal prenatal stress and other developmental risk factors for adolescent depression: Spotlight on sex differences. *Journal of Abnormal Child Psychology*, doi:10.1007/s10802-017-0299-0 (2017).

McIntosh, J. Postpartum depression: Women's help-seeking behaviour and perceptions of cause. *Journal of Advanced Nursing* **18**, 178–184 (1993).

Monk, C. et al. Distress during pregnancy: Epigenetic regulation of placenta glucocorticoid-related genes and fetal neurobehavior. *The American Journal of Psychiatry*, appiajp201515091171, doi:10.1176/appi.ajp.2015.15091171 (2016).

Monk, C. et al. Maternal stress responses and anxiety during pregnancy: Effects on fetal heart rate. *Developmental Psychobiology* **36**, 67–77 (2000).

Monk, C. et al. Fetal heart rate reactivity differs by women's psychiatric status: An early marker for developmental risk? *Journal of the American Academy of Child and Adolescent Psychiatry* **43**, 283–290 (2004).

Monk, C. et al. Effects of maternal breathing rate, psychiatric status, and cortisol on fetal heart rate. *Developmental Psychobiology*, n-a–n/a, doi:10.1002/dev.20513 (2010).

Moog, N. K. et al. Maternal exposure to childhood trauma is associated during pregnancy with placental-fetal stress physiology. *Biological Psychiatry* **79**, 831–839, doi:10.1016/j.biopsych.2015.08.032 (2016).

Moog, N. K. et al. intergenerational effect of maternal exposure to childhood maltreatment on newborn brain anatomy. *Biological Psychiatry*, doi:10.1016/j.biopsych.2017.07.009 (2017).

Muller, C. L. et al. Impact of maternal serotonin transporter genotype on placental serotonin, fetal forebrain serotonin, and neurodevelopment. *Neuropsychopharmacology* **42**, 427–436, doi:10.1038/npp.2016.166 (2017).

Nemoda, Z. & Szyf, M. Epigenetic alterations and prenatal maternal depression. *Birth Defects Research* **109**, 888–897, doi:10.1002/bdr2.1081 (2017).

Nolvi, S. et al. Maternal prenatal stress and infant emotional reactivity six months postpartum. *Journal Affect Disorders* **199**, 163–170 (2016).

Oberlander, T. F. et al. Prenatal exposure to maternal depression, neonatal methylation of human glucocorticoid receptor gene (NR3C1) and infant cortisol stress responses. *Epigenetics: Official Journal of the DNA Methylation Society* **3**, 97–106 (2008).

O'Connor, T. G., Heron, J., Glover, V. & Alspac Study, T. Antenatal anxiety predicts child behavioral/emotional problems independently of postnatal depression. *Journal of the American Academy of Child and Adolescent Psychiatry* **41**, 1470–1477, doi:10.1097/00004583-200212000-00019 (2002).

O'Connor, T. G., Heron, J., Golding, J. & Glover, V. Maternal antenatal anxiety and behavioural/emotional problems in children: A test of a programming hypothesis. *Journal of Child Psychology and Psychiatry* **44**, 1025–1036 (2003).

O'Connor, E., Rossom, R. C., Henninger, M., Groom, H. C. & Burda, B. U. Primary Care Screening for and treatment of depression in pregnant and postpartum women: Evidence report and systematic review for the US preventive services task force. *JAMA* **315**, 388–406, doi:10.1001/jama.2015.18948 (2016).

O'Donnell, K. J., Glover, V., Barker, E. D. & O'Connor, T. G. The persisting effect of maternal mood in pregnancy on childhood psychopathology. *Development and Psychopathology* **26**, 393–403, doi:10.1017/S0954579414000029 (2014).

O'Donnell, K. J. & Meaney, M. J. Fetal origins of mental health: The developmental origins of health and disease hypothesis. *The American Journal of Psychiatry* **174**, 319–328, doi:10.1176/appi.ajp.2016.16020138 (2017).

O'Donnell, K., O'Connor, T. G. & Glover, V. Prenatal stress and neurodevelopment of the child: Focus on the HPA axis and role of the placenta. *Developmental Neuroscience* **31**, 285–292 (2009).

O'Donnell, K. J. et al. Maternal prenatal anxiety and downregulation of placental 11beta-HSD2. *Psychoneuroendocrinology* **37**, 818–826, doi:S0306-4530(11)00284-8 [pii] 10.1016/j.psyneuen.2011.09.014 (2012).

O'Donnell, K. J., Glover, V., Holbrook, J. D. & O'Connor, T. G. Maternal prenatal anxiety and child brain-derived neurotrophic factor (BDNF) genotype: Effects on internalizing symptoms from 4 to 15 years of age. *Development Psychopathology* **26**, 1255–1266, doi:10.1017/s095457941400100x (2014).

O'Mahony, S. M., Clarke, G., Dinan, T. G. & Cryan, J. F. Early-life adversity and brain development: Is the microbiome a missing piece of the puzzle? *Neuroscience* **342**, 37–54, doi:10.1016/j.neuroscience.2015.09.068 (2017).

Orleans, C. T., Johnson, R. W., Barker, D. C., Kaufman, N. J. & Marx, J. F. Helping pregnant smokers quit: Meeting the challenge in the next decade. *The Western Journal of Medicine* **174**, 276–281 (2001).

Paquette, A. G. et al. Placental epigenetic patterning of glucocorticoid response genes is associated with infant neurodevelopment. *Epigenomics* **7**, 767–779, doi:10.2217/epi.15.28 (2015).

Pearlstein, T., Howard, M., Salisbury, A. & Zlotnick, C. Postpartum depression. *American Journal of Obstetrics and Gynecology* **200**, 357–364, doi:10.1016/j.ajog.2008.11.033 (2009).

Pearson, R. M. et al. Maternal depression during pregnancy and the postnatal period: Risks and possible mechanisms for offspring depression at age 18 years. *JAMA Psychiatry* **70**, 1312–1319, doi:10.1001/jamapsychiatry.2013.2163 (2013).

Pearson, R. M. et al. Maternal perinatal mental health and offspring academic achievement at age 16: The mediating role of childhood executive function. *Journal Child Psychology Psychiatry* **57**, 491–501, doi:10.1111/jcpp.12483 (2016).

Plant, D. T., Jones, F. W., Pariante, C. M. & Pawlby, S. Association between maternal childhood trauma and offspring childhood psychopathology: Mediation analysis from the ALSPAC cohort. *British Journal of Psychiatry* **211**, 144–150, doi:10.1192/bjp.bp.117.198721 (2017).

Posner, J. et al. Alterations in amygdala-prefrontal circuits in infants exposed to prenatal maternal depression. *Translational Psychiatry* **6**, e935, doi:10.1038/tp.2016.146 (2016).

Pressman, E., DiPietro, J., Costigan, K., Shupe, A. & Johnson, T. Fetal neurobehavioral development: Associations with socioeconomic class and fetal sex. *Development Psychobiology* **33**, 79–91 (1998).

Qiu, A. et al. Effects of antenatal maternal depressive symptoms and socio-economic status on neonatal brain development are modulated by genetic risk. *Cereb Cortex*, 1–13, doi:10.1093/cercor/bhx065 (2017).

Radloff, L. S. The CES–D scale: A self–report depression scale for research in the general population. *Applied Psychological Measurement* **1**, 385–401 (1977).

Radtke, K. M. et al. Transgenerational impact of intimate partner violence on methylation in the promoter of the glucocorticoid receptor. *Translation Psychiatry* **1**, e21, doi:10.1038/tp.2011.21 (2011).

Raikkonen, K. et al. Maternal depressive symptoms during pregnancy, placental expression of genes regulating glucocorticoid and serotonin function and infant regulatory behaviors. *Psychological Medicine*, 1–10, doi:10.1017/S003329171500121X (2015).

Raikkonen, K. et al. Maternal licorice consumption during pregnancy and pubertal, cognitive, and psychiatric outcomes in children. *American Journal of Epidemiology* **185**, 317–328, doi:10.1093/aje/kww172 (2017).

Rakers, F. et al. Transfer of maternal psychosocial stress to the fetus. *Neuroscience and Biobehavioral Reviews*, doi:10.1016/j.neubiorev.2017.02.019 (2017).

Reynolds, R. M. et al. Maternal depressive symptoms throughout pregnancy are associated with increased placental glucocorticoid sensitivity. *Psychological Medicine* **45**, 2023–2030, doi:10.1017/S003329171400316X (2015).

Robinson, M. et al. Pre- and postnatal influences on preschool mental health: A large-scale cohort study. *Journal Child Psychology Psychiatry* **49**, 1118–1128 (2008).

Rodriguez, A. & Waldenstrom, U. Fetal origins of child non-right-handedness and mental health. *Journal Child Psychology Psychiatry* **49**, 967–976, doi:10.1111/j.1469-7610.2008.01923.x (2008).

Sandman, C. A. et al. Maternal hypothalamic-pituitary-adrenal disregulation during the third trimester influences human fetal responses. *Developmental Neuroscience* **25**, 41–49 (2003).

Sarkar, P., Bergman, K., Fisk, N. M. & Glover, V. Maternal anxiety at amniocentesis and plasma cortisol. *Prenatal Diagnosis* **26**, 505–509 (2006).

Serpeloni, F. et al. Grandmaternal stress during pregnancy and DNA methylation of the third generation: An epigenome–wide association study. *Translational Psychiatry* **7**, e1202, doi:10.1038/tp.2017.153 (2017).

Siu, A. L. et al. Screening for depression in adults: US preventive services task force recommendation statement. *JAMA* **315**, 380–387, doi:10.1001/jama.2015.18392 (2016).

Smith, M. V. et al. Success of mental health referral among pregnant and postpartum women with psychiatric distress. *General Hospital Psychiatry* **31**, 155–162, doi:10.1016/j.genhosppsych.2008.10.002 (2009).

Spielberger, C. D. & Gorsuch, R. L. *Manual for the State-Trait Anxiety Inventory (Form Y): ("self-evaluation questionnaire")*. Rev. edn (Consulting Psychologists Press, Inc., 1983).

Spinelli, M. G. Interpersonal psychotherapy for depressed antepartum women: A pilot study. *The American Journal of Psychiatry* **154**, 1028–1030 (1997).

Spinelli, M. G. & Endicott, J. Controlled clinical trial of interpersonal psychotherapy versus parenting education program for depressed pregnant women. *The American Journal of Psychiatry* **160**, 555–562 (2003).

Suh, D. I., Chang, H. Y., Lee, E., Yang, S. I. & Hong, S. J. Prenatal maternal distress and allergic diseases in offspring: Review of evidence and possible pathways. *Allergy Asthma Immunology Research* **9**, 200–211, doi:10.4168/aair.2017.9.3.200 (2017).

Tau, G. Z. & Peterson, B. S. Normal development of brain circuits. *Neuropsychopharmacology* **35**, 147–168, doi:npp2009115 [pii] 10.1038/npp.2009.115 (2010).

Tibu, F. et al. Evidence for sex differences in fetal programming of physiological stress reactivity in infancy. *Development and Psychopathology*, 1–10, doi:10.1017/S0954579414000194 (2014).

Togher, K. L., Treacy, E., O'Keeffe, G. W. & Kenny, L. C. Maternal distress in late pregnancy alters obstetric outcomes and the expression of genes important for placental glucocorticoid signalling. *Psychiatry Research* **255**, 17–26, doi:10.1016/j.psychres.2017.05.013 (2017).

Urizar, G. G., Jr. et al. Impact of stress reduction instructions on stress and cortisol levels during pregnancy. *Biological Psychology* **67**, 275–282 (2004).

Urizar, G. G., Jr. & Munoz, R. F. Impact of a prenatal cognitive-behavioral stress management intervention on salivary cortisol levels in low-income mothers and their infants. *Psychoneuroendocrinology* **36**, 1480–1494, doi:10.1016/j.psyneuen.2011.04.002 (2011).

van den Bergh, B. R. H. et al. Prenatal developmental origins of behavior and mental health: The influence of maternal stress in pregnancy. *Neuroscience and Biobehavioral Reviews*, doi:10.1016/j.neubiorev.2017.07.003 (2017).

Van den Bergh, B. R. & Marcoen, A. High antenatal maternal anxiety is related to ADHD symptoms, externalizing problems and anxiety in 8–9 year olds. *Child Development* **75**, 1085–1097 (2004).

Van den Bergh, B. R., Van Calster, B., Smits, T., Van Huffel, S. & Lagae, L. Antenatal maternal anxiety is related to HPA-axis dysregulation and self-reported depressive symptoms in adolescence: A prospective study on the fetal origins of depressed mood. *Neuropsychopharmacology* **33**, 536–545 (2008).

van Os, J. & Selten, J.-P. Prenatal exposure to maternal stress and subsequent schizophrenia: The May 1940 invasion of The Netherlands. *The British Journal of Psychiatry*, 324–326, doi:10.1192/bjp.172.4.324 9715334 (1998).

Varcin, K. J., Alvares, G. A., Uljarevic, M. & Whitehouse, A. J. O. Prenatal maternal stress events and phenotypic outcomes in Autism Spectrum Disorder. *Autism Research: Official Journal of the International Society for Autism Research*, doi:10.1002/aur.1830 (2017).

v Ballestrem, C. L., Strauss, M. & Kachele, H. Contribution to the epidemiology of postnatal depression in Germany—implications for the utilization of treatment. *Archives of Women's Mental Health* **8**, 29–35, doi:10.1007/s00737-005-0068-x (2005).

Walsh, K. et al. Associations among child abuse, depression, and interleukin-6 in pregnant adolescents: Paradoxical findings. *Psychosomatic Medicine* **78**, 920–930, doi:10.1097/PSY.0000000000000344 (2016).

Werner, E. et al. Higher maternal prenatal cortisol and younger age predict greater infant reactivity to novelty at 4 months: An observation-based study. *Developmental Psychobiology* **55**, 707–718, doi:10.1002/dev.21066 (2013).

Werner, E. A. et al. Prenatal predictors of infant temperament cognitive-behavior therapy for reduction of persistent anger. *Developmental Psychobiology* **49**, 474–484, doi:10.1002/dev.20232 (2007).

Werner, E. A. et al. PREPP: Postpartum depression prevention through the mother-infant dyad. *Archives of Women's Mental Health*, doi:10.1007/s00737-015-0549-5 (2015).

Werner, E., Miller, M., Osborne, L. M., Kuzava, S. & Monk, C. Preventing postpartum depression: Review and recommendations. *Archives of Women's Mental Health* **18**, 41–60, doi:10.1007/s00737-014-0475-y (2015).

Whitton, A., Warner, R. & Appleby, L. The pathway to care in post-natal depression: Women's attitudes to post-natal depression and its treatment. *The British Journal of General Practice: The Journal of the Royal College of General Practitioners* **46**, 427–428 (1996).

Yali, A. M. & Lobel, M. Coping and distress in pregnancy: An investigation of medically high risk women. *Journal of Psychosomatic Obstetrics & Gynecology* **20**, 39–52 (1999).

Zijlmans, M. A., Korpela, K., Riksen-Walraven, J. M., de Vos, W. M. & de Weerth, C. Maternal prenatal stress is associated with the infant intestinal microbiota. *Psychoneuroendocrinology* **53**, 233–245, doi:10.1016/j.psyneuen.2015.01.006 (2015).

Zung, W. W. A self-rating depression scale. *Archives of General Psychiatry* **12**, 63–70 (1965).

Part II
Procreation, Pregnancy, and Delivery

3

'A Precipice in Time' – Reproductive Biotechnology

Psychosocial Impact and Unintended Consequences

Joan Raphael-Leff

Around the world, infertility inflicts self-blame and suffering, and has painful social consequences:

> *"The man planted his seed in me, but the soil inside me could not make it grow into a plant"* says an African farm-worker in her native language Shona: *"Haunting and being haunted. Bad dreams, bad words, bad food, everything took on the colour of blood. And I thought I would cry for ever inside me. Right inside the inside of my heart. Then names came … you witch, you day-witch, you who ate the roots of your own womb"*.
>
> [Chenjerai Hove, <u>Bones</u>, 1989]

'Haunted', suffering and stigmatised for inability to bring a desired baby to fruition, worldwide women consult experts – herbalists, midwives or exorcists – for explanations and magical potions, and seek solace in local beliefs and customs. Often, the emotional processes involved are too great to work through alone. In industrialised societies, we increasingly turn towards science for answers. However, while it offers amazingly novel solutions, its enigmatic forces also have a profound emotional effect on parents, donors and offspring. In addition, it impacts on society at large, In this chapter, I shall trace some psychosocial, ethical, legal and emotional implications, as well as effects on generative identity and unforseen consequences of the biotechnology revolution in reproduction.

Generative Identity

I will begin with the idea that an unconceived baby's power to 'haunt' lies in the significance given to *generativity* in that particular location. I maintain that the greater the centrality granted to procreation, the more traumatic the impact on personal and sociocultural identity, if the baby-wish is thwarted.

Cross-cultural observations suggest that before sexual distinction sets in, a very young child naively believes s/he can be and do everything. Toddlers identify indiscriminately with the capacities of both sexes and a little boy sticks out his belly pretending to be pregnant. But in most societies, this 'over-expansive' view is re-evaluated with increasing awareness of sexual divisions.

Freud posited that the primal question is: *Where do babies come from?* (1905). The startling answer to this anthropogenic puzzle – that *we are not self-made*, but come from a two-sex coupling – initiates a new developmental process.

The growing child is confronted by various restrictions:

- s/he can be only one specific sex;
- each sex has distinct reproductive capacities;
- adults can make babies; children cannot;
- parents have an adult (sexual/baby-making) relationship from which children are excluded.

Coming to terms with these facts of life involves loss of the early sense of omnipotence. To Freud, the turning point comes when the oedipal child eventually submits to the incest taboo, giving up hope of ever receiving or giving the parent a baby. Compensation lies in the promise of eventually finding an exogamous mate, with whom to have a future baby of one's own.

I argue that becoming aware of the potential to create a family of one's own constitutes a momentous shift for the little girl or boy – a shift from being someone else's creation to becoming a procreator. Acceptance of these facts of life fosters a sense of '*Generative identity*'which I proposed as a fourth component of Gender Identity along with 'Sexual Embodiment', 'Gender Role Representation' and 'Erotic Desire' (Raphael-Leff, 2007).

In Freud's day, females were devalued as 'lacking', and seen to need a baby as a substitute penis. But due to both Freud's innovative idea of 'psychic bisexuality' and Feminism's challenge to the power structure of binary difference, today we recognise that while male or female sex is anatomical, our normative gender constructs are socially determined.

If sexed difference confronts us with what we are not and cannot have, gender instigates greater awareness of who we are. Self-ascriptions and 'performance' of feminine or masculine roles, even sexual choices, rest on the amount of leeway each society allows – whether it enforces strict heterosexuality and a polarity between the sexes or permits choices on a spectrum of desire, behaviours and characteristics which overlap across males and females. *Gender is not a physical fact – but a social power relation that varies historically and culturally.*

In societies where free-expression prevails, a young person's sense of generativity need not remain in abeyance until future procreation of a *real baby*. A child or adolescent can consciously actualise his or her agency in imaginative play, or in artistic or intellectual productions. This instigates a further shift in those who can imaginatively forge mental freedom from constraints of sex, age, race and birth order through creativity, inventiveness and cross-identifications. If confrontation with the facts of life reduces the young child's unrealistic sense of omnipotence, using the imagination to exceed reality's restrictions contributes to greater intentionality and complexity of self.

However, *in recent decades, innovations of science and technology have altered eternal facts of life!* Today, we no longer need to use our imaginations to transcend absolute limitations: our wildest fantasies can be actualised in reality – leaving us feeling omnipotent once more.

No Limits

So, what happens when there are no absolutes? Who do we become when we anticipate no fixities? What are the unintended psychological consequences of scientific innovations which signify that personal constraints of mono-sexuality, two-person genesis and inevitable finitude can be eliminated?

In this chapter, I explore some effects of biotechnologies which have altered generative facts of life that have been around since primates evolved. Given the rapidity of these changes, I argue that we must look to the unintended consequences for the future when in the field of *generativity* the once de-limiting parameters of *gender, generation* and *genesis* are undone by a seemingly infinite array of new facts:

- *A person is no longer bound to his or her specific birth sex.*
  Transitioning goes beyond transgender fantasies and cross-dressing – males and females can be bodily exchanged. London's Tavistock Gender Identity Disorder Clinic has children as young as four demanding to become the other sex.
- *Sexual relations are no longer restricted to the adult generation.*
  Onset of puberty has dropped to age ten or even nine. Exposed to pornography, numerous pre-teen children are already sexually active.
- *As for Genesis, many children's parents did not engage in a reproductive union.*
  Some begetters are not heterosexual. Even the fundamental fact that it takes *two sexes* to conceive and that each sex has a distinct reproductive capacity, is being annulled by incredible scientific phenomenon – of three-person conception, auto-genesis by cloning and the feasibility of using primordial germ cells (PGCs) from a male to produce an egg, thus allowing an infant to have two biological fathers.
- *Assisted, conception no longer rests on an arbitrary conjunction* of a single sperm and egg but is annulled by artificial selection of the best fertilised eggs, requisitioned embryos, ICSI and genetic engineering.
- *Ethical conundrums that occupied generations of philosophers are commonplace.*
  Every Western woman who undergoes routine antenatal tests is in effect engaged in a form of *'soft eugenics'*. Medical techniques and recommendation to abort flawed babies calibrate our standards of acceptable disability.[1] Screening tools also root out defective embryos in the pre-implantation stage.
- *Biotechnology also seems to invalidate the irreversibility of life's trajectory.*
  Time's ravages are revoked by Botox or cosmetic surgery or enhanced by breast and penile implants. Hormonal supplements delay menopause, and medical procedures like knee or hip replacements correct wear and tear. Implants derived from embryonic stem cells can regenerate lost brain functions after neurological injury or disease. Electronic devices can replace or augment injured neural circuits.[2] With artificial respiration death itself seems to retreat! As science changes the human-scape, entropy and decay slow down – and one of three babies born in 2020 will live to be 100! For 21st-century adults, death can be averted by organ transplants, pacemakers, life-support machinery, synthetic biology and 3D printing to name but a few. A dead person's genome has been reconstructed without extracting DNA from their remains but rather pieced together from fragments of his DNA found in hundreds of his modern-day descendants.

These are incredible times, when every day, we encounter biblical reproductive miracles – of asexual immaculate conception, virginal births and post-menopausal childbearing. In this new reality ancient legends come alive. Like the ancient Egyptian Goddess Isis, a widow can be posthumously impregnated by her dead husband – but now she is medically assisted with semen mechanically removed from the comatose man before his death. Today, a grandmother can carry her daughter's babies in her own womb. Sibling rivalry can be avoided by foetal 'reductions' and twins are often born years apart. A donated frozen embryo may be older than its pregnant mother. But we must ask what fantasies do these children carry about their own identities?

As imaginative fictions become ordinary possibilities in actuality, are we so focused on the technological marvels that we overlook the relational intricacies of surrogacy, gamete donation or lesbian egg-swapping? We complacently accept the idea of prenatal surgery, the cultivation of ova or stem cells from aborted or discarded embryos, artificially cultured parthenogenetic human embryos grown to the blastocyst stage, sheep gestated in artificial wombs, or even of extra–uterine male gestations.

Unintended Consequences

Do not get me wrong! I find technological inventions wonderfully exciting. It is their unintended consequences that worry me. All around us fantastic contrivances materialise, but we ourselves no longer know how to fix the most basic gadgets. Undoubtedly, we all benefit tremendously from helpful appliances and our science-enriched social fabric is ever-more complex, variegated and advanced. For instance, just this week a mother devised an innovation in our own perinatal field – a breast pump contained within the working mother's bra enables her to bridge both domains with less disruption thus reducing conflict between maternal and employee demands.

However, to our sorrow, we know that the most well-meaning medical interventions can have unforeseen and far-reaching repercussions. Remember the effects of Thalidomidegiven to expectant mothers in the 1950s to reduce nausea and morning sickness? Or effects that only emerged a generation later of Diethylstilbestrol prescribed from the 1940s in the mistaken belief that it would reduce the risk of pregnancy complications but was eventually stopped in 1971 when shown to cause vaginal tumours and infertility in females who had been exposed to DES in utero? The anti-epilepsy drug sodium valproate/Epilim which caused malformations in 20,000 children since it was prescribed during pregnancy from the 1970s onwards is now found to provoke trans-generationally transmitted symptoms in unexposed grandchildren.

But even our everyday electronic devices hold unanticipated risks. We have become addicted to our cell phones. Our dependency is such that cognitive skills like mental arithmetic have atrophied with ever-accessible calculators. We are just learning the effects of being available on call and connected to others at all times of the day, which disrupts even mother–baby intimate moments. It seems we can no longer tolerate not knowing or just musing. It must be rectified immediately by access to the vast international reference library or the interactive gaming technology in our pockets!

In the 21st century, data proliferate exponentially and our culture is changing precipitously. We all dip into vast tranches of new knowledge – yet our wisdom lags behind. For instance, we are only just beginning to grapple with moral dilemmas such as the long-term effects on future sexual relations of youth's unrestricted access to pornographic imagery. We understand little about the psychosocial significance of everyday friendships that are always filtered through social media communication. And we are yet to discover the unforeseen consequences of augmenting our sensual experiences by virtual reality. And, in our own field, as the bizarre becomes commonplace, we tend to normalise biotechnological interventions rather than trying to fathom what the emotional impact of the unknown might be on those we induce to allow their bodies to undergo inexplicable medical and fertility treatments.

In trying to explore some of the meanings and fantasies involved in this ever-changing reality I can only touch on the subjective disorientation of persons caught up in, or those produced by, heterologous assisted reproduction which alters a family's affective climate and genetic lineag. I focus specifically on emotional issues of (non)conception, fertility investigations, diagnosis and treatment

A Precipice in Time

'...a precipice in Time... a sudden bringing of ancient and modern into absolute contact...'[3]

I argue that today we humans dangle over a formidable precipice in Time when our most 'ancient' activity – that of sexual reproduction with all its erotic imagery and sensual connotations is juxtaposed with the most 'modern' forms of clinical reproduction. We cannot halt the technological avalanche – but we must acknowledge our human vulnerabilities. As one of my patients exclaims:

> *These scientific procedures cast strange shadows – invading our sex-life, our privacy and even my inner-most sense of femininity. Doubts creep insidiously right into my body and mind – no wonder I feel quite crazy! Becoming parents once seemed simple.* <u>*Now technology forces us into unknown realms with no guiding precedents*</u>.

The woman in my consulting room is a 45-year-old university lecturer with a rare gift for language. Until her late 30s she devoted herself to considerable academic achievement within an exacting discipline, rising rapidly and feeling fulfilled, with no interest in childbearing. However, when after several unsatisfactory relationships, she eventually met and married her 'soul mate' who had always wanted children, she conceded to his wish for a baby.

She expected to fall pregnant as soon as her contraceptive coil was removed. Devastated by a taxing year of unsuccessfully trying to conceive the couple eventually resorted to medical investigations, followed by intensive fertility treatments to boost their ageing reproductive systems. Like the biblical Rachel's exclamation, "Give me a baby or I will die!" my 21st-century 'Rachel' says: "*I didn't use to think so but now life seems unendurable without a baby! However much it costs physically and financially, we must go on trying!*". But she adds: "*I yearn to be a mother but I'm also so afraid…*".

The Revolution

Fear comes from uncertainty. Since prehistoric times, humanity has always replicated itself through copulation. From time immemorial every single person anywhere on the planet was born of sexual intercourse. Yet no long ago, technology restructured the eternal mode of procreation – by engendering *asexual reproduction*!

The revolution has uncanny and surreal aspects but as it happened in intersecting stages, each became a 'new normal', contributing to our omnipotent belief that we have the power to control it all. Although artificial insemination with fresh sperm had been used discreetly for over 100 years, our reproductive reality altered dramatically in 1953 when the first successful pregnancy using frozen sperm *disconnected the sexual protagonists* in time as well as space. Then, from the late 1960s efficient female contraception further *uncoupled sex from conception*, and in the 1970s safe abortion *detached conception from motherhood*. Just a few years later, in 1978, Assisted Reproductive Technology (ART) took off, *disengaging conception from sex*. If 'banked' frozen sperm had displaced the primal scene from bedroom to laboratory, with birth of the first IVF baby, the gamete's meeting place shifted from uterine tubes to the 'test tube'.

Then, the first successful egg donation in 1983 disconnected the biological mother from the genetic mother; and a year later, the space-time continuum was further ruptured as the 'freeze-thaw baby' *disconnected conception from birth* – having conceived, a woman could freeze the foetus washed from her body for future reimplantation (or donation). The first child born following pre-implantation genetic diagnosis (PGD) in 1990 heralded genetic 'engineering' and, finally, in 1997 a successful birth using frozen eggs opened up an international market of ova transactions, and further improvements in long-term cryation also permitted young women to *pause time* by freezing their own eggs for use when ready to become mothers.

So, over a very short period of time, we have traversed chronological, spatial, inter-corporeal and, above all, *conceptual frontiers*. Like last century's watershed of the Hiroshima atom bomb, we now live with the knowledge that scientific innovations can alter our most fundamental axioms. I argue that our conscious (let alone non-conscious) understanding cannot grasp the unprecedented implications of these galloping innovations – and conversely, that scientific wonders are now catching up with ancient myths and fantasies, actualising our fictions in reality. To me, *transformation of mental representations* is the most profound impact of this incredible biotechnological revolution. A case in point is the altered conceptualisation of *femininity*: historically defined by our reproductive function, from earliest times we women conceived, gestated, gave birth and spent the bulk of our adult lives in repeated pregnancy and babycare. Relatives were defined by blood and marriage. Women who transgressed sexually or those who proved barren were condemned to a secondary position, banished from their husband's domain, or even stoned and killed. But in the handful of decades since I was a young woman, a fundamental paradox has been revealed:

For the species, reproduction is a necessity.
For an individual woman it is neither instinct nor feminine destiny – but an option!

Survival of the Species

In Patriarchal cultures, women are still ruled by a broad spectrum of social constraints to ensure legitimate offspring. Religious prohibitions, genital mutilation and 'honour'-violence are employed to control their sexuality. In many lower-income countries, female generative identity is still restricted to childbearing and childrearing functions. Worldwide, 130 million girls still have no entry to education although when they do have access to school they tend to excel. Even in very affluent societies extremist religions require girls to do household chores rather than study, and many are married off to older men and compelled to become mothers at a very young age.

But nonetheless, where female-based contraception is available, both in high- and lower-income countries, *young women around the world are having fewer babies than their mothers*. In some Western societies the birth rate has now fallen below the critical replacement rate of 2.2 – currently 1.9 in the UK and 1.34 in Italy![4] Elsewhere, I suggested that one unanticipated consequence of small families is our difficulty in working-through primary experience while growing up. Over the last few decades in stratified societies, an only child has few opportunities to actively process his/her own infantile feelings in the presence of a baby sibling or cousin. This generation of parents has had little contact with infants. They are unprepared for the emotional impact of their own baby and are therefore more susceptible to perinatal disturbance (see Raphael-Leff, 1991, 2015).

Furthermore, if species survival depends on reproduction, its extinction is heralded by *loss of the ability to reproduce*. We now face an unprecedented crisis: a 2017 meta-study of 43,000 men found that in Australia, North America and Europe sperm count declined by more than 50% in less than 40 years – dropping from an average concentration of 99 million sperm per millilitre to 47 million. Below 40 million, reproduction is less likely to occur. Due to environmental toxicants, lifestyle changes with excessive drug or alcohol intake, obesity and rising comorbidities, geographical areas of accelerated industry and advanced agriculture (including China and Japan) now show this *steep decline in sperm quantity* (albeit not yet Africa or the Far East). Researchers predict that if this trend continues, by 2050 the sperm count of Western men will be *zero* (Levine et al., 2017)!

But it is not only quantity; *sperm quality is declining too*. In addition to exposure to non-ionising radiation (from cell phones, coloured TV or laptops), pathogens such as pesticides and industrial oestrogen are blamed. Specifically, a group of widely used EDCs (endocrine disrupting chemicals) is linked to weakened reproductive systems in both men and women – a clear-cut case of unintended consequences.[5] In recent years, reduced fecundity is also ascribed to sexually transmitted diseases or infections (STD or STI), a very common and preventable cause of infertility. But besides pathogens, another psychosocial factor intervenes in our technologically sophisticated societies: *generative agency can now be expressed by both women and men across a wider variety of choices outside of reproduction.*

In fact, emancipation of women's creative capacities from the procreative template (and from female self-deprecation) has brought about a demographic transformation, especially in higher-income countries. *In Europe, some 12–25% of women now decide to remain childless by choice.* As a result, under-populated societies such as Spain, Italy and Germany must offer procreative incentives or swell their growth with immigrants to ensure their continuity.

Female-based contraception (i.e. pills, reversible sterilisation, patches, depo-provera injections) as well as the 'morning-after pill' safe abortion, selective feticide and own-egg freezing all offer women more control over their fertility, and real choices such as men have always had – *of whether, when, with whom and how to have a baby.* Benefitting from educational parity, marketplace participation and increased longevity, many women suspend reproduction to partake of exciting new opportunities. Maternity itself may feel less enticing when career women who do become mothers experience a high level of discordance between their work culture and ambitions (which have changed so dramatically since the second wave of feminism), and the needs of their babies which have changed not at all since we lived in caves!

However, delayed childbearing – whether for emotional, practical, financial or career reasons – also comes at a cost. *Fertility reduces with age.* But if for centuries we heard the female biological clocks ticking loudly, we now know that male reproductive postponement affects fertility too, as sperm quantity decreases and semen quality declines after men's mid-30s.[6]

Like Superman, ART swooped in to the rescue! Since then a whole biotechnological industry has materialised to combat rising subfertility, generating ever-more innovative ways of conceiving, gestating, enhancing and sustaining pregnancy with enormous and often unknown ramifications for all concerned – society, parents, offspring, donors and others.

ART and the 'Time Bomb'

Back to my patient:

To Rachel, inability to conceive seems to prove her failure as a woman. Painfully, she experiences her recalcitrant body letting her down as it did when she tried to diet in adolescence. Over the past few years, she feels increasingly drained by the emotional 'roller coaster' of hope and despair, unrealistic expectations and frustratingly dashed plans, within a never-ending round of numerous IUI, IVF and ICSI cycles. Rachel wonders how much the undiminished intensity of her wish for a baby is due to the tantalising promise of an ever-new invention just around the corner. Now, as a last-ditch attempt, the couple is told to contemplate donor egg, or even donated embryo:

> Last night I dreamed I was pregnant and gave birth – but when I came to breast feed, it was a monster with sharp little teeth. I know I'm worried about having a stranger's baby. <u>An alien being growing inside my body</u>, genetically unrelated to me – an unknown species, different genus… Should we continue or give up?

A few weeks later, still haunted by the idea of breeding an 'alien', Rachel bursts into tears, grieving her never-to-be genetic baby:

> "I'm so aware of Time working against me. Seeing my friends' kids grow up I realise I've missed out on a whole generation. Sometimes I wonder if I'm being punished, not entitled to a baby … Our dream of a joint baby is vanishing. We have this new bizarre idea to digest. <u>What is a donor to us and who is my baby to her?</u> I worry about the long-term effect of such origins. How can a child ever come to terms with being 'manufactured', and by three, or even four parents?!
>
> Is this a baby or a dangerous Time-bomb we're considering?"

She is not alone in her misgivings. In the perinatal field, we have already been using technological advances for many years without consistently toting up the unintended consequences, such as ultrasound abuse in female feticide, the impact of unprecedented kinship relations in new modes of family formation, and the potential subclinical effects of incubated 24-week preemies.

Now, after a hundred thousand years of random mutation and natural selection for robustness a further revolution is fomenting: *genetic technology provides the means to control evolution!*

It is no longer a matter of 'survival of the fittest' when specialists have the technological expertise to artificially select one high-powered sperm to be micro-injected into a chosen egg cell. Since the human genome was sequenced, a new technique now allows genetic codes to be manipulated, modified, inserted or deleted. It is only recently that the technique using CRISPR (clustered regularly interspaced short palindromic repeats) was implemented for genome editing, and it is now being applied to human reproduction. Many scientists agree that while gene editing has positive potentialities, it also poses an unprecedented danger. In fact, it has been described as 'a biological bomb' of unintended consequences (see Cobb, 2017). *Once again it is a matter of no absolute constraints.*

In our human aspiration for perfection can we draw a line between corrective remedial action and enhancement? Indeed, recent cracking of genetic sequences associated with certain physical characteristics and new refinements in micro-array technology raise justified concerns: not only about cherry-picking of specific embryos selected for transfer, but fear that future technology will permit the manipulation of genetic material *within* an embryo. Many scientists worry that while eradicating some of the 10,000 genetic disorders and diseases caused by a mutation that is passed down the generations, zealous colleagues will succumb to an extremely powerful, indeed 'irresistible' wish to *improve* capabilities (see Doudna & Sternberg, 2017; Heine, 2017; Rochman, 2017).

Genetic 'engineering' has long raised the spectre of 'designer babies'. For decades would-be parents have perused catalogues to choose the optimal sperm donor with suitable talents and intellectual or sporting prowess. Today, procreators are closer than ever to choosing or indeed, fabricating the characteristics of their own unconceived child. In addition to moral issues about granting parental wishes, there are ethical concerns about a potential demographic bias should such chosen mental and physical capacities be available only to the wealthier strata of the population who can afford the procedure. And the flip side of this apprehension is an anxiety about us devaluing those born with lesser talents and disabilities, even blaming their parents for *not* aborting them.

These concerns are no longer hypothetical.

While the moral principles prohibiting cloning are clear cut, those of mitochondrial replacement therapy are less so. As of last year, the UK allowed the creation of 'three-parent babies' to prevent diseases being passed on.[7] We are just beginning to realise the implications of donated gametes changing the future hereditary germlines of an individual family's descendants. But CRISPR goes further – it permanently alters distribution of genes *in the population*. In fact, the immense power of gene editing and the relative ease of its application actually led President Obama's Director of National Intelligence James Clapper to describe CRISPR as a 'weapon of mass destruction' in 2016 (cited by Cobb, 2017). Again, it is a matter of unintended consequences.[8] No one is sure what will happen when a gene drive is altered – since its frequency *increases exponentially* with each generation, thereby rapidly 'flooding' the whole population! Many thoughtful writers, philosophers and, indeed, even the inventors of CRISPR, have expressed their anxieties warning that heritable human genetic modifications pose serious risks, and the therapeutic benefits are tenuous (e.g. Lanphier et al., 2015). And they too reiterate the need for global regulation of gene drives (e.g. Baltimore et al., 2015).

Joan Raphael-Leff

The Dark Side

Caution is apparent on an individual level too, since reproductive technology provides hope but also has a down side, both foreseen and unexpected:

- Living with the process of ongoing failure to conceive or experiencing repeated miscarriage despite scientific intervention not only lays bare our powerlessness but provokes darker dimensions sparking disillusionment in the magic of technology.
- A lost baby is now a baby known, scanned since the follicles ripened. Miscarriage, leaves would-be parents bewildered and bereft.
- Early scans also disclose previously undiscovered twin conceptions, in which one sibling fails to develop and vanishes when absorbed after 14 weeks' gestation, and the other serves as a reminder of inter-woven life-giving/death-dealing forces inherent in maternity.
- Ultrasound misuse has led to feticide of millions of female babies.
- Where state regulation is lacking, ovarian hyper-stimulation raises the number of eggs rises significantly. In the absence of restrictions, rates of multi-foetal pregnancies increase dramatically and women conceive a high rate of twins, triplets and even unprecedented viable 'litters' of octets.[9]
- Replacement of more than one fertilised egg also introduces cruel dilemmas about foetal 'reduction'. Selection may be driven by sexual preference and/or guilt-inducing disposal decisions about how many embryos to kill off, which baby to retain and what the survivor will feel in years to come.
- Similar questions arise about the fate of stored frozen embryos, especially those who outlive the relationship but not the genomes of their progenitors.

Importantly, such science fiction-like interventions do not take place in outer space, but, as my patient says, are inserted into 'the innermost interior' of a female body, infiltrating into the woman's feminine identity, and the inner sanctum of a couple's relationship.

Finally, when a baby is produced rather than reproduced, conception is no longer an intimate body-to-body two-person coupling. The centralised process may involve three or more genitors, including one or two donors, possibly a surrogate or gestational carrier, and multiple practitioners – the team of medical experts and their various helpers. Although it purports to empower women, many aspects of reproductive biotechnology still tend to *commodify* women's bodies and gametes, ignoring the psychological accompaniments. But human emotions are paramount. How does it feel to know that anonymous donor and recipient's menstrual cycles are synchronised in the process of transferring eggs? What does it mean to us that embryos, ovaries and even wombs can be transplanted from one body into another? Although a rare occurrence, fantasies about having the wrong couple's embryo transplanted 'haunt' many in assisted pregnancy. And what does a woman feel when some of the eggs she produced by ovarian hyper-stimulation are given to another woman to fund the donor's own fertility treatment? How does she cope with the fact that donated eggs have a greater chance of 'taking' in the recipient and may not implant in the chemically overdosed woman who provided them? And if she, the donor, fails to conceive, will she be haunted by the thought that her baby grows in another woman's womb? What explanatory systems do we evolve when carefully chosen perfect embryos die inexplicably in a receptive womb? Or when a surrogate decides to keep the baby? These are painful questions that must be considered.

As many sceptical feminists have pointed out, over the decades the scientific establishment has remained preponderantly male, white, upper-middle class and corporate. Sperm donation is painless, and sometimes lucrative. Egg donation is painful and possibly dangerous. ART offers new hope to infertile people, but also has a potential for exploitation of less fortunate women as egg donors, or womb providers, in exchange for medical care. Ethical concerns arise when wealthy clients and celebrities travel to less privileged places to purchase babies, embryos, eggs or sperm. Or when women who are unable to conceive, or who prefer to avoid pregnancy borrow a womb. Even legitimate reproductive tourism is emotionally fraught – unregulated, commercialised and unpredictable.[10]

Ironically, 'first world' expenditure on fertility treatments vastly exceeds investment in reproductive healthcare in low-income countries, where 90% of the world babies are born. In many societies where fertility is literally a life or death matter, ART may not be available at all. Not only is there an unequal global distribution of technological resources but investment in HIV prevention and prophylactic medical care is often lacking, or else financial foreign aid is withdrawn on dubious moral grounds, from clinics that also offer abortions. This despite the fact that in vast parts of Africa, the only continent where the young outnumber the old much subfertility is potentially avoidable (and due to treatable STDs such as chlamydia and gonorrhoea). By contrast, in high-income countries technology provides hope not only for infertile couples but for same-sex partners, lone men as well as single women. Some residents in low- and middle-income countries question whether these reproductive policies are determined solely by economics or may be rooted in a nexus of discriminatory power and prejudicial ends.

Furthermore, popular Western mass media sustains persistent misconceptions.[11] The very low 'take-home-baby' rate of assisted reproduction is concealed or overlooked, raising false hopes and heartache, aggravated by post hoc revelations of human or digital error.

Human Liberties and Moral Claims

In conclusion, centralised reproduction must grapple with basic philosophical issues. In this age when we recognise no absolute restrictions, do we each have a fundamental right to procreate? And if so, are such rights grounded in wishful thinking and desire, or in the sanctity of autonomous control over one's body?

Is treatment to be free on the National Health Service, and fairly distributed, or determined by postal-code lottery? Are private clinics entitled to pick and select clients for the sake of a statistically high success rates? How ethical is egg sharing to pay for a donor's fertility treatment if it stacks the odds against her?

This is a moral maze. We recognise violations of an individual's reproductive rights when they involve direct physical intimidation – rape, or transgressions like forced abortion or sterilisation. But what about governmental population control that interferes with personal reproductive decisions or sexual activity?[12] There are multiple perspectives. Assisted reproduction is an ethical challenge involving the legalities, rights and responsibilities of donors and surrogates,[13] as well as the rights and feelings of donor-conceived or surrogate-gestated children. A biotechnologically produced child's self-image incorporates science fictional realities: '*It is a bit weird to think I was once a ball of cells in a freezer*' said Emily Boothroyd, the first IVF baby born from a frozen embryo. Three specific developmental tasks have been delineated for therapeutic work with children who were not 'brought by the stork' – confronting one's sense of uniqueness, establishing a sense of belonging and forging an identity based on assisted-conception origins (Ehrensaft, 2007). In such nontraditional family formations it is suggested that engaging together in a 'family reverie' about conception and wantedness facilitates the child's sense of belongingness (Corbett, 2001). But intrapsychic conflicts and emotional defensiveness may impact on the relationship and parents often choose not to disclose the child's origins. When children born of assisted reproduction unconsciously fathom family secrets, they may disparage their parents' cowardice, or incapacity, inducing a mental split between idealised fertile donor and ineffective parental imagoes. But as ever, it is *the quality* of the specific relationship that matters, rather than the number, gender, sexual orientation or biological relatedness of parents. A comparative study finds that children born of reproductive technologies are well-adjusted, and, if anything, their parents are more attentive (Golombok, 2017b). But needless to say, *why* the child was conceived is as important as *how*.

Conscious and Unconscious Motivations to Conceive

For many fertile people natural conception occurs unintentionally – through ignorance or abnegated consequences of desire. For them, unprotected sex may reflect an unconscious wish and/or magical 'dicing' with outcome. In others, the conscious decision to have a baby arises once they have met the ideal partner. They wish to meld their genetic material together, or to create a baby that conjures up the other's unknown childhood. Overcome by the biological clock's urgency, some women decide to have a child on their own, wishing to flesh out a long-held fantasy baby before it is too late.

But when fertility treatment intervenes, the nature of the process of ongoing determination to conceive reveals in 'slow motion' that in addition to a conscious sense of readiness to give [*"I have so much to offer"*] it may be driven by several other less conscious incentives:

- Need for proof of undamaged fertility [*"Am I normal?"*] which may even result in abortion following conception.
- Response to social/family/peer pressures [*"Everybody keeps on asking…"*]
- Desire to be pregnant rather than to mother [*"That belly is so awesome…"*]
- Wanting to keep or 'fire up' a failing relationship [*"…a baby would improve things between us"*]
- Seeking a purpose or identity [*"Everyone else has children"*] or loneliness [*"I feel so alone"*]
- Compulsion to vicariously recapture lost aspects of the (baby) self [*"I'll provide everything I ever wanted"*]
- A wish to rewrite history and actively control what was passively encountered [*"<u>This</u> family will be a loving one"*]
- An unconscious need to resolve incomplete childhood mourning [*"…compensation for my mother's dead baby"*]
- A desire to repair, or repay old debts of generosity or wreak revenge [*"I'll show them!"*], and/or to meet or refute internalised parental ascriptions [*"He always said I'd be a terrible mother"*]
- A fantasy of recapturing lost aspects of one's baby-self and/or renegotiating incomplete developmental tasks [*"My toilet training was messed up – she still tyrannises my bowels. There'll be no holding back or straining for <u>my</u> baby!"*]

Or possibly a need to articulate further maturation, or, defiance in the face of traumatic life events:

- Cheating death of its finality [*"I'll leave a living testimony of my existence"*].
- Perpetuating the genealogical lineage [*"I can't let infertility win! I will not have sperm donor! It's not just <u>a</u> baby I want, but my own <u>genetic</u> child"*]

'Be fruitful and multiply'

Paradoxically, a great division occurs once a heterosexual couple suspend their mode of contraception to make a hybrid baby. Even the most egalitarian partners begin to diverge dramatically. At the very moment of male/female unification their differently sexed bodies polarise – each to their own respective reproductive apparatus and substances. His concerns with erection, virility, potency, magnitude of sperm or fantasies of their super-active or 'sluggish' quality contrast with her centripetal anxieties, focused on her monthly egg, her enigmatic interior, and its vague organs and lubricants. Quintessentially feminine, she is undertaking what only members of her sex can do, engaging with the *female mysteries of implantation, formation, transformation and sustenance* (Raphael-Leff, 1993, 2015). But conception can occur only if one bold sperm among many finds its way to meet and penetrate her receptive ovum, encountering no obstacles on the way. If all goes well, her womb will be the one to nurture their baby; her body will carry it, give birth and lactate. If not, the failure to conceive, complications or miscarriage will occur in *her* body, with all the accompanying culpability and guilt. In many societies, childlessness is ascribed to the woman although male factors are just as common in infertility.

Once obsessed with conception, each partner becomes both observer and observed in their own coupling. Their sex life may suffer under the strain of domination by her ovulation. To those yearning for a baby, recurrent loss or failure to conceive can seem like punishment by a malevolent force, for untold sins.

In Westernised societies, when sexual activity fails to produce the desired outcome, people may go to therapy or the gym; some consult the internet, or begin supplementing their diets with fertility-boosting foods or potions advertising their energising, moistening or nourishing qualities in glossy magazines. As uncertainty mounts superstitions flourish. People resort to ever-more magical compulsive actions and avoidances. Dreams focus on the withheld baby and desperation increases the wish to believe in anything that offers solace, however wild the rationalisation.

In traditional or religious subcultures, community prayers are supplemented by gifts to pacify annoyed gods, goddesses or ancestors. Ceremonial rituals draw on associative procedures like untying knots, or eating special herbs and rich milk products, seed pods, garlic cloves. An array of symbolic talismans encourages fecundity, from wearing special threads or beads, to dolls, or a bit of placenta to be kept under a pillow during sleep. Where non-conception is ascribed to a curse, in addition to blessings, incantations remedial activities involve exorcism, and usually some form of sacrifice (money, poultry, goats, etc.) to appease powerful spirits. Similarly, if conception results in recurrent miscarriage, interventions may include special nourishment, wearing a consecrated amulet, massaging the recalcitrant belly with plant extracts, application of medicinal concoctions to aid the vaginal outflow of impurities, and even manual trans-vaginal repositioning of the womb.

Similarly, in London and other mega-cities around the world, weekend 'Fertility Shows' are held in massive halls, advocating organic diets and medications, and holistic complementary activities with explanatory systems that promise to enhance fertility, and reduce anxiety, 'stress' and despair.

Investigations

Invention of the 'pill' endorsed an illusion of control over our female reproductive bodies. Therefore, prolonged failure threatens our inner security, evoking irrational explanations:

> *"I'm bleeding again. [It] just confirms that I'm not good enough to have a baby. My womb feels rotten, full of rubbish and yucky things inside which won't let a baby grow"* wails one of my patients.

Usually, after about a year of unsuccessfully trying to conceive most Western couples seek medical help. In time, this leads them to undertake a time-consuming range of laboratory tests and complex investigations which affect their love-making.[14] Not only their insides but their sex life is now on show. They must report to authority figures how often, when and how they have intercourse. These strangers intrude into their private space, highlighting their failures and inadequacies. When the focus turns to male problems it is often accompanied by a sense of shame and emasculation. Men undergoing fertility evaluation may feel judged, potency is erroneously conflated with virility, and sexual disturbances, including transient impotence, are not uncommon.

Unexpected reproductive failure is a major life event. In an age that proclaims certainty and personal choice, inability to reproduce constitutes an *existential crisis*. It undermines confidence, challenging a person's most fundamental belief in that old infrangible promise of his or her own future generativity, taken for granted since toddlerhood. For most of us, our first intimately known adults were parents. If this inextricable unconscious link between adulthood and parenthood is strong a childless state may be associated with childishness. Transferential issues increase the scrutinised couple's feeling infantilised by their doctors, like pre-fecund children in the hands of prodding, probing fertile adults.

Diagnosis – and Treatment Decisions

Given the primordial nature of the issues involved, diagnosis has far-reaching repercussions. Whether the verdict is the shocking outcome of a medical emergency, such as an ectopic pregnancy, or a gradual realisation that something is wrong; whether it comes after extensive investigations or surgical intervention, ascribed to damage or biochemical causes – to most people, the diagnosis involves intense suffering and a severe blow to self-esteem. But it can also provide relief and an explanation of their mysterious difficulties.

Specialists draw distinctions between irreversible *sterility* (resulting from defects, scarring or other damage to one or both of their reproductive systems), *infertility* due to a combination of causes including ageing, and *subfertility* attributed to a correctable single cause or several factors in one or both partners or their particular combination (such as cervical mucus incompatibility), which can produce problems at any stage before, during or after the successful meeting of sperm and ovum.

In some 30% of cases infertility remains unexplained (UI), sometimes due to undiagnosed conditions such as endometriosis, tubal disease, premature ovarian ageing (POA) or immunological infertility.

> *"…I feel isolated and lonely"* says one of my patients after many weeks of investigations and an eventual inconclusive diagnosis *"Left out. As if I am stuck in a box of my own horrible feelings…awful, miserable, unhappy, envious, angry feelings that have been flooring me. I have lost my femininity. There is no forgetfulness. This pain and loss are constant. I am so full of my rage! Hurt by other people's rude health and gross insensitivity. Even my mother wounds me with her casual remarks. My empty pocket is invisible. No one, not even my partner has any conception of my grief. We might as well be on different planets".*

People need a sense of closure. As we saw in the initial quote, all over the world it is in the nature of human beings to seek relief from helplessness and uncertainty by constructing reasons for their predicament. In the absence of a diagnosis they may ascribe infertility to past sexual misdemeanours, bad thoughts, nightmares or stress, or even to ill-will – the 'evil eye' of jealous colleagues, or malicious spirits.

For a diagnosed couple who feel up against uncontrollable forces, unsurprisingly, fertility experts take on the aura of omnipotent saviours. But as time passes with chemically exacerbated cycles of elation and deflation on the helter skelter of increasingly strange, emotionally and financially depleting treatments, their doctors may seem like *withholding* parents. Puzzlement about the origin of babies and wild theories of how they are made or destroyed resurface as godlike specialists pick and choose, deciding on treatment courses, and which, and how many laboratory-grown fertilised eggs to transfer to an artificially primed receptive uterus.

Acknowledging the emotional stress experienced by their patients while awaiting conception – some major fertility clinics now offer psychotherapy or counselling, alongside ongoing investigations and treatment interventions they sometimes in conjunction with alternative therapies and natural remedies, including yoga, mindfulness or mind-body stress-reducing groups.

Couples

Today, we recognise that infertility strikes indiscriminately, so failure to conceive is no longer attributed to psychogenic factors. Nonetheless, emotions are paramount. Even in cases of clear cut physiological or biochemical obstructions to fertility, the protracted period of failing to conceive exacerbates internal conflicts and fantasies. Repeated disillusionment heightens a person's psychological vulnerability, and sense of partnership. Lack of control over one's own generative agency undermines a basic sense of hegemony, permeating life on every level, lowering self-esteem and affecting life style, work and social relationships, professional competence and especially their sex life:

"When he wants to make love I feel murderously angry. What for? It can't lead anywhere. We can't make a baby ourselves. I can't bear him to touch me – it's just a reminder that we're <u>useless</u>" says a woman in couple therapy.

In a world now divided starkly into *haves* and *have-nots* fertile friends may be resented. A couple may choose to keep their situation a secret, fleeing out of shame or superstition into self-chosen social isolation to protect themselves from sympathetic family, friends or even pregnant strangers in the supermarket. Some partnerships are torn apart while seeking ways to render the unbearable bearable; others draw closer in their joint sorrow.

One partner may experience searing self-recriminations over a previous abortion. Another may blame the other's sexual indiscretions or lack of fitness. Bottled-up emotions often burst out, holding each other responsible for infertility due to the many years of postponed childbearing. Some couples manage to brave bitter accusations and uncontrollable outbursts with compassionate understanding. Others fail to break the thick silence between them or may find relief in discharging their feelings with a trusted confidante. Couple therapy enables partners to channel their chaotic emotions into a fruitful discussion.

Yet even in a close loving heterosexual marriage profound alienation can prevail because of their different male and female reproductive functions. Medical solutions affect them differently, especially when one needs help from a gamete donor, and not the other. In couples where intensity of desire for a child is asymmetrical, or if one partner feels cheated and let down by the other's failure, the relationship is liable to deteriorate and without couple therapy, separation may feel inevitable. Profoundly affected people come up with drastic solutions. A man may take a mistress. A fertile wife may secretively indulge in an impregnating 'fling'. A sterile husband may feel so guilt-ridden that he self-sacrificingly suggests divorce. In some cases where only one partner is afflicted, they may choose to settle for a surrogate, sperm or egg donor so as to have a baby who is genetically related to at least to one of them. Involving a third generates bitter-sweet mixed feelings of enormous gratitude yet acrimony invoking fantasies and/or paranoid ideas about the mythical unknown yet real fertile provider. To some partners, offering hospitality to foreign sperm or embryo seems like adultery. Other couples deny the significance of a donor, and it is not unknown for unscrupulous doctors to collude by proposing to mix in some of the husband's sperm with the donor's or even contribute a sample of their own.

Re-Evaluation of Generativity

Finally, the crisis of identity at finding oneself unable to reproduce when ready to do so compels revaluation of one's generative agency. A diagnosis of sterility affects people in many different ways, depending on the centrality of parenthood to their generative identity. Feelings of despair and desperation are especially intensified in people who for a variety of reason during their early childhood or after have retained their self-esteem and sense of creativity rooted in physical procreativity. Also, those who historically suffered reproductive complications in their families of origin. Finding that s/he is the *final link* rather than middle of an ongoing genealogical chain may threatens the very core of a person's being – posing another form of precipice! When life loses its meaning an insecure individual may feel that the very epistemological centre of his or her world has collapsed. If no solution seems available to forge a meaningful way of life, suicide is contemplated. Another person remains determined to defy fate. Feeling compelled to fight s/he enlists different clinics and new doctors in the hope of changing the pessimistic prognosis. Yet another grieves but recovers, refusing to pursue treatment that seems fruitless, and resolved to continue living a fulfilling life, even if childless. Some people will use their ingenuity to find another avenue to lavish their love and to engage with young children in a parental, social, creative or educational way.

To some the prospect of alternate solutions, be it sublimation, childlessness, adoption or fostering, having a baby by surrogacy or donated gametes may seem absolutely untenable as long as there is felt to be any glimmer of hope of an infant of their own. Now that menopause is no barrier, a devastated woman is so determined to be pregnant herself that she resolves to go to any lengths to actualise her sense of feminine generativity, no matter what the verdict and how long it takes, and despite the financial and emotional cost.

The protracted process of trying to conceive against the odds becomes increasingly multifactorial. Whilst ART offers hope, success rates are still disappointingly low. The treatment process is often fraught with conflict, heartache and painful disillusionment. But getting off the roundabout of an ongoing treatment regimen is complicated, and there is always a suggestion that increasingly sophisticated diagnostic techniques will eventually locate the difficulty and resolve it. At numerous nodal points, the experts' own determination to succeed interacts with less conscious co-existing motivations in the patient, affecting their decisions to continue, alter or discontinue treatment. Many people continue to put their lives on hold for many years as the rapidly changing scene of ever-new advances tantalises with a promise of future success. *In sum, when science has no limits, treatment has no natural cut off.*

As we teeter over our own 'precipice in Time', the 'transit-line' between the eternal and the unprecedented widens a break in the continuum of our human story inviolable since the Stone Age, altering our relation to the world and to ourselves. We can no longer afford to ignore the inevitability of manifold unintended consequences of biotechnological innovation, and their as yet unknown emotional, ethical, sociocultural and legal implications for future generations.

Notes

1 A new non-invasive genetic test for Down syndrome has already increased the number of babies aborted. This test which detects tiny amounts of foetal DNA in the mother's bloodstream is rapidly replacing the widespread use of alternatives (such as amniocentesis or chorionic villous sampling) that involve a risk of miscarriage.

2 Neuro-modulation can actually write signals into the brain. Between them, they can restore lost sensation or defunct sight, imparting communication to enhance brain activity or to control prostheses. As technology races unstoppably ahead, subcutaneous radio-frequency GPS-enabled micro-chips are predicted to become as common as cell phones. And there are probably already more robots than humans on earth.

3 My title 'A precipice in Time' is borrowed from a phrase by English novelist Thomas Hardy who thus described the 1851 Great Exhibition in London ...'an extraordinary chronological frontier or transit-line, at which there occurred what one might call a precipice in Time. As in a geological "fault" ... a sudden bringing of ancient and modern into absolute contact...' [In 'The Fiddler of the Reels', Scribner's Magazine, May 1893].

4 Even in Norway the figure is now down to 1.71, having dropped every year since 2009. Among the EU member states, France had the highest fertility rate in 2015, with 1.96 live births per woman. By contrast, the lowest fertility rates in 2015 were recorded in Portugal (1.31 live births per woman), Poland and Cyprus (both 1.32). In most of the EU member states, the total fertility rate declined considerably between 1980 and 2000–2003: by 2000, values had fallen *below 1.30* in Bulgaria, the Czech Republic, Greece, Spain, Italy, Latvia, Slovenia and Slovakia. After this the total fertility rate increased in most member states and by 2015, all of them reported total fertility rates that were above 1.30.

5 Called phthalates, they are widely influential — applied to make plastic more flexible, used as coating for medicines and food supplements and also found in construction materials, detergents, medical devices, food products, textiles, carpets, cleaning materials, nail polish, liquid soap, electronic products, meat,

milk, etc. Phthalates also threaten *future* reproduction. Known to pass through the placenta they reach the embryo. In the first trimester of pregnancy, this is especially critical for the development of the reproductive system. Phthalates may also be associated with the falling age of puberty and accelerated sexual maturation in girls.

6 For instance, the Beth Israel Deaconess Medical Center found that of thousands of IVF attempts in the Boston area, women under the age of 30 with a male partner between 40 and 42 were significantly less likely to give birth than those whose male partner was between 30 and 35.

7 Three-parent babies are conceived in '*pronuclear transfer*', when the nucleus of a donor's fertilised egg is replaced with that of the would-be mother's fertilised egg or again in '*spindle nuclear transfer*' when the father's sperm can fertilise an egg containing mitochondrial DNA from a known or anonymous donor, in addition to the recipient's nuclear DNA.

8 CRISPR technology which permits genetic codes to be 'edited' has many extraordinary uses in clinical practice (for instance implants derived from embryonic stem cells are used to restore lost brain functions after neurological injury or disease, to regenerate brain cells in stroke cases, release insulin when needed to manage blood sugar levels in diabetics, or even cancer-seeking skin cells or organs cultivated for replacement). DNA derived from one species of flora or fauna has long been spliced into the genome of another. But since completion of the international project to sequence the human genome in 2000, the quest to perfect ourselves has begun despite concerns such as the possibility of commercial exploitation of genetic information, or medical-insurance discrimination against people because of their genes. Already, many people have inexpensive access to their own genome charts, and have even begun to self-experiment. In a recent lecture about human genetic engineering streamed live on Facebook, a presenter injected himself to boost his strength by removing the gene for myostatin, which regulates muscle growth despite including possible tissue damage, cell death, or an unforeseen self-attacking immune response. Ignoring potential unintended consequences, other 'biohackers' are beginning to tinker with their own genes.

9 As noted by Wischmann, in this volume, if we leave out the six countries in which in over half of the treatment cycles only one embryo was transferred back (so-called 'elective single-embryo transfer'), the rate of twins following assisted reproduction is 15 times greater in comparison with births after spontaneous conception, and the rate of triplets 36 times higher. Regarding feticide, in the 1980s ten years after ultrasound became a routine antenatal practice its widespread misuse became apparent in India and China, where scanning was being used to detect and destroy female foetuses. Coupled with infanticide this led to many millions of missing girls, and eventually, a lack of brides for two whole generations of men. This resulted in celibacy or men marrying down a caste, but also, I would venture, resulted in unforeseen social after-effects such as the increasingly vicious gang rapes, and ferocious female kidnapping seen in India today.

10 Egg donors have begun to claim their right to be paid or at least forewarned about the discomfort and possible dangers of ovarian hyper-stimulation syndrome and increased risk of ovarian/uterine cancer as well as psychological after-effects of giving up their eggs (Kenney & McGowan, 2010). Hopeful parents travel the globe, at the mercy of a changing scene (e.g., having to seek help elsewhere, now that Cambodia closed down its surrogacy industry which had flourished due to the neighbouring countries of India, Nepal and Thailand outlawing it).

11 A recent study by NYU School of Medicine examined 416 issues of celeb magazines from 2010 to 2014. It found that only two out of 240 older celebs mentioned that their pregnancies were the result of fertility treatment. But despite the media hype, scientists say that out of 100 fertilised eggs on average fewer than 50 reach the blastocyst stage, 25 implant into the womb and only some 13 develop beyond three months.

12 'WHO's proclamation stresses recognition of the

> basic right of all couples and individuals to decide freely and responsibly the number, spacing and timing of their children and to have the information and means to do so, and the right to attain the highest standard of sexual and reproductive health … free of discrimination, coercion and violence'.
> (see www.who.int//reproductive-health/gender/index.html).

Yet the Chinese implemented a one-child per family rule that enforced abortions, and resulted in a massive surplus of males (and scarcity of brides). Conversely, Ceausescu instituted draconian policies to increase Romania's very low birth rate to four or even five children per woman, by subjecting them to humiliating mandatory monthly gynaecological examinations, forbidding contraception, abortion and divorce under strict state control that included taxation of childless men and women. This resulted in scores of thousands of unwanted babies institutionalised in orphanages by families who could not afford to bring them up. [Ironically, in today's Romania, one motivation for women's widespread sale of their eggs is said to be a defiant celebration of autonomous bodily ownership (see Nahman, 2008).]

13 In the USA where marriage, not biology, underpins the legal relation, a pregnant woman's husband is automatically presumed to be her child's father. But this clause has faced legal challenges from genetic 'fathers'. Conversely, in the UK, use of sperm obtained privately or from unlicensed clinic will deem the *donor* the father. However, parenthood can be transferred by parental order or adoption. There is a debate about awarding donors recognition. Some go as far as to suggest that registered egg or sperm donors should have visitation rights. Surrogacy, too, poses a conundrum. UK law treats the woman who gives birth as the mother with the right to keep the baby, even if not genetically related, and contracts are unenforceable. And regarding offspring, campaigners claim the right for donor-conceived people to know their origins. However, international studies reveal that many parents do not tell the child about their donor origins (e.g. Golombok, 2017a). In the UK, the HFEA no longer allows anonymity for gamete providers to a fertility clinic. At 18 years of age, children are entitled to break the register code to seek data or contact. In the US fertility treatment, practices are currently largely self-regulated. But thinking ahead to the eventuality of a donor register, the American Society for Reproductive Medicine (ASRM) promotes two-part guidelines for distinguishing between disclosure to a child that s/he was conceived with donor gametes, and providing information about the medical history and identity of a donor. But in today's digital world, savvy donor offspring often discover their ancestry and first-degree relatives, through DNA testing and internet sleuthing on donor-sibling websites (which unethically may find that up to 50 half-siblings were sired by a single donor across many families).

14 They use ovulation kits, temperature charts, expensive tablets and partake of a cocktail of injections. Diagnostic procedures may involve post-coital tests, semen evaluation, technological assessments such as ovarian reserve tests and more or less invasive procedures from ultrasound imaging (to look for uterine fibroids or polyps), scrotum sonography or X-ray hysterosalpingogram using a radiographic dye to check whether the fallopian tubes are clear of blockages or scarring for insertion of a minute camera (laparoscopy or hysteroscopy) to examine the interior of the uterus.,

References

Baltimore, D. et al. (2015). A Prudent Path Forward for Genomic Engineering and Germline Gene Modification. *Science*, 348(6230): 36–38.

Cobb, M. (2017). The Brave New World of Gene Editing. *New York Review of Books*, July 13. Issue.

Corbett, K. (2001). Nontraditional Family Romance. *Psychoanalytic Quarterly*, 70: 599–624.

Doudna, J.N., & Sternberg, S.H. (2017). *A Crack in Creation: Gene Editing and the Unthinkable Power to Control Evolution*, New York: Houghton Mifflin Harcourt.

Ehrensaft, D. (2007). The Stork Didn't Bring Me, I Came from a Dish: Psychological Experiences of Children Conceived through Assisted Reproductive Technology. *Journal of Infant, Child & Adolescent Psychotherapy*, 6: 124–140.

Golombok, S. (2017a). Disclosure and Donor-Conceived Children. *Human Reproduction*, 32(7): 1532–1533.

——— (2017b). Parenting in New Family Forms. *Science Direct, Current Opinion in Psychology*, 15: 76–80.

Heine, S.J. (2017). *DNA Is Not Destiny: The Remarkable, Completely Misunderstood Relationship Between You and Your Genes*, New York: Norton.

Kenney, N.J., & McGowan, M.L. (2010). Looking Back: Egg Donors' Retrospective Evaluations of their Motivations, Expectations, and Experiences during their First Donation Cycle. *Fertility & Sterility*, 93(2): 455–466.

Lanphier, E., Urnov, F., Haecker, S.E., Werner, M., & Smolenski, J. (2015). Don't Edit the Human Germ Line, *Nature International Journal of Science*, 519: issue 7544, 12 March 2015.

Levine, H. et al. (2017). Temporal Trends in Sperm Count: A Systematic Review and Meta-Regression Analysis. *Human Reproduction*, Update. 23(6): 646–659.

Nahman, M. (2008). Nodes of Desire: Romanian Egg Sellers, 'Dignity' and Feminist Alliances in Transnational Ova Exchanges. *European Journal of Women's Studies*, 15: 65–82.

Raphael-Leff, J. (1991). *Psychological Processes of Childbearing*, London: Chapman & Hall, 4th edition Anna Freud Centre, 2011.

——— (1993). *Pregnancy – The Inside Story*. London: Karnac, New York: Other Press 2001.

——— (2007). Femininity and Its Unconscious 'Shadows': Gender and Generative Identity in the Age of Biotechnology. *British Journal of Psychotherapy*, 23(4): 497–515.

——— (2015). *The Dark Side of the Womb – Pregnancy, Parenting & Persecutory Anxieties*, London: Anna Freud Centre.

Rochman, B. (2017). *The Gene Machine: How Genetic Technologies Are Changing the Way We Have Kids—and the Kids We Have*, New York: Scientific American/Farrar, Straus and Giroux.

4

Psychological Impact of Infertility and Assisted Reproduction[1]

Tewes Wischmann

Infertility and Assisted Reproduction – Basic Facts and Figures

Definitions and Basic Facts

According to the WHO's (clinical) definition, it is appropriate to speak of infertility when despite regular unprotected sexual intercourse a couple has been waiting one year or more for pregnancy (Zegers-Hochschild et al., 2009). The demographic definition extends the period in question to two years. If the woman has previously given birth to a living child, the term "secondary infertility" is used, and all other instances are cases of "primary infertility." In 2010, 1.9% of women between 20 and 44 years of age who were exposed to the eventuality of pregnancy displayed primary infertility and 10.5% were unable to have another child (secondary infertility) (Mascarenhas, Flaxman, Boerma, Vanderpoel, & Stevens, 2012). In the investigation of a sample of over 15,000 individuals, a recent study indicates that the clinical definition of infertility (see above) applies to one out of eight women and one out of ten men (Datta et al., 2016). Approximately 57% of the women and 53% of the men with fertility problems in this sample had sought medical or other professional help for their disorder. It has to be mentioned clearly that the majority of studies on psychosocial aspects of infertility had been conducted on women and men seeking medical treatment for infertility, so little is known about short- and long-term development of infertile individuals outside the medical system (Greil, Slauson-Blevins, & McQuillan, 2010). This could also help to distinguish the experience of infertility from the experience of infertility treatment.

The lifetime prevalence of fertility disorders (the probability of being affected by such a disorder once or more at any point in one's life) is higher. Between a third and a quarter of all women have had to wait a year to become pregnant (McQuillan, Greil, White, & Jacob, 2003; Schmidt, 2006) without necessarily regarding themselves as unintentionally childless. After two years of unprotected intercourse, 11% of all couples are still waiting for pregnancy (Slama et al., 2012). There are various factors that make it difficult to supply more precise figures on infertility prevalence. For many couples, the transition from intentional childlessness (for professional reasons, lack of partner, etc.) to unintentional childlessness is gradual. And how are couples to be assessed on the basis that one of the partners wants a child but the other does not (or not yet)? The desire for a child is postponed until the relevant parameters involve a lower (usually professional/vocational) risk for the couple (and particularly for the woman!) (Mills et al., 2011). When the couple finally feels that the time is ripe, the biological restrictions may already have taken decisive effect.

It is still true to say that standard medical values on which to base female or male infertility diagnoses are conspicuous by their absence, and where they do exist (e.g. in the WHO manual on semen analysis (WHO, 2010)), they have been redefined so frequently that they cannot be properly compared across a number of decades. For example, before 1987 oligozoospermia was diagnosed if sperm concentration was lower than 40 million spermatozoa per milliliter of ejaculate. Later the threshold value fell to 20 million, and since 2015 it has been 15 million. An American study found that of 982 men whose fertility was classified as subnormal in accordance with the WHO criteria of 1999, 380 (=38.7%) would be considered "normal" in terms of the 2010 criteria (Esteves et al., 2011).

Potentialities and Risks of ART

The term assisted reproductive techniques (ART) encompasses all forms of treatment and all procedures brought to bear on human egg cells, sperm, or embryos with a view to bringing about pregnancy and the birth of a child. The procedures employed in assisted reproduction (medically induced pregnancy) are in vitro fertilization (IVF) and intracytoplasmic sperm injection (ICSI), somewhat less frequently intrauterine insemination (IUI) after previous hormone stimulation for the woman. These procedures can be briefly described as follows. *IVF*: after previous hormone stimulation, oocytes are removed from the woman's ovaries and fertilized by the (processed) sperm of the male partner in a Petri dish in the laboratory. After a number of days in the incubator, the fertilized oocytes are transferred to the uterus. *ICSI*: aspiration and back–transfer as with IVF, but here insemination is done via microinjection of one single sperm into an egg cell. *IUI with previous hormone stimulation*: the sperm is injected into the uterus with a catheter (after hormone stimulation in the female partner to enhance maturation of egg cells). Gamete donation (treatment with donor sperm or oocyte donation) can be combined with all three procedures. The psychosocial aspects of this particular kind of family planning require special consideration that goes beyond the concerns associated with ART procedures affecting couples only. Use can be made either of "freshly" obtained gametes (so-called "fresh" cycle) or of semen/egg cells that were initially frozen and later thawed (so-called "cryo" cycle).

In 2013, some 685,000 ART treatment cycles were carried out in Europe, of which approximately 145,000 were IVF cycles, 330,000 ICSI cycles, 40,000 cycles with egg-cell donation, 150,000 cryo cycles with embryos, and 6,600 cryo cycles with egg cells (Calhaz-Jorge et al., 2017). For the same year we have reports of about 175,000 inseminations with partner semen and approximately 44,000 with donor semen. It is unclear how reliable these figures are, as in about half of the countries participating in the register by no means all the reproductive medicine centers had reported data for the year in question (e.g. only about two-thirds of the 198 IVF centers and only half of the 314 IUI clinics in Spain). Accordingly, it is difficult to assess the success rates actually achieved, i.e. the live birth rate per treatment cycle carried out (subsequent to aspiration/ thawing of egg cells). The average birth rates reported in the European register are 20.9% per IVF/ ICSI cycle (taken together) and 18.0% per cryo cycle. As per insemination cycle, the birth rates listed are 8.6% (with partner semen) and 11.1% (with donor semen). In the case of oocyte donation (fresh and cryo cycle combined), a birth rate of 53% per aspiration has been reported.

From the birth rates per treatment cycle, we can calculate the cumulative birth rate, which is of particular interest for the relevant couples. After three cycles with IVF/ICSI (taken together), some 50% of the couples are still unsuccessful in terms of the target outcome ("live birth of a child"), and after six attempts the figure is still approximately 25%. For cryo treatments and IUIs the cumulative rates are little lower, for egg-cell donation the cumulative rates are substantially higher. This means that a large majority of couples in Europe undergoing treatment with ART have to face up to the fact that the undertaking is likely to remain unsuccessful unless four or more treatment cycles are financially viable. Accordingly, they need to devise "plan B" in good time (Van den Broeck, Emery, Wischmann, & Thorn, 2010). In Germany, for instance, fewer than 20% of the women in question undergo four or more treatment cycles (DIR (Deutsches IVF-Register), 2015, p. 531).

One of the most important risks involved in ART treatment is the likelihood of multiple births. In Europe in 2013, 17.5% of all births following "fresh" IVF/ICSI cycles were twin births and 0.5% triplet births (Calhaz-Jorge et al., 2017). In comparison with births after spontaneous conception, the rate of twins is 15 times higher and the rate of triplets 36 times higher. If we leave out the six countries in which in over half of the treatment cycles only one embryo was transferred back (so-called "elective single-embryo transfer"), the share of twin births rises to 20% and that of triplets to 0.9%. Despite greatly improved obstetric intervention resources, the health risks for multi-birth progeny should not be underestimated. Compared with singletons, the risk of cerebral palsy is four times higher in twins and 18 times higher in triplets, while the risk of death by age 1 year is seven times higher for twins and 20 times higher for triplets. Half of the twins and almost 90% of the triplets born after ART treatment in Europe are premature. In the meantime, however, other risks associated with ART like the ovarian hyperstimulation syndrome, bleeding, or infection have become very rare (Calhaz-Jorge et al., 2017).

Causes of Infertility

Fertility disorder diagnoses are distributed more or less equally across women and men. In approximately 40% of cases, both partners have fertility disorders, in about a third of them the cause is associated exclusively with the woman partner, in about a fifth of them exclusively with the man, and in fewer than 10% no cause of infertility can be detected in either partner (Wischmann, 2012). Chief among the causes of infertility in women are ovulation disorders in about one-third of all cases, damage to the fallopian tubes in about a quarter of such instances, and – more rarely – endometriosis or cervical factors. In men, the OAT syndrome is the most frequent culprit (impaired sperm concentration, motility, morphology) followed by asthenozoospermia (sperm motility defect) and teratozoospermia (abnormal sperm morphology).

In contrast to earlier psychosomatic models, evidence-based scientific research (Apfel & Keylor, 2002; Wischmann, 2003) has established that the psyche has no direct influence on the causes of infertility – for example unconscious anxieties about pregnancy and/or parenthood or a conflictual attitude to the child (Kainz, 2001). Unintentionally childless couples are unremarkable in psychopathological terms – whether medical causes can be identified for their situation or not (Gameiro et al., 2015; Wischmann, Stammer, Scherg, Gerhard, & Verres, 2001). Indirect influence by the psyche can only be assumed to play a role in the context of behaviorally conditioned infertility (Schilling, Toth, Rosner, Strowitzki, & Wischmann, 2012). A behaviorally conditioned fertility disorder – with potentially psychosocial (part-)causes – is present when (a) despite counseling by a doctor a couple continues to display behavior detrimental to fertility (eating habits, especially overweight/underweight and eating disorders, competitive sport, overindulgence in alcohol/tobacco, abuse of medicines, etc.), (b) a (heterosexual) couple refrains from sexual intercourse on fertile days or displays a non-organic sexual function disorder, or (c) a couple expressly concedes the necessity of medical therapy in fulfilling their desire for a child but fails to embark on such therapy even after a lengthy period of deliberation, e.g. constantly postponing tube blockage tests (Hysterosalpingography) or a sperm analysis. A pilot study suggests that the prevalence of behaviorally conditioned infertility is approx. 9% in women and 3% in men (Schilling et al., 2012).

The influence of everyday stress or emotional strain (over-anxiety, depressive states, etc.) on the inception of pregnancy should not be overrated either (Boivin, Griffiths, & Venetis, 2011). Relaxation techniques (autogenic training, progressive muscle relaxation, yoga, etc.) can usually be confidently recommended to women (and their partners) as a way of coping with unintentional childlessness and treatment with reproductive medicine, but only in very rare cases do they heighten the probability of pregnancy (Wischmann, 2008; Pasch et al., 2012). Even extreme stress, e.g. after the Fukushima disaster in Japan, does nothing to lower pregnancy rates after ART (Hayashi, Fujimori, Yasumura, & Nakai, 2017).

Psychological Impact of Infertility and Diagnosis

In a much-cited earlier study, 48% of the women and 15% of the men said that for them infertility was the worst crisis in their lives (Freeman, Boxer, Rickels, Tureck, & Mastroianni, 1985). For many women, the effects of this crisis are sometimes just as severe as those caused by a serious illness (HIV infection, cancer, etc.) or the loss of a close relative (Domar, Zuttermeister, & Friedman, 1993), so playing down the significance of the unfulfilled desire for a child ("There are worse things that can happen") is likely to be counterproductive. Counselors providing psychosocial advice for couples wanting a child should bear this in mind and proceed accordingly (Cousineau & Domar, 2007). On average, the desire for a child – and the stress associated with unintentional childlessness – is likely to be more pronounced in women. Up to menopause, they are (regularly) confronted every month with the fact that they are still not pregnant, whereas the men involved are not so directly affected by this experience (Wischmann & Thorn, 2013).

The unfulfilled desire for a child is frequently perceived as a potential loss that in its wake can set off various stages of mourning familiar from other mourning processes (from "shock" through "despair" to "acceptance"). On the surface, men and women appear to express their mourning in stereotypically different ways. Whereas women give emotional expression to their grief and will readily talk about it, men tend to avoid the overt expression of emotions and assume the role of the "stoical partner" (Hudson & Culley, 2013). Probably all individuals, male or female, have at their disposal, albeit to different degrees, both loss-oriented and recovery-oriented coping styles not necessarily bound up with traditional gender roles (Jaffe & Diamond, 2010).

Depending on the diagnosis, men and women experience a fertility disorder differently. Various studies indicate that if the diagnosis of the cause of infertility is "woman only," "both partners," or "unclear" (idiopathic infertility), the woman involved will be more likely to feel "responsible" for the situation. Only a "man only" diagnosis will clear the female partner of all "blame." In such cases, men will frequently suffer more from unintentional childlessness than women, though the studies on this issue are not unanimous. But if the diagnosis is "azoospermia," the men in almost all these studies feel this to be a source of considerable stress, particularly when insemination by donor is addressed as a potential therapy option (Wischmann, 2013b; Hammarberg, Collins, Holden, Young, & McLachlan, 2017).

From a purely medical point of view, the diagnosis "idiopathic infertility" may seem to hold out a good prognosis, but the couples involved frequently find the situation extremely stressful because of the absence of a well-defined organic cause that can be tackled medically (Wischmann et al., 2001). This often prompts the couples involved to start brooding about the question of the extent to which psychic factors may be responsible for the diagnosis. In counseling, it is important to address such subjective cause-ascriptions proactively and intervene with a view to reducing stress (Van den Broeck et al., 2010).

Coping Strategies of Infertile Couples

The capacity to adapt to infertility-related stress depends to a large extent on both partners' coping strategies. The coping strategies resorted to by infertile couples are usually classified into four groups: active-confronting (e.g. asking friends and relatives for advice), active-avoidance (e.g. not sharing feelings, avoiding children or pregnant women), passive-avoidance (e.g. hoping for a miracle or believing that waiting is the only solution), and meaning-based coping (e.g. belief that both the man and the woman have "grown" significantly as a result of the experience or that it has had a beneficial effect on their marriage/partnership) (Wischmann & Kentenich, 2016). Various studies agree that some coping strategies are more useful than others in coming to terms with infertility-specific stress (Peterson, Pirritano, Christensen, & Schmidt, 2008; Volmer, Rösner, Toth, Strowitzki, & Wischmann, 2017). In terms of emotional adjustment, active-avoidance coping appears to be the least effective strategy and meaning-based coping the most favorable alternative (Gameiro et al., 2015).

In couples, these coping strategies are reciprocal in their effects. If both the woman and the man opt for active-avoidance, this option is associated with a higher risk of emotional stress for both partners. But the reciprocal effect is stronger still. Active-avoidance coping in the woman is associated with high risk of stress in the male partner (partner effect), while vice versa the effect is even more marked (Volmer et al., 2017). A high degree of meaning-based coping in the woman is associated with a low risk of stress both for herself and her partner (partner effect). Psychological counseling can then help to promote recourse to positive coping strategies such as meaning-based coping and train couples to avoid using negative coping strategies such as active-avoidance (Peterson et al., 2012). Because of the importance of partner effects on psychological risks, psychological infertility counseling should be predominantly angled at the couple rather than the individual partner (Volmer et al., 2017).

Psychological Impact of ART on Women and Men

In most cases, treatment with reproductive medicine is felt by both women and men to be a severe emotional strain (Boivin et al., 2012). The typical pattern here is the "emotional roller coaster." Phases of optimistic anticipation and hope after insemination or embryo transfer are followed by periods of disappointment and frustration when menstruation sets in again (Van den Broeck et al., 2010). Accordingly, the waiting period prior to the pregnancy test is felt to be emotionally the most stressful time in the course of ART treatment (Boivin & Lancastle, 2010). This treatment-specific stress is also referred to by many couples as a major reason for prematurely terminating ART treatment, even if the medical prognosis is favorable (Gameiro, Boivin, Peronace, & Verhaak, 2012).

In itself, an infertility diagnosis may have substantial effects on the sex life of the couple in question, and if this is the case, infertility treatment may represent an additional source of stress (Wischmann, 2013a; Wischmann, 2010). Women frequently report loss of libido and impaired sexual satisfaction (Millheiser et al., 2010), while men suffer more from erectile dysfunction and ejaculation problems. Both partners complain especially about the loss of spontaneous sexual desire as a result of scheduled sexual activity designed to fulfill the wish for a child ("baby-making" instead of "love-making") (Wischmann et al., 2014). These sexual "lows" do not normally require treatment and in most cases they will soon disappear again of their own accord. However, sexual dysfunction and covert sexual problems may themselves be a part cause of infertility. The study by Schilling and colleagues (2012) cited earlier refers to rates of 7% reduced sexuality and 2% functional sexual disorders in women at the beginning of infertility treatment (over and against 1% of the men in each case). Another study reports that in every 16th ART treatment cycle the man was unable to achieve ejaculation via masturbation and the cycle in question had to be discontinued as a result (Pottinger, Carroll, & Mason, 2016).

Specific Aspects of Third-Party Reproduction

Founding a family with gametes or embryos donated by others (and sometimes also via surrogacy) involves specific psychological aspects of its own. As one other person is involved in the process (or two in the case of embryo donation), the genetic origins of the child are a significant factor

(Thorn & Wischmann, 2009). If the ovarian reserves of the female partner are exhausted, oocyte or embryo donation becomes an option. In the case of male infertility, embryo donation and semen donation (as for lesbian couples or single mothers "by choice" too) are the available alternatives. The special genetic links (potentially) created in this way make engagement with two topics unavoidable: (a) the question of when the child should be enlightened on the subject and (b) the question of the identifiability of gamete donors. Scientific studies indicate that there is hardly any doubt that a child born as a result of third-party gamete or embryo donation should be apprised of his/her genetic origins in an appropriate way at an early stage and provided with access to reliable information about his/her genetic origins and the existence of siblings or half-siblings, if any (Peterson et al., 2012). The implication of this is that for psychosocial and ethical reasons couples wanting a child should be strongly advised against availing themselves of *anonymous* gamete donation (although at present in Europe the vast majority of treatments with oocyte donations are solely and exclusively feasible on an anonymous basis).

Development of Pregnancies, Children, and Families after ART

In terms of the subjective experience of pregnancy and birth following ART, overall apprehension in women is no higher than in the case of "normal" pregnancy, but specific anxieties in connection with damage to, or loss of, the child are more marked, particularly if there have been miscarriages in the past. In comparison with controls, men entertain higher anxieties about these pregnancies but like the women display the same prenatal attachments. Many women are disappointed by the frequency of caesarean section after ART (36% even with singletons), and after birth this may lead to complications like increased maternal anxiety and breastfeeding problems (Hammarberg, Fisher, & Wynter, 2008). Pregnancy following oocyte donation appears to be associated with higher medical risks for mother and child (Savasi, Mandia, Laoreti, & Cetin, 2016).

A good overview of the psychosocial development of children born after ART in different kinds of family building can be found in Susan Golombok's book on the subject (2015). With regard to singletons born following ART, the number of studies on the situation in families with heterosexual and lesbian parents and with single mothers "by choice" can be regarded as satisfactory. In the vast majority of cases, children growing up in families of this kind display a development somewhere between unremarkable and unusually good, particularly as most of them are "wanted." Relationships of the parents are also unremarkable. Restrictions have to be made in connection with the situation of older single mothers "by choice", as the demands involved in looking after handicapped children or progeny from multiple births may represent a challenge for them in case of restricted social support.

The state of research on the psychosocial aspects of family planning via embryo donation, surrogate motherhood, and anonymous oocyte donation is inadequate. Alongside the medical risks referred to earlier, families with higher birth multiplicity also display psychosocial risks (e.g. higher parent separation rate, retarded development in the children, etc.). Singletons after ART are more likely to be premature and have a lower average birth weight (in comparison with their spontaneously conceived counterparts) (Kamphuis, Bhattacharya, van der Veen, Mol, & Templeton, 2014; Wennberg et al., 2016). After "fresh" ICSI cycles, they also display a higher average malformation rate (compared with IVF cycles/spontaneous conceptions) (Davies et al., 2012).

Long-Term Effects of Involuntary Childlessness

There have been a number of studies (including the long-term variety) investigating couples who have remained childless against their will. For couples who have been able to set themselves other life goals than parenthood and who are not socially isolated, the prognosis is good. Women with a persistent desire for pregnancy three to five years after unsuccessful treatment may experience more anxiety and depression than women who find new life goals or women who become mothers (Gameiro et al., 2015). On average, there are no long-term differences in sexual satisfaction identifiable between ART mothers, adoptive mothers, and women (or men) who have remained childless (Sydsjö, Svanberg, Lampic, & Jablonowska, 2011). In one study, the separation rate 10–14 years after infertility treatment was 17%, which is significantly lower than the separation percentage for this length of partnership in the population as a whole (25–30%) (Wischmann, Korge, Scherg, Strowitzki, & Verres, 2012). Other studies found a higher risk of separation for childless couples five/twelve years after ART (in comparison with parents), but here again the separation rates were lower than in the general population (Johansson et al., 2010; Kjaer et al., 2014). More than half the women and a third of the men in the study by Wischmann and co-workers (2012) referred to social support, frank communication, an open attitude, and active confrontation as positive coping factors in the period when they were trying to have a child. Twenty percent of the women and 12% of the men referred to new life goals, termination of treatment, acceptance, and developing other interests as helpful in this connection.

Psychological Interventions for Infertile Couples

Counseling Needs of Infertile Couples and Individuals

In one German study (Wischmann, Scherg, Strowitzki, & Verres, 2009), couples were investigated at the beginning of treatment at a center for reproductive medicine. Of those who indicated an openness to counseling, almost half actually attended infertility counseling, and two groups, "no counseling" and "taking up counseling," were therefore compared. The main results were: more couples with stressful life events were found in the counseling group. For women taking up counseling, psychological distress, in the form of suffering from childlessness and depression as well as subjective excessive demand (as a potential cause for infertility), was higher in comparison to women not counseled. The higher distress for men in the counseling group was indicated by relative dissatisfaction with partnership and sexuality and by accentuating the women's depression. The authors came to the following conclusions: infertile couples seeking psychological help are characterized by high levels of psychological distress, primarily in women. The women's distress seems to be more important as a reason for attending infertility counseling than that of the men.

Notably the following constellations urgently necessitate infertility counseling, which in these cases should not only be offered on a take-it-or-leave-it basis but explicitly recommended:

- Vulnerable individuals/couples (e.g. earlier psychiatric disorders, abuse of addictive substances, special physical or mental needs and requirements, restricted capacity for "informed consent")
- Presence of a behaviorally conditioned fertility disorder (Schilling et al., 2012)
- Response in the form of individual crisis (e.g. massive self-esteem problems, depressive response with a sustained and pronounced obsession with the desire for a child and neglect of other life goals)
- Response in the form of a crisis in couple dynamics (e.g. sexual problems, prolonged ambivalence or indecision with respect to potential medical treatment)
- Prior to invasive medical interventions (e.g. transition from IUI to IVF/ICSI)
- Prior to pre-implantation or prenatal diagnostic measures during or after (successful) ART
- During multiple pregnancy (especially before fetal reduction)
- In the case of (repeated) miscarriage or stillbirth (Toth et al., 2015)
- Before, during, and after treatment with gamete/embryo donation or surrogate motherhood

- Before treatment with reproductive medicine abroad in another country (Thorn & Wischmann, 2012)
- Donors and surrogate mothers should also be urgently advised to avail themselves of psychosocial counseling before, during, and after treatment (Thorn & Wischmann, 2009).

To underline the pertinence of psychosocial infertility counseling, it is advisable to document in writing the couples' decision either to embark on counseling or to (initially) reject it. By contrast, experienced psychosocial counselors working in this field are unanimous in advising against *mandatory* infertility counseling, as among other things this would interfere with the couple's reproductive autonomy and contradict the low-threshold principle in psychosocial counseling.

Types of Counseling

Internationally, it is customary to distinguish the following kinds of psychosocial counseling in terms of subject matter: "implications counseling," "decision-making counseling" (frequently amalgamated as "implications and decision-making counseling"), "support counseling," "crisis counseling," and "therapeutic counseling." These are frequently preceded by "information gathering and analysis." Table 4.1 indicates the essential differences between various forms of counseling (Peterson et al., 2012).

In general, these different types of infertility counseling are entrusted to different groups of professionals specializing in infertility diagnosis or treatment. Always provided, of course, that there are sufficient resources available, "information gathering" and "implications and decision-making counseling" can safely be allotted to ART practitioners and other fertility staff in the framework of "patient-centered care." "Support counseling" can normally be provided by psychosocial counseling specialists not involved in the treatment itself. Much the same is true of "crisis counseling." "Therapeutic counseling," however, normally requires a psychotherapist specifically trained for the purpose. These distinctions are not however cast in stone. Psychosocial counseling specialists will also provide counseling on information gathering, the effects of

Table 4.1 Different forms of psychosocial infertility counseling (after Wischmann, 2012)

Information gathering and analysis	Collecting or providing information on the medical and psychosocial aspects of infertility counseling (e.g. obtaining a "second opinion")
Implications counseling	Counseling on the repercussions of all treatment options on the individual involved, on partners and family members, and on the unborn child, particularly prior to invasive treatment
Decision-making counseling	Thorough discussion of the specific effects of decisions on the individual involved, on partners and family members, and on gamete donors/surrogate mothers and their partners
Support counseling	Emotionally supportive counseling, notably in psychologically stressful situations and processes (e.g. after a miscarriage)
Crisis counseling	Targeted and focused psychosocial counseling in the case of critically exacerbated stress response (e.g. after ART failure or termination of unsuccessful treatment)
Therapeutic counseling	Specific psychotherapeutic assistance in connection with infertility treatment, e.g. when partner conflicts (including disturbances of sexual functions) materialize or threaten to become chronic, or when depression looks like setting in

different stages of treatment, and decision-making, so that the patients involved have counseling at their disposal that is independent of the treatment itself. They will also be called upon to provide counseling in crisis situations if a psychotherapeutic specialist is either unnecessary or unavailable. Concerning ethical dilemmas in ART, fertility counseling *independently* of the medical treatment is essential (Horowitz, Galst, & Elster, 2010).

Objectives of Infertility Counseling

The following is a list of the central aims pursued by psychosocial infertility counseling:

- normalization, depathologization, externalization
- greater flexibility (couple communication, "roadmaps")
- maximizing the couple's active involvement in the proceedings
- impartiality and open-mindedness in the interests of the couple and the (unborn) child
- decision-making on the basis of best possible information status
- decision-making in the spirit of greatest possible authenticity

Normalization and *depathologization* mean making clear to the client(s) that feelings like helplessness, envy of pregnant women, or guilt feelings are entirely understandable and completely normal as a response to an infertility diagnosis. *Externalization* means switching from the subjective view "I'm infertile" to the attitude "My sperm count is seriously inadequate." "Feeling guilty" is not automatically identical with "being guilty." Counseling should also seek to achieve greater *flexibility*, notably by keeping couple communication "alive" even though it may seem as if everything has already been said on the subject of unintentional childlessness. Another aim in connection with couple communication is to give adequate scope and expression both to ambivalence(s) in the desire for a child and to life "outside" the unfulfilled desire for a child. In a situation of the kind represented by a course of reproductive medicine, the influence of the couple on the course of events is minimal, and the doctors themselves can do no more than optimize the preconditions for successful pregnancy. This makes it doubly important to maximize the active involvement of the couples involved (e.g. working out roadmaps).

Another important aspect of infertility counseling is to encourage acceptance of a life without biological children and in the counseling process to explicitly include from the outset the possibility that infertility treatment may turn out to be unsuccessful. Couples should also be supported in identifying alternative perspectives ("plan B"). Although we know from experience that many couples find this difficult, "plan B" should be elaborated either before or at the beginning of reproductive medicine. The success of the medical treatment does not depend on the extent to which the couple "believes" in it ("positive thinking"). In counseling, one recommendable way of convincing the couple of the importance of working out plan B at an early stage is the following: if after (possibly) a number of years, the treatment with reproductive medicine should turn out to be unsuccessful and the couple had to fall back on this plan B, then they would already have it "in the drawer." And if the infertility treatment was ultimately successful, then that's where it could stay (Wischmann, 2012).

For the greater benefit of the couple and the (unborn) child, counseling should be *impartial* and "*open-minded*," i.e. it should not be for or against a specific infertility treatment option from the outset and should be mindful of the perspective of the potential child. Closely bound up with this is the importance of ensuring that decisions can be made on the basis of the *best possible information status*. Providing such a basis is a crucial task in psychosocial infertility counseling. Adequate, trustworthy, up-to-date information on all therapeutic aspects of fertility disorders can today be found in books on the subject or on the Internet (Covington, 2015).

Decision-making on the basis of *greatest possible authenticity* refers especially to treatment with gamete donation and the anonymity or identifiability of the donor. In enlightening the child at a later stage, it may be important to convey to him/her that at the point of time in question, *anonymous* gamete donation was the only viable course of action, either for legal reasons or because the emotional stress for the parents-to-be had become too great.

Content in Infertility Counseling

The subject matter addressed in infertility counseling has been widely discussed (Boivin & Kentenich, 2002; Covington & Burns, 2006; Van den Broeck et al., 2010; Wischmann, Stammer, Gerhard, & Verres, 2002). The following is an outline of typical elements:

- *Assessment of medical diagnosis and therapy by the couple.* Explicit reference is made to the fact that the man and the woman may assess potential treatment success differently and to the hopes or the resignation associated with that fact. The question of guilt ascription is also addressed. If there are one-sided "accusations" of guilt, it is important that counselors display an understanding, impartial, open-minded attitude (see above).
- *Subjective ascription of causes.* Notably, couples with idiopathic infertility tend to assume that the causes of the fertility disorder are (partly) psychological. In this connection, the word "stress" is usually employed, particularly, as the majority of (medical) guides to the issue still suggest that psychic stress is one of the prime causes of infertility. Normally, it will suffice in counseling to point out that everyday stress definitely has no impact on fertility – unless stress causes people to adopt behaviors detrimental to fertility – and that only in wartime (if then) will stress play a causal role in the unfulfilled desire for a child. Naturally, discussing the subjective ascription of causes will also involve exploration of fantasies about reasons for infertility, e.g. that unintentional childlessness is a "retribution" for an earlier induced abortion. Here again, it is usually enough to point out that a competently performed abortion with no complications involved does nothing whatsoever to lower the chances of another pregnancy.
- *Coming to terms with childlessness and the treatment for it.* Having a child cannot be regarded as an distinct indicator for an intact, resilient, and sexually fulfilling couple relationship. But not having children is frequently regarded as a flaw, and childless couples usually avoid talking about the subject because they are ashamed. Men talking openly about their infertility problem may indeed have to put up with snide remarks from colleagues or acquaintances, and this is by no means restricted to the less well-educated strata of society. In counseling, the balance between "hiding" the desire for a child (or the relevant treatment) and unprotected openness can be redefined. The subjective experience of reproductive therapy ("emotional roller coaster") and the planning of further stages of treatment are also discussed here. Frequently, it is appropriate to inquire about the individual values and especially the ethical and religious/spiritual background of both partners, as these may affect both the way the couple comes to terms with the situation psychologically and their potential acceptance of the ART options (Greil et al., 2010).
- *Present life situation and job(s).* The discussion of the couple's vocational situation serves to identify potential fertility-relevant stressors affecting the man and/or the woman. One example is shift work for either or both partners (Gaskins et al., 2018). Other detrimental factors such as lack of money or care for a bedridden parent can also be addressed here. During treatment with reproductive medicine, it is certainly a good idea to put potentially divisive or stressful topics on the "back burner" or to deal with them conclusively before therapy reaches a more invasive stage.

- *Motivation for wanting a child.* Some changes that come with the arrival of a child are things that the couple can take an active hand in at an early stage, independently of the success of therapy (e.g. quitting uncongenial employment, clearer demarcation between the couple and parents/parents-in-law). After years of fertility treatment, couples may hardly be aware of the ambivalences bound up with the desire for a child itself or with the treatment they are undergoing. Here, counselors need to play the role of "advocates of (negative) emotions," gently reminding the couple of these ambivalent feelings. Conscious awareness of, and engagement with, these ambivalences frequently leads to greater critical detachment and hence to greater inner freedom over and against the desire for a child and the medical therapy (Wischmann et al., 2002).
- *Families of origin.* Couples who went through stressful or traumatic experiences in childhood/adolescence frequently link the desire for a child with the (unconscious) desire for reconciliation and the fear of re-actualization. A child can give the couple a new identity (as a "proper" family) and thus change the relationship to the family or families of origin. In this connection, psychotherapists Janet Jaffe and Martha Diamond use the term "reproductive trauma" to underline the fact that in many cases infertility crises may have a traumatic effect (Jaffe & Diamond, 2010).
- *Social environment.* The social pressure many couples feel exposed to particularly when they have reached a certain age ("the biological clock is ticking") may lead to a defensive attitude in connection trying for a child. Friends and parents are left in the dark about the couple's desire for a child or the treatment they are undergoing, and for some couples an evasive strategy appears to be the best course ("white lies"). In the meantime, however, by no means small percentage of couples have learned that a frank and open attitude to this issue will encourage others to report on their own experiences with unintentional childlessness (temporary or definitive). Time and again, couples will find that a couple with no children among their (possibly distant) relations will turn out to be involuntarily childless. Examples like this can serve to bring home to the couple the long-term effects of infertility, which may have a reassuring effect. In most cases, permanently childless couples will report that overcoming this crisis has "welded them together" rather than estranging them from one another (Wischmann et al., 2012).
- *Couple relations.* Infertility treatment is sometimes challenging and frequently long-drawn-out, and this may impose considerable strain on the partnership. As a result, the couple may lose sight of the differences between their standpoints and wishes. In counseling, both partners are encouraged to mutually (re-)perceive and recognize these differences. Frequently, counselors will witness polarization between the partners ("depressive woman" vs. "helpless man"), which may hinder communication between them and restrict their ability to come to terms with the situation (Van den Broeck et al., 2010). In counseling, the couple is encouraged to tell positive stories about themselves, thus changing the perspective from what is "missing" to the satisfactory things in life. Useful in this connection is homework in the form of a "positive diary" in which every day both partners "have to" enter (at least) one positive event they have experienced.
- *Sexuality and body awareness.* In those stages of medical treatment in which the couple is instructed to have "scheduled" intercourse, the carefree nature of spontaneous love-making may be more or less entirely forfeited. It is also conceivable that the pressure to "perform" will become so strong that functional sexual disorders ensue and (against their conscious will) the couple will no longer have intercourse on fertile days. With a view to reducing such pressure, it may be a good idea here to discuss with the couple a division into "purpose-oriented" sex on fertile days and "pleasure-oriented" sex the rest of the time.
- *Alternative life plans.* At the beginning of treatment, most couples cannot envisage a meaningful perspective in which a biological child does not figure. Addressing this idea jointly at as

early a stage of counseling as possible will frequently enable the couple to start with a "work of mourning" through which they can take their leave of something they have failed to achieve. This facilitates the timely emergence of new life perspectives, e.g. via active engagement with the prospect of adoption or foster parenthood, the creation of a new vocational or social identity, or intensification of couple relations against the background of different values and new goals. It is an aspect of counseling that revolves around confrontation with the possible failure of medical treatment. This work of mourning can however only begin when conception has proved to be not merely improbable but definitively impossible. As long as there is still the slightest chance of pregnancy, this chance will be associated with a spark of hope that militates against active mourning. Accordingly, couples on the way to abandoning their desire for a child once and for all should be advised to practice contraception (e.g. use condoms) so as not to unnecessarily delay the mourning process.

Effects of Infertility Counseling

An older overview (Wischmann, 2008) of the effects of psychosocial infertility counseling comes to the following conclusions: providing procedural information concerning the technical aspects of infertility investigation will probably facilitate coping with infertility itself and the techniques of assisted reproduction. This information can be given in the form of booklets or educational films. Using the Internet is a fast and easy way to obtain information on infertility and its treatment, albeit with the risk of coming across erroneous or misleading information. Telephone counseling can be helpful in providing specific information about the infertility workup, but it cannot replace face-to-face counseling on distressing psychosocial issues. Attendance of support groups can be recommended to strengthen coping abilities. Psychosocial counseling and psychotherapy are definitely effective in reducing negative affects, mostly within a short period of time (fewer than ten sessions). Pregnancy rates are unlikely to be affected by psychosocial interventions.

A recent survey of five reviews and three meta-analyses on psychosocial infertility counseling (Wischmann, 2017) indicates that we still cannot make any reliable statements about the effects of such interventions. The immense heterogeneity and the methodological defects of available studies make it impossible to undertake a summarizing evaluation in the form of systematic reviews or meta-analyses. Analyses taking account of ART as a moderator variable show hardly any effects for the target variables "quality of life" and "pregnancy" in infertile women and men. As is customary in psychotherapeutic research, future studies in this field should facilitate making specific statements about "what works for whom," i.e. which psychosocial interventions (emotional support, cognitive restructuring, etc.) are likely to cause which effects (quality of life and partnership quality, stress reduction, pregnancy rates, etc.) in which setting (by phone, in the group) for which person(s) (woman, man, couple) at which stage of treatment (before embryo transfer, after pregnancy test, after termination of ART without live birth) and with which repercussions and side effects (treatment-induced distress, sexual problems, miscarriages, etc.). In terms of subject matter, the interventions should be angled more systematically at the couple and strengthen their joint and individual resources and coping capacities.

In dealing with infertility disorders, scientifically well-founded psychosocial interventions are highly unlikely to have a detrimental effect, and the reviews and meta-analyses indicate at least a probability of improvement in life quality following counseling and/or psychotherapy. Accordingly, low-threshold access to such assistance should be made available to all couples requiring it. It should however be borne in mind that the latest scientific research on the subject indicates that such interventions do nothing to improve the prospects of pregnancy (except in instances of behaviorally conditioned infertility).

Interventions for the Mental Health Professional

First Interview

The first interview serves to define the task in hand. What do the clients have on their minds, what are their aims in seeking counseling? What can counseling do for them (and what not), who else might be better able to help them with their concerns? The following are typical subjects to be addressed at the first interview:

- Establishing the importance of the desire for a child for her/him (see above). One useful exercise is the "empty chair" on which the desired child is placed. The prospective parents then talk to him/her about concrete wishes and experiences or apprehensions. But one "parent" can also take a seat on this chair so that the subject of anticipated role changes for the parents can be addressed. Stammer and co-workers (2002, p. 76) recommend an exercise (also suitable for individual counseling) in which the couple draws up a "cake diagram" as a way of identifying the partners' (possibly different) perceptions and also of defining frontiers in connection with the fertility issue. Each of the partners draws a circle and divides it up into a cake diagram, allotting slices of the cake to the most important things in their present lives: the fertility problem and its treatment, work, leisure time and hobbies, friends, partnership, sexuality, parents and siblings, etc. When the slices have been allocated, the partners ask themselves for each individual thing they have mentioned to what extent it is more of a pleasure/gratification or more of a stress factor. They draw a green line round the "positive" areas and a red line around the "negative" ones. Then they put the diagrams next to each other and talk about the results: what status do the respective segments have for the individual partners, and which of them have been designated as congenial or as a stress factor?
- Identifying subjective cause theories, especially in cases of idiopathic infertility (so that if necessary the counselor can intervene to alleviate any guilt feelings that may be operative).
- If the child is idealized, it is best not to be confrontative but to include the experience of other couples in the equation: "What makes you so sure that in terms, say, of sleepless nights, things will be so different with you than with your colleagues/neighbors/friends?"
- Ensure basic knowledge on sexuality and reproduction: pregnancy chances are highest – max 30% – if sexual intercourse takes place two days before ovulation. Sex exclusively at the time of ovulation reduces these chances to 6–8%, one day later they are down to 1–2%. Intercourse only once a week entails a high risk of missing out on the fertility window.
- Indicate reliable available information material, e.g. on the Internet at www.ESHRE.eu, www.ASRM.org, www.NICE.uk. Several relevant Internet links can be found in Covington (2015).
- Find out how the couples relate to their social environment, and point out that "at the bottom line" a more outgoing, but at the same time more self-detached attitude to others is less effort than constant "white lies."
- Encourage couple communication. The subjective experience of unintentional childlessness is frequently different in the two partners. This should be borne in mind but not value-judged. It is important to identify unhelpful role play (e.g. "depressive woman – helpless man") and achieve greater flexibility in that respect. Confronted with a crushing fertility verdict, women will want to talk about their pain and anguish, while men feel helpless to intervene and withdraw into themselves. This circular pattern can lead to polarization and isolation, at a time when both partners need each other more than ever. Women tend to believe their partner to be less affected and far less depressive than the men assess themselves as being, while

men may overrate their partners' depressive moods and feel them to be more dramatic than they actually are. In counseling, it may be helpful to call attention to this polarizing effect.

- Normalizing and depathologizing "negative" feelings. Intensely, "negative" feelings such as despair after a negative test result, or rage at the unfairness of the situation, possibly also guilt feelings and/or partner blaming (e.g. for years of indecision about the desire for a child), are completely normal, understandable, and acceptable.
- "Give space to the desire for a child, and restrict that space at the same time" is the central tenet in psychosocial infertility counseling. Normally, the desire is omnipresent and should be estimated as such. But it should not dominate everyday life entirely. As long as the desire for a child exists, it will remain a topic, but it is important to actively go in search of a life "outside" the desire for a child and to cultivate it. Key questions here include: "In what situations do you manage to forget that your desire for a child is unfulfilled?" "How exactly do you recharge your batteries?"

Counseling after Diagnosis

Typical counseling topics after diagnosis are:

- If the diagnosis is "idiopathic infertility" (but also in cases of organic indications), many couples start asking themselves why there should be this "inner blockade," a question frequently motivated by comments from their social environment ("Do not get all uptight about it, stop thinking so much, then it's bound to work"). Here, stress-reducing interventions are essential ("psychogenic sterility myth") (Jacobs & O'Donohue, 2007).
- Independently of this, it is of course necessary to investigate whether the fertility disorder is behaviorally conditioned. Asked about the influence of stress, the counselor should phrase his/her answer along these lines:

   Everyday stress quite definitely has no influence on unintentional childlessness. The only way it might make itself felt is by exacerbating behaviors that condition infertility (such as smoking or indulgence in other bad-for-you's) or by causing a decrease in sexual contact.

- Before embarking on "third-party reproduction," the problem of donor anonymity needs to be addressed at all costs. From a psychodynamic viewpoint, the participation of a third party is bound up with a host of fantasies. These may be idealizing in nature, but they can also be distressing for the child, and they can massively interfere with the engagement with, and the requisite separation process from, the social parents.

Counseling during ART

The most common themes addressed in the course of treatment with ART are the following:

- For many women, the psychic stress they experience during the waiting period after embryo transfer is harder to take than all the medical interventions involved in IVF treatment. Couples can be apprised of this *before* the onset of IVF treatment. Usually, however, the issue is not addressed until after the first unsuccessful attempt.
- Despite lack of success, about half of all couples desist from taking advantage of all the treatment cycles offered to them, largely because of the emotional stress that ART brings with it. Here, the couple should be advised to actively prepare themselves for further attempts and their possible outcomes: who calls the IVF lab and when? How can we take care of ourselves, as a couple and individually, if it has not worked out?

- As long as the desire for a child persists, disappointments will be part and parcel of that desire and the "emotional roller coaster" will go through all its ups and downs. Its worst effects can be mitigated, but it cannot be evened out altogether. There are no "psycho-tricks" for avoiding it in its entirety (Jacobs & O'Donohue, 2007).
- Before the first IVF cycle, mention should be made in counseling of the general overestimation of the "baby-take-home" rate. Frequently, however, the couple will have no ears for this before at least one attempt has failed. A realistic assessment of the likelihood of success will make it easier to contemplate the elaboration of "plan B." Concrete indications on drawing up roadmaps can be found in Van den Broeck et al. (2010, p. 424):

Box 4.1 Working Out Roadmaps for ART

- First establish a "lifeline of satisfaction" from the beginning of the partnership up to (and including) now. Integrate the ups and downs in the partnership (e.g. wedding and couple crises) into this line. Attempt to outline the dimensions of the clients' life satisfaction as a couple in the near and remoter future, both with and without a child.
- Central elements of this schedule are flow diagrams with the different options (no pregnancy, miscarriage, live birth).
- Work out "plan B," "plan C," etc., from the outset.
- Initially, each partner works out his/her own schedule, but later they are placed on top of one another and aligned.
- If necessary, roadmaps can be rewritten (e.g. after a first unsuccessful attempt at IVF), but the couple should always impose a limit on infertility treatment.

- Most couples go through (temporary) impairments of their sex lives. Hence, the normalization of changes in the couple's love life is essential. Common implicit conjectures in connection with this sector ("My wife only wants to sleep with me because we're trying for a child." "My husband is less interested in sex; does he really want a child with me?") should be actively addressed in counseling and normalized accordingly. It may also be a good idea to relinquish the idea that intercourse should always be "ideally romantic." Occasionally, it is also helpful to "prescribe" time out from infertility therapy. The couple temporarily interrupts treatment and/or practices contraception so as to decouple the "reproductive act" from sexual intimacy (Wischmann, 2010). This of course is only possible if the biological clock is not ticking too loudly.
- Counseling should reassure clients about the development of children born after ART, particularly as prejudices on this point are obstinate. Of course, neither the likelihood of multiple births nor the higher probability of malformations should be played down. But in terms of psychosocial development, the minds of the prospective parents can be put almost entirely at rest.

Counseling on Alternative Medical Support

- After abortive ART cycles, couples frequently avail themselves (additionally) of alternative medicine. Counseling will need to indicate the highly contradictory study situation with regard to the efficacy of alternative medicine. In most alternative approaches, couples wanting a child are advised to keep to a healthy diet (with weight reduction where necessary) and to avoid luxury bad-for-you's (alcohol, caffeine, nicotine). If pregnancy ensues, this is then attributed exclusively to healthier living. In most cases, these procedures do not represent a genuine alternative because most fertility disorders are organically caused in nature. As long as there are no medical counter-indications and the couple have adequate (financial and emotional) resources, there are no objections to additional alternative medical treatment, as long as the couple in question is happy with it psychologically (Wischmann, 2012).

Counseling after Successful Treatment

- When the desired baby has arrived, the mother may have difficulty with breastfeeding. This happens of course with spontaneously conceived children as well. After such a long period waiting for the child to come, it may be distressing for the mother to experience her body as "failing on the job" once again. She should be advised to apprise the midwife/child nurse of the circumstances she has been through, so that her personal breastfeeding experience can be better understood.
- After successful treatment, counseling may be required in some cases because the desired number of children has not been achieved. Despite the success of the treatment, active "mourning work" may then need to take place.

Counseling after Unsuccessful Treatment

- It needs to be clearly stated that there are only slight differences in life quality between persistent childless couples and parents. Prognoses are favorable if couples are able to positively re-evaluate and accept the situation and actively search for alternatives and social contacts. Bad for the prognosis is brooding and avoidance coping, feelings of helplessness, and an unremittingly strong focus on children as a life goal. Notably, social isolation is a risk factor militating against success in coping with unintentional infertility. The couple should however be informed that the process may leave a "scar" that may break open again later in life when friends become grandparents.
- If one member of the couple wants to terminate infertility treatment more quickly than the other, the following advice is useful: the partner wanting to terminate treatment should wait for other partner who cannot as yet decide what to do.
- When treatment has finally been discontinued, the couple should if necessary be advised to practice contraception, pointing out that the mourning process cannot begin as long as there is still a chance of pregnancy, however remote. At all events, it is helpful (perhaps in conjunction with an expert on such matters) to induce the couple to work out some kind of farewell ritual (planting a tree, lighting candles and floating them down the river, leaving special stones on a mountain summit, writing the unborn child a letter and keeping it, etc.). This will support the work of mourning (Jacobs & O'Donohue, 2007).

Counseling in the Transition to Psychotherapy/Psychiatric Treatment

- If depression threatens, it will be necessary to refer the patient to a medical/psychological psychotherapist. The tell-tale symptoms are the following: all life sectors are affected, enjoyment has become impossible, increasing lethargy is recognizable, the patient reports quick fatigue and/or sleep disorders, increasing withdrawal from society.
- In the case of patently behavior-conditioned infertility, the patient should be referred accordingly (e.g. addiction counseling, psychotherapy for eating disorders, or sex therapy).
- Before referring a patient for psychotherapy, it is a good idea to point out that while for a majority of patients even low-threshold psychotherapy significantly reduces emotional stress.

Pregnancy rates are normally not affected by psychosocial interventions during ART treatment (exception: behavior-conditioned infertility).

Special Topics in Psychosocial Infertility Counseling

The following specific topics may prove to be important for counseling, hence the indications included for further reading.

- Counseling in the case of endometriosis (Dunselman et al., 2014), counseling prior to use of cross-border reproductive services (Thorn & Wischmann, 2012), counseling prior to PGD, PND, and fetal reduction (see Chapter 5 in this book), culture-sensitive counseling (Sexty et al., 2016), and counseling in the case of late parenthood (Zweifel, Covington, & Applegarth, 2012).

Concluding Remarks and Summary

Today, many (but of course not all) cases of unintentional infertility can be remedied with the help of reproductive medicine. But independently of the outcome, restricted fertility and its treatment are sources of stress that most couples experience as a major life crisis. Precisely because of this stress, many couples are prepared to try out new procedures, sometimes crossing national borders to do so (Neri, Turillazzi, Pascale, Riezzo, & Pomara, 2016). If all attempts fail, this may exacerbate the crisis, particularly as in most cases specialists in reproductive medicine will not be in a position to help couples cope with the ensuing mourning and despair. Low-threshold psychosocial counseling should be made available to couples before, during, and after reproductive medicine so that they can individually assess the benefits and risks involved and engage adequately with the various options available. One of these options is "child-free living."

The large number of offers available for reproductive medicine and the wide range of unconventional family constellations plus the growing attention given to them by the media make it increasingly difficult for couples (and individuals) to set limits to the fulfillment of their desire for a child and develop realistic alternative options before it is too late (Burns, 2004). As things stand, the requisite realistic assessment of the success rates of ART and the elaboration of "plan B" are frequently only possible in the framework of psychosocial infertility counseling, as is also the case with counseling on the decision for or against (further) reproductive measures or opting for such measures abroad in other countries. The complexity of present-day reproductive medicine and its measures in terms of their medical, legal, psychological, and ethical aspects make full-scale counseling for couples or individuals struggling with unintentional infertility absolutely essential. Ideally, this counseling should be interdisciplinary in nature and provided by professionals specifically trained for the purpose. Treatment with ART should never be offered without optional psychosocial infertility counseling to go with it.

The expectable (and sometimes feared) progress in reproductive medicine in the coming decades will improve the chances of success (i.e. a higher rate of live births). Very probably, we will be witnessing developments in genetic diagnosis that will need to be carefully and critically scrutinized from a societal and ethical viewpoint. The CRISPR/Cas gene-editing system makes for easy modification of human stem cells and embryos, the consequences of which cannot be adequately assessed because they will be affecting the generations to come. Deriving viable gametes from stem cells will be another important research goal, though it is questionable whether in the next few decades the "biological clock" can be halted so as to produce a time-limited phase of fertility within an individual's lifespan, quite apart from the question of whether this is desirable in the first place, and, if so, for whom. Psychosocial counseling on social egg freezing will increase in the coming years. But at present the question remains whether this will (a) open up a new option for women, (b) lead to a medicalization of societal ills, or (c) turn out to be a development that cannot be reliably assessed. At present, we do not have enough scientific studies on the issues to make any cogent statements about long-term child development (beyond adolescence) after ART and various new family forms (e.g. families with "solo fathers" and families established with embryos from third persons). Further research is still indispensable.

Note

1 The content of this chapter is taken partly from Wischmann (2012).

References

Apfel, R. J., & Keylor, R. G. (2002). Psychoanalysis and infertility – Myths and realities. *International Journal of Psychoanalysis, 83*, 85–103.

Boivin, J., Domar, A. D., Shapiro, D. B., Wischmann, T. H., Fauser, B. C. J. M., & Verhaak, C. (2012). Tackling burden in ART: An integrated approach for medical staff. *Human Reproduction, 27*(4), 941–950. doi: 10.1093/humrep/der467

Boivin, J., Griffiths, E., & Venetis, C. A. (2011). Emotional distress in infertile women and failure of assisted reproductive technologies: Meta-analysis of prospective psychosocial studies. *British Medical Journal, 342*, d223. doi: 10.1136/bmj.d223

Boivin, J., & Kentenich, H. (Eds.). (2002). *Guidelines for Counselling in Infertility*. Oxford: Oxford University Press.

Boivin, J., & Lancastle, D. (2010). Medical waiting periods: Imminence, emotions and coping. *Women's Health, 6*, 59–69.

Burns, L. H. (2004). Exit counseling. *International Congress Series, 1266*, 264–269. doi: 10.1016/j.ics.2004.01.085

Calhaz-Jorge, C., de Geyter, C., Kupka, M. S., de Mouzon, J., Erb, K., Mocanu, E., … Goossens, V. (2017). Assisted reproductive technology in Europe, 2013: Results generated from European registers by ESHRE. *Human Reproduction, 32*(10), 1957–1973.

Cousineau, T. M., & Domar, A. D. (2007). Psychological impact of infertility. *Best Practice & Research Clinical Obstetrics & Gynaecology, 21*(2), 293–308.

Covington, S. N., & Burns, L. H. (Eds.). (2006). *Infertility Counseling. A Comprehensive Handbook for Clinicans* (2nd ed.). Cambridge, London, New York: Cambridge University Press.

Covington, S. N. (Ed.). (2015). *Fertility Counseling: Clinical Guide and Case Studies*. Cambridge: Cambridge University Press.

Datta, J., Palmer, M. J., Tanton, C., Gibson, L. J., Jones, K. G., Macdowall, W., … Wellings, K. (2016). Prevalence of infertility and help seeking among 15 000 women and men. *Human Reproduction 31*(9), 2108–2118. doi: 10.1093/humrep/dew123

Davies, M. J., Moore, V. M., Willson, K. J., Van Essen, P., Priest, K., Scott, H., … Chan, A. (2012). Reproductive technologies and the risk of birth defects. *New England Journal of Medicine, 366*(19), 1803–1813. doi: 10.1056/NEJMoa1008095

DIR (Deutsches IVF-Register). (2015). D.I.R. Annual 2014 – The German IVF-Registry. *Journal of Reproductive Medicine and Endocrinology, 12*(6), 506–547.

Domar, A., Zuttermeister, P., & Friedman, R. (1993). The psychological impact of infertility: A comparison with patients with other medical conditions. *Journal of Psychosomatic Obstetrics & Gynecology, 14 Suppl*, 45–52.

Dunselman, G. A., Vermeulen, N., Becker, C., Calhaz-Jorge, C., D'Hooghe, T., De Bie, B., … Nelen, W. (2014). ESHRE guideline: Management of women with endometriosis. *Human Reproduction, 29*(3), 400–412. doi: 10.1093/humrep/det457

Esteves, S. C., Zini, A., Aziz, N., Alvarez, J. G., Sabanegh, E. S., Jr., & Agarwal, A. (2011). Critical appraisal of world health organization's new reference values for human semen characteristics and effect on diagnosis and treatment of subfertile men. *Urology, 7*, 7.

Freeman, E. W., Boxer, A. S., Rickels, K., Tureck, R. W., & Mastroianni, L. (1985). Psychological evaluation and support in a program of in vitro fertilisation and embryo transfer. *Fertility and Sterility, 43*, 48–53.

Gameiro, S., Boivin, J., Dancet, E., de Klerk, C., Emery, M., Lewis-Jones, C., ... Vermeulen, N. (2015). ESHRE guideline: Routine psychosocial care in infertility and medically assisted reproduction—a guide for fertility staff. *Human Reproduction, 30*(11), 2476–2485. doi: 10.1093/humrep/dev177

Gameiro, S., Boivin, J., Peronace, L., & Verhaak, C. M. (2012). Why do patients discontinue fertility treatment? A systematic review of reasons and predictors of discontinuation in fertility treatment. *Human Reproduction Update, 18*(6), 652–669. doi: 10.1093/humupd/dms031

Gaskins, A. J., Sundaram, R., Buck Louis, G. M., Chavarro, J. E. (2018): Predictors of Sexual Intercourse Frequency Among Couples Trying to Conceive. *The Journal of Sexual Medicine, 15*(4), 519–528.

Golombok, S. (2015). *Modern Families: Parents and Children in New Family Forms.* Cambridge: Cambridge University Press.

Greil, A., McQuillan, J., Benjamins, M., Johnson, D. R., Johnson, K. M., & Heinz, C. R. (2010). Specifying the effects of religion on medical helpseeking: The case of infertility. *Social Science & Medicine, 71*(4), 734–742. doi: 10.1016/j.socscimed.2010.04.033

Greil, A. L., Slauson-Blevins, K., & McQuillan, J. (2010). The experience of infertility: A review of recent literature. *Sociology of Health & Illness, 32*(1), 140–162.

Hammarberg, K., Collins, V., Holden, C., Young, K., & McLachlan, R. (2017). Men's knowledge, attitudes and behaviours relating to fertility. *Human Reproduction Update, 23*(4), 458–480. doi: 10.1093/humupd/dmx005

Hammarberg, K., Fisher, J. R. W., & Wynter, K. H. (2008). Psychological and social aspects of pregnancy, childbirth and early parenting after assisted conception: A systematic review. *Hum Reprod Update, 14*(5), 395–414. doi: 10.1093/humupd/dmn030

Hayashi, M., Fujimori, K., Yasumura, S., & Nakai, A. (2017). Impact of the Great East Japan Earthquake and Fukushima Nuclear Power Plant Accident on Assisted Reproductive Technology in Fukushima Prefecture: The Fukushima Health Management Survey. The Journal of Clinical Medicine Research, 9(9), 776–781.

Horowitz, J. E., Galst, J. P., & Elster, N. (2010). *Ethical Dilemmas in Fertility Counseling.* Washington: American Psychological Association.

Hudson, N., & Culley, L. (2013). 'The bloke can be a bit hazy about what's going on': Men and cross-border reproductive treatment. *Reproductive BioMedicine Online, 27*(3), 253–260. doi: 10.1016/j.rbmo.2013.06.007

Jacobs, N. N., & O'Donohue, W. T. (2007). *Coping with Infertility: Clinically Proven Ways of Managing the Emotional Roller Coaster.* New York: Routledge.

Jaffe, J., & Diamond, M. O. (2010). *Reproductive Trauma. Psychotherapy with Infertility and Pregnancy Loss Clients.* Washington: American Psychological Association.

Johansson, M., Adolfsson, A., Berg, M., Francis, J., Hogström, L., Janson, P. O., ... Hellström, A.-L. (2010). Gender perspective on quality of life, comparisons between groups 4–5.5 years after unsuccessful or successful IVF treatment. *Acta Obstetricia et Gynecologica Scandinavica, 89*(5), 683–691. doi: 10.3109/00016341003657892

Kainz, K. (2001). The role of the psychologist in the evaluation and treatment of infertility. *Women's Health Issues, 11*(6), 481–485.

Kamphuis, E. I., Bhattacharya, S., van der Veen, F., Mol, B. W., & Templeton, A. (2014). Are we overusing IVF? *British Medical Journal, 348*, g252. doi: 10.1136/bmj.g252

Kjaer, T., Albieri, V., Jensen, A., Kjaer, S. K., Johansen, C., & Dalton, S. O. (2014). Divorce or end of cohabitation among Danish women evaluated for fertility problems. *Acta Obstetricia et Gynecologica Scandinavica, 93*(3), 269–276. doi: 10.1111/aogs.12317

Mascarenhas, M. N., Flaxman, S. R., Boerma, T., Vanderpoel, S., & Stevens, G. A. (2012). National, regional, and global trends in infertility prevalence since 1990: A systematic analysis of 277 health surveys. *PLOS Medicine, 9*(12), e1001356. doi: 10.1371/journal.pmed.1001356

McQuillan, J., Greil, A. L., White, L., & Jacob, M. C. (2003). Frustrated fertility: Infertility and psychological distress among women. *Journal of Marriage and Family, 65*(4), 1007–1018.

Millheiser, L. S., Helmer, A. E., Quintero, R. B., Westphal, L. M., Milki, A. A., & Lathi, R. B. (2010). Is infertility a risk factor for female sexual dysfunction? A case-control study. *Fertility and Sterility, 94*(6), 2022–2025. doi: 10.1016/j.fertnstert.2010.01.037

Mills, M., Rindfuss, R. R., McDonald, P., te Velde, E., (2011). Why do people postpone parenthood? Reasons and social policy incentives. *Human Reproduction Update, 17*(6), 848–860. doi: 10.1093/humupd/dmr026

Neri, M., Turillazzi, E., Pascale, N., Riezzo, I., & Pomara, C. (2016). Egg production and donation: A new frontier in the global landscape of cross-border reproductive care: Ethical concerns. *Current Pharmaceutical Biotechnology, 17*(4), 316–320. doi: 10.2174/1389201017666160118103418

Pasch, L. A., Gregorich, S. E., Katz, P. K., Millstein, S. G., Nachtigall, R. D., Bleil, M. E., & Adler, N. E. (2012). Psychological distress and in vitro fertilization outcome. *Fertility and Sterility, 98*(2), 459–464. doi: 10.1016/j.fertnstert.2012.05.023

Peterson, B., Boivin, J., Norre, J., Smith, C., Thorn, P., & Wischmann, T. (2012). An introduction to infertility counseling: A guide for mental health and medical professionals. *The Journal of Assisted Reproduction and Genetics, 29*(3), 243–248. doi: 10.1007/s10815-011-9701-y

Peterson, B. D., Pirritano, M., Christensen, U., & Schmidt, L. (2008). The impact of partner coping in couples experiencing infertility. *Human Reproduction, 23*(5), 1128–1137. doi: 10.1093/humrep/den067

Pottinger, A. M., Carroll, K., & Mason, G. (2016). Male attitude towards masturbating: An impediment to infertility evaluation and sperm parameters. *Andrologia, 48*(7), 774–778. doi: 10.1111/and.12511

Savasi, V. M., Mandia, L., Laoreti, A., & Cetin, I. (2016). Maternal and fetal outcomes in oocyte donation pregnancies. *Human Reproduction Update, (22)*5, 620–633. doi: 10.1093/humupd/dmw012

Schilling, K., Toth, B., Rosner, S., Strowitzki, T., & Wischmann, T. (2012). Prevalence of behaviour-related fertility disorders in a clinical sample: Results of a pilot study. *Archives of Gynecology and Obstetrics, 286*(5), 1307–1314. doi: 10.1007/s00404-012-2436-x

Schmidt, L. (2006). *Infertility and Assisted Reproduction in Denmark. Epidemiology and Psychosocial Consequences.* Copenhagen: Lægeforeningens Forlag.

Sexty, R., Hamadneh, J., Rosner, S., Strowitzki, T., Ditzen, B., Toth, B., & Wischmann, T. (2016). Cross-cultural comparison of fertility specific quality of life in German, Hungarian and Jordanian couples attending a fertility center. *Health and Quality of Life Outcomes, 14*(1), 27.

Slama, R., Hansen, O. K. H., Ducot, B., Bohet, A., Sorensen, D., Giorgis Allemand, L., … Bouyer, J. (2012). Estimation of the frequency of involuntary infertility on a nation-wide basis. *Human Reproduction, 27*, 1489–1499. doi: 10.1093/humrep/des070

Stammer, H., Wischmann, T., & Verres, R. (2002). Counseling and couple therapy for infertile couples. *Family Process, 41*(1), 111–122. doi: 10.1111/j.1545-5300.2002.40102000111.x

Sydsjö, G., Svanberg, A. S., Lampic, C., & Jablonowska, B. (2011). Relationships in IVF couples 20 years after treatment. *Human Reproduction, 26*(7), 1836–1842. doi: 10.1093/humrep/der131

Thorn, P., & Wischmann, T. (2009). German guidelines for psychosocial counselling in the area of gamete donation. *Human Fertility (Camb), 12*(2), 73–80.

Thorn, P., & Wischmann, T. (2012). German guidelines for psychosocial counselling in the area of "cross border reproductive services". *Archives of Gynecology and Obstetrics (287)*, 599–606. doi: 10.1007/s00404-012-2599-5

Toth, B., Würfel, W., Bohlmann, M. K., Gillessen-Kaesbach, G., Nawroth, F., Rogenhofer, N., … von Wolff, M. (2015). Recurrent miscarriage: Diagnostic and therapeutic procedures. guideline of the DGGG (S1-Level, AWMF Registry No. 015/050, December 2013). [Diagnostik und Therapie beim wiederholten Spontanabort. Leitlinie der DGGG (S1-Level, AWMF-Registernummer 015/050, Dezember 2013)]. *Geburtshilfe und Frauenheilkunde, 75*(11), 1117–1129. doi: 10.1055/s-0035-1558299

Van den Broeck, U., Emery, M., Wischmann, T., & Thorn, P. (2010). Counselling in infertility: Individual, couple and group interventions. *Patient Education and Counseling, 81*(3), 422–428. doi: 10.1016/j.pec.2010.10.009

Volmer, L., Rösner, S., Toth, B., Strowitzki, T., & Wischmann, T. (2017). Infertile partners' coping strategies are interrelated – Implications for targeted psychological counseling. [Wechselbeziehungen bei den Bewältigungsstrategien unfruchtbarer Partner – Implikationen für eine zielgerichtete psychologische Beratung]. *Geburtshilfe und Frauenheilkunde, 77*(01), 52–58. doi: 10.1055/s-0042-119200

Wennberg, A. L., Opdahl, S., Bergh, C., Aaris Henningsen, A.-K., Gissler, M., Romundstad, L. B., … Wennerholm, U.-B. (2016). Effect of maternal age on maternal and neonatal outcomes after assisted reproductive technology. *Fertility and Sterility, 106*(5), 1142–1149.e1114. doi: 10.1016/j.fertnstert.2016.06.021

WHO. (2010). *WHO Laboratory Manual for the Examination and Processing of Human Semen* (5th ed.). Geneva: World Health Organization.

Wischmann, T. (2003). Psychogenic infertility – Myths and facts. *Journal of Assisted Reproduction and Genetics, 20*(12), 485–494.

Wischmann, T. (2008). Implications of psychosocial support in infertility – A critical appraisal. *Journal of Psychosomatic Obstetrics and Gynecology, 29*(2), 83–89. doi: 10.1080/01674820701817870

Wischmann, T. (2012). *Einführung Reproduktionsmedizin: Medizinische Grundlagen – Psychosomatik – Psychosoziale Aspekte* (Vol. 3757: Psychologie, Medizin). München: Reinhardt.

Wischmann, T. (2013a). Sexual disorders in infertile couples: An update. *Current Opinion in Gynecology and Obstetrics, 25*(3), 220–222. doi: 10.1097/GCO.0b013e328360e507

Wischmann, T. (2013b). 'Your count is zero'—Counselling the infertile man. *Human Fertility (Camb), 16*(1), 35–39. doi: 10.3109/14647273.2013.776179

Wischmann, T. (2017). Effekte psychosozialer Interventionen auf Lebensqualität und Schwangerschaftsraten bei infertilen Frauen und Männern – eine aktuelle Übersicht. *Journal für Reproduktionsmedizin und Endokrinologie, 14*(1), 8–13.

Wischmann, T., & Kentenich, H. (2016). A couple who cannot conceive naturally (Coping of infertile couples). In K. M. Paarlberg & H. B. M. van de Wiel (Eds.), *Bio-psycho-social Obstetrics and Gynaecology. A Competency-oriented Approach* (pp. 249–261). Cham: Springer International.

Wischmann, T., Korge, K., Scherg, H., Strowitzki, T., & Verres, R. (2012). A 10-year follow-up study of psychosocial factors affecting couples after infertility treatment. *Human Reproduction, 27*(11), 3226–3232. doi: 10.1093/humrep/des293

Wischmann, T., Scherg, H., Strowitzki, T., & Verres, R. (2009). Psychosocial characteristics of women and men attending infertility counselling. *Human Reproduction, 24*(2), 378–385. doi: 10.1093/humrep/den401

Wischmann, T., Schilling, K., Toth, B., Rösner, S., Strowitzki, T., Wohlfarth, K., & Kentenich, H. (2014). Sexuality, self-esteem and partnership quality in infertile women and men. *Geburtshilfe und Frauenheilkunde, 74*(8), 759–763. doi: 10.1055/s-0034-1368461

Wischmann, T., Stammer, H., Gerhard, I., & Verres, R. (2002). Couple counseling and therapy for the unfulfilled desire for a child – The two-step approach of the "Heidelberg Infertility Consultation Service". In B. Strauß (Ed.), *Involuntarily childlessness – Psychological assessment, counseling and psychotherapy* (pp. 127–149). Seattle: Hogrefe International.

Wischmann, T., Stammer, H., Scherg, H., Gerhard, I., & Verres, R. (2001). Psychosocial characteristics of infertile couples: A study by the 'Heidelberg Fertility Consultation Service'. *Human Reproduction, 16*(8), 1753–1761.

Wischmann, T., & Thorn, P. (2013). (Male) infertility: What does it mean to men? New evidence from quantitative and qualitative studies. *Reproductive BioMedicine Online, 27*(3), 236–243. doi: 10.1016/j.rbmo.2013.06.002

Wischmann, T. H. (2010). Sexual disorders in infertile couples. *The Journal of Sexual Medicine, 7*(5), 1868–1876. doi: 10.1111/j.1743-6109.2010.01717.x

Zegers-Hochschild, F., Adamson, G. D., de Mouzon, J., Ishihara, O., Mansour, R., Nygren, K., ... van der Poel, S. (2009). The International Committee for Monitoring Assisted Reproductive Technology (ICMART) and the World Health Organization (WHO) revised glossary on ART terminology, 2009. *Human Reproduction, 24*(11), 2683–2687. doi: 10.1093/humrep/dep343

Zweifel, J. E., Covington, S. N., & Applegarth, L. D. (2012). "Last-chance kids": A good deal for older parents—but what about the children? *Sexuality, Reproduction & Menopause, 10*(2), 4–12.

5

Prenatal Diagnosis

Psychological Impact and the Parents' Experience in the Presence of Fetal Anomalies

Joann Paley Galst

The rapid expansion in prenatal testing – particularly non-invasive screening methods which identify fetal cell-free DNA from the placenta in a pregnant woman's blood as early as ten weeks into a pregnancy, carrying no risk of fetal damage or loss and with high sensitivity and specificity – has changed the landscape of the pregnancy experience. Women (and their partners if part of a couple) are now offered increasing amounts of information regarding the health and well-being of the fetus being carried. If a prenatal screening test indicates a high risk of an anomaly, worry, uncertainty, and feelings of being out of control can be generated in the recipient parents. While earlier studies suggested that women may try to distance themselves from their pregnancy (i.e., putting the pregnancy on hold) upon receiving this implication of risk (Georgsson-Ohman, Sissel, Waldenstrom, Grunewald, & Olin-Lauritzen, 2006), a more recent study of Danish couples awaiting results of more definitive prenatal diagnostic testing found a more varied approach to waiting while they worried (Lou, Nielsen, Hvidman, Petersen, & Risor, 2016). Couples often withdrew from social interactions and everyday activities to be together, gather information, and discuss their situation multiple times, taking control and building a sense of agency by trying to understand medical information. Some couples chose not to share their situation with others while others sought input and advice from family and friends. Some also reported periodically seeking to distract themselves through social engagement to help them cope with the waiting period. In addition, couples used methods of emotion-focused coping to help them control their emotional distress and maintain hope (e.g., reassuring interpretations of their uncertain situation including selective recall of clinical information, a belief that their good health and the positive personal experience of the pregnancy thus far increased the likelihood of a good outcome, and gratitude for the good things in their life). These researchers found couples reported surprisingly little discussion of what they would do in the case of an abnormal result, possibly because most expressed certainty that they would terminate the pregnancy or consciously decided to postpone a final decision until receiving more definitive results.

While every pregnancy carries an approximately 3% risk of a birth defect regardless of whether the pregnancy was conceived naturally or through assisted reproductive technology (Hoyert, Mathews, Menacker, Strobino, & Guyer, 2006), few parents are prepared to receive news that they carry a genetically or structurally imperfect child. Most have been found to undergo prenatal testing because it is the social norm at present and their obstetrician recommended the screening, but most expected to see the baby if an ultrasound was involved, possibly determine the sex, and receive reassuring news, unprepared to receive input of anything being wrong with their baby (McCoyd, 2013). This reinforces the importance of comprehensive patient education prior to pursuing prenatal screening to ensure that patients have adequate understanding of possible test results. If a diagnosis of anomaly is received and the condition cannot be treated or corrected through fetal surgery, parents face the monumental task of deciding to continue the pregnancy with a fetus that may not survive the pregnancy, may have a shortened life expectancy or compromised quality of life, or terminate the pregnancy. There is typically a level of uncertainty about the precise phenotypic manifestation of the disorder in the child being carried, as information regarding the severity of the anomaly is often limited and cannot be ascertained prenatally. The time to decide is also limited as most states within the USA and countries throughout the world that allow abortion restrict the gestational time frame within which a termination can be performed. This often leaves the parents anxious to collect as much medical input as possible yet still riddled with uncertainty, being torn between an attachment to their unborn child and the desire to prevent the child's suffering, referred to by one set of researchers as an experience of "chosen losses and lost choices" (Sandelowski & Barroso, 2005).

Bernhardt et al. (2013) found that many patients struggled enormously in making decisions after receiving poor prenatal genetic screening results, some even regretting having pursued prenatal testing at all. These researchers concluded that patients would benefit from a genetic counselor's determination of their tolerance for uncertainty as well as discussing their values, views toward abortion, and attitudes regarding parenting a disabled child in pre-test counseling. Another study found that if patients had the opportunity to deliberate the advantages and disadvantages of prenatal screening in advance, they had less adverse emotional reactions and less difficulty making decisions after an abnormal result than patients who were uninformed of potential negative results prior to screening (Kleinveld, Ten Kate, van den Berg, van Vugt, & Timmermans, 2009).

Any indication of a problem with the fetus can transform the experience of pregnancy. False-positive prenatal diagnoses are also possible and have been found to increase levels of anxiety and depression in women for the remainder of the pregnancy even after demonstrated to be incorrect through further testing, i.e., "watchful waiting" (Bernhardt et al., 2013). Concerns are not totally alleviated by normal sonograms or even by delivery of a child who appears normal at birth and during infancy, as concerns for the child's health and development can continue long after birth (Redlinger-Grosse, Bernhardt, Berg, Muenke, & Biesecker, 2002). Viaux-Savelon et al. (2012), in a small French study comparing mothers who received what turned out to be false-positive results to control mothers, found mother-infant interactions were affected in that fewer infants inaccurately diagnosed prenatally with a fetal anomaly (based on soft markers) were breastfed. Additionally, mothers expressed fewer positive emotions toward their infants, less sensitivity to and greater difficulty perceiving their infants' signals, and higher maternal intrusive behaviors, as well as experiencing higher infant avoidance of mothers. Efforts need to continue to reduce false diagnoses to the greatest extent possible to minimize these negative psychological effects on mother-infant attachment. Medical providers also need to try to present clear and reassuring information to parents while awaiting final results and help manage longer-term maternal reactions to input that is then proven to be a false positive. These researchers suggested screening for anxiety and depression during obstetric follow-up visits and during later pediatric visits with their infants in mothers who had received a soft marker screening detection that had subsequently been found to be inaccurate.

Prevalence Rates of Termination of Pregnancy for Fetal Anomaly (TOPFA)

Approximately 150,000 women are diagnosed with a fetal anomaly each year in the USA (ACOG, 2007). Overall, termination rates for fetal anomaly have been found to range from 43% to 100%, with variability depending on both the severity and type of anomaly. Schechtman, Gray, Baty, and Rothman (2002) found that 72.5% of pregnancies were terminated if the impairment was deemed to have a serious impact on the fetus's quality of life, with the highest rates if the central nervous system was involved. Mansfield, Hopfer, and Marteau (1999) compared termination rates for five anomalies (Down syndrome, spina bifida, anencephaly, Turner syndrome, and Klinefelter syndrome) and found the highest termination rate for Down syndrome (92%) and the lowest for Klinefelter syndrome (58%). In a study reviewing articles published between 1995 and 2011, Natoli, Ackerman, McDermott, and Edwards (2012) found an average termination rate of 67% for Down syndrome in population-based studies and 85% in hospital-based studies, suggesting that parents may not always accurately report a pregnancy termination when queried by researchers.

Variability in termination rates for sex chromosome anomalies also exists, ranging from 42% for mosaicisms to 58–74% for Klinefelter syndrome and 70–100% for Turner syndrome (Hamamy & Dahoun, 2004; Johnson et al., 2012). Taken together, these studies suggest that the majority of parents who receive a diagnosis of a serious fetal anomaly decide to terminate rather than continue the pregnancy, although multiple factors appear to be involved in this decision, for example, religion, maternal age, gestational age, number of existing and/or desired children, and history of induced abortion (Choi, Van Riper, & Thoyre, 2012; Jeon, Chen, & Goodson, 2012; Mezei, Pepp, Toth, Beke, & Papp, 2004). The decisional process has been found to be most influenced by the partner's views and much less by healthcare providers, family, or friends (Korenromp et al., 2005b).

Psychological Impact of Decisions after the Diagnosis of a Prenatal Fetal Anomaly

A recent prospective study, the Turnaway study (Biggs, Upadhyay, McCulloch, & Foster, 2016), interviewed and assessed anxiety, depression, self-esteem, and life satisfaction in women eight days after receiving or being denied an abortion and continuing every six months for five years thereafter. The researchers concluded that undergoing a wanted abortion for an unwanted pregnancy was not associated with either initial or long-term adverse psychological outcomes. Women who were denied an abortion, however, especially those who later miscarried or had to travel elsewhere to have an abortion, were the most adversely impacted, although both groups eventually converged on psychological well-being over time, indicating the requirement of pre-abortion counseling in some states of the USA regarding adverse emotional outcomes is providing blatantly inaccurate information to women. This study, however, specifically excluded those with known fetal anomalies, fetal demise, or maternal health indications for abortion. Those women/couples facing an unexpected diagnosis of fetal anomaly in a typically very wanted pregnancy may follow a very different emotional trajectory.

As indicated above, the majority of women who learn of a fetal anomaly during pregnancy choose to terminate the pregnancy. A pregnancy termination due to fetal anomaly jars the recipient's assumptive world, replacing the normative expectation of a normal healthy baby with a pregnancy characterized by risk and anticipation of death. Multiple losses are experienced by the recipients of such news, for example, a wanted baby, future hopes and dreams, and the innocence of the "just world belief" (i.e., if I follow the rules and do good things, good things will happen to me). It also changes the anticipated role of parent to that of a bereaved parent. Feelings of grief may be accompanied by conflicting feelings of relief, guilt, and doubt. Self-esteem can suffer on multiple fronts: biologically for creating an imperfect pregnancy, morally for being responsible for ending a wanted pregnancy when the parents have been the self-expected protectors of their baby, and socially both for feeling inadequate to take on parenting a disabled child and alienated from others, as parents often fear condemnation by others and thus often secretly carry feelings of shame regarding the termination (White-Van Mourik, Connor, & Ferguson-Smith, 1992).

Undergoing a TOPFA is frequently experienced as a traumatic event, as significant a loss as other pregnancy losses (Maguire et al., 2015), with feelings of emotional distress often lingering for a substantial number of women (Lafarge, 2016). Diagnostic symptoms of post-traumatic stress (PTS) have been found in 67% of women at six weeks post-termination, 41% of women at one year (Davies, Gledhill, McFadyen, Whitlow, & Economides, 2005), 20% at 16 months (Korenromp, Page-Christiaens, van den Bout, Mulder, & Visser, 2009), and 17% at two to seven years post-termination (Korenromp, Christiaens, & van den Bout, 2005a). Depression was reported by 30% of women at six weeks, 39% at six months (Davies et al., 2005), and 13% at 16 months post-termination (Korenromp et al., 2009). Grief symptoms are reported by 47% of women at six weeks and 27% at one year post-termination (Davies et al., 2005). Korenromp et al. (2009) found that 14–20% of women demonstrated a complicated grief disorder at 12–14 months post-TOPFA. This is somewhat higher than that shown by a longitudinal study of the loss of a close relative that found a prevalence of 11% at nine months post-loss, with lack of preparedness for the death being associated with complicated grief both at baseline (four months post-loss) and at the nine-month follow-up (Barry, Kasl, & Prigerson, 2002), but quite a bit higher than 2.4–4.8% of the population reported experiencing a persistent complex bereavement disorder in DSM V (American Psychiatric Association, 2013).

Women are required to provide informed consent for a pregnancy termination. In addition, men may defer to their partner out of respect for her right to make decisions involving her body. Together these factors can result in a woman feeling greater responsibility for the decision and possibly increased feelings of guilt. Since a woman's feelings may appear more intense, men's emotional reactions to a TOPFA are often overlooked. They may be expected by others and themselves to be taking care of their partner's emotional distress, instead (Doka & Martin, 2010). Men's losses are often not acknowledged by others, with friends and family more frequently inquiring about how their partner is faring after a loss. This further reinforces the notion that men should concern themselves more with their partner's feelings than their own. Although generally lower in distress than women, men have been found to experience a high degree of psychological morbidity as well, i.e., 22% demonstrated symptoms of PTS and 16% of depression post-TOPFA. Nevertheless, despite enduring levels of distress reported by parents for one year or more post-termination of their pregnancy with a fetal anomaly, only 2–2.7% of women and 1% of men regretted their decision to interrupt the pregnancy (Korenromp et al., 2007).

When confronted with loss, women's grief tends to be more loss-oriented while men's is more restoration-oriented (Stroebe & Schut, 1999). As indicated above, however, men, too, experience negative feelings after a TOPFA, although they tend to internalize their feelings more quickly than women and focus on practical matters such as arranging a funeral, caring for other children if their wife is unable to do so, and returning to work (Kaasen et al., 2013; Locock & Alexander, 2006; White-van Mourik et al., 1992). Male stoicism can be misunderstood by their partners, however, as not caring and being unaffected by the pregnancy loss. Clinically, this author has also found that men may fear that expressing their emotions will exacerbate their wife's sadness. Unfortunately, this stoic gender-socialized role runs the risk of alienating his partner, leaving her feeling isolated from her spouse while wanting to emotionally experience their loss together. This underlines the importance of including both parents in support services and psychological counseling. Educating grieving parents of these common gender differences can help reduce misunderstandings between partners.

Since the majority of prenatally diagnosed fetal anomalies end with pregnancy termination, there are few studies examining the experience and needs of parents who decide to continue a pregnancy with either a lethal or serious non-lethal anomaly. Korenromp et al. (2005a) found that approximately one-third of women they studied recalled being counseled only about the option to terminate and not continue a pregnancy with a Down syndrome baby, although this may have reflected the strength of couples' intent to terminate the pregnancy. Patient's frustration at the lack of balanced information on Down syndrome and at the lack of referral to Down syndrome support groups has also been reported (Skotko, 2005).

Parents choosing to continue their pregnancy enter a new life path, mourning the loss of the baby they expected, readjusting their expectations about the future of their child, and learning to cope with the challenges that face both their child and themselves (Hickerton, Aitken, Hodgson, & Delatycki, 2012). Cope, Garrett, Gregory, and Ashley-Koch (2015) studied 158 women and 109 men, all of whom lost a pregnancy to anencephaly, a lethal neural tube defect. Of these participants, 41% terminated the pregnancy. Their pregnancies ended from one month to 32 years prior to participation in the study (median = 3 years). A selection bias may have existed in this study, however, as this was only approximately half of that reported by other literature reviews, including the 84% termination rate for anencephaly found by Mansfield et al. (1999) and 83% by Johnson et al. (2012). Women who terminated their pregnancy reported higher levels of despair, avoidance, and depression than women who continued the pregnancy, as did those whose losses were in the more recent past, although there was much individual variability in psychological outcomes (24% of women and 11% of men scored in the pathogenic range for grief, 20% of women and 13% of men scored in the pathogenic range for PTS, 34% of women and 19% of men scored within the range for depression). The method of termination for this lethal anomaly (induction termination or dilation and evacuation) did not significantly influence psychological outcomes in women or men. For 59% who continued the pregnancy, there were no significant differences in psychological outcomes between those delivering a live-born baby or a stillborn. In contrast, men whose partners continued the pregnancy reported greater difficulty coping than men whose partner terminated the pregnancy. Participation in organized religion was associated with less grief in parents but had no impact on PTS or depression. While no differences were found between women who terminated the pregnancy in the first trimester and second trimester, men whose partners terminated in the second trimester reported significantly higher grief, PTS intrusions, and depression than men whose partners terminated in the first trimester. This may be attributable to women forming a stronger emotional bond earlier in the pregnancy than men.

A small study was conducted with 24 parents who chose to continue a pregnancy after a diagnosis of a non-lethal anomaly (i.e., holoprosencephaly [HPE], a defect in the midline of the forebrain) in which the prognosis was poor but uncertain as the level of severity often could not be determined in utero. Parents were interviewed anywhere from 6 months to 12 years after their pregnancy experience (Redlinger-Grosse et al., 2002). They described the decision to continue the pregnancy as an evolving one that they revisited multiple times throughout the pregnancy. Decisions were influenced by religious beliefs, the uncertainty involved in the diagnosis, parents' perceptions of the diagnosis, feelings regarding pregnancy termination, and previous personal experience (e.g., with relatives having a disability, infertility). Multiple coping strategies, both task- and emotion-focused, were used by parents throughout the pregnancy to cope with their decision. Parents reported needs for both information and emotional support, including referral to organizations and families living with a child with HPE, and family, friends', and healthcare providers' support, respect, and acceptance of their decision to continue the pregnancy rather than imposing their beliefs and judgments on them. Considerable ambivalence toward the pregnancy, with parents being torn between the possibility that their baby may die and secretly hoping their baby would not survive, was also expressed when parents were specifically asked about these feelings and given nonjudgmental space for their expression.

It is important that healthcare professionals listen carefully to how parents perceive and interpret the diagnosis their baby receives. Parents' conflicted needs, for example, for specific information regarding the potential severity of the disability while simultaneously wanting hopeful input in the case of a non-lethal anomaly present a difficult challenge for healthcare providers. Bolstering parents' confidence in their ability to make and carry out the best decision for their baby and their family under recognized conditions of uncertainty may be a way to offer support in the face of these conflicting parental needs.

Differences in psychological outcomes between parents terminating and those continuing a non-viable pregnancy may be impacted by the fact that those women who continued the pregnancy typically had more time between diagnosis and ending of their pregnancy to grieve and prepare for an impending loss prior to delivery, whereas women who terminate often have little time to prepare for their loss. Women who continued the pregnancy may also receive more support for their decision from family (McCoyd, 2007) and have the opportunity to find meaning and create memories (e.g., by taking photos, creating keepsakes, offering organs for donation), although it is also possible that women who continued a pregnancy aware of a fetal anomaly after prenatal testing may be seen as more to blame and less deserving of sympathy than those parents who were never offered the option to test the fetus (Lawson, 2003). Women continuing a viable pregnancy with an anomaly have also reported the opportunity to grieve before the birth of their child which appeared to help them bond with their child when they were born (Hickerton et al., 2012). Both patients who make the decision to continue a pregnancy that is expected to end in death, either before birth or shortly thereafter, and those who choose to terminate a pregnancy with a fetal anomaly may benefit from anticipatory counseling to prepare them for potential psychological reactions, determine whether or not to view the fetus, help them negotiate their way through additional medical visits and others' reactions to their decision, help them understand they may encounter disagreement to their decision whatever that decision regarding a pregnancy with fetal anomaly, and be given information about local and online resources for support and individual/couples' counseling.

Clinically, this author has found that both receiving a diagnosis of fetal anomaly and making a subsequent decision to terminate the pregnancy are traumatic. Women report experiencing intense grief whether they chose to terminate the pregnancy or chose to arrange for palliative or perinatal hospice care for their pregnancies (Wool, 2011). Parents who make the decision to interrupt their pregnancy may initially react with acute PTS and later suffer from post-traumatic stress disorder (PTSD), depression, grief, and/or persistent complex bereavement disorder (American Psychiatric Association, 2013). With few, if any, rituals available to them and without tangible memories, parents are frequently left on their own to grieve, often questioning whether they even have the right to grieve because of their role in ending the pregnancy. Subsequent pregnancies may also be affected by uncertainty and anxiety, as parents come to view pregnancy through a lens of risk, conditioned to expect bad news and potential loss (Turton, Hughes, Evans, & Fainman, 2001).

Risk Factors for Continued Emotional Distress after a TOPFA

While most individuals experience receiving news of a fetal anomaly and being confronted with having to decide whether to terminate or continue a pregnancy as traumatic, a number of risk factors have been found to be associated with longer lasting and higher levels of distress. These include high decisional conflict, high distress immediately after the termination, lack of partner support, incongruent grief and coping with partner, low perceived social support and isolation, more advanced gestational age of fetus, a non-lethal anomaly, prior history of mental health issues or trauma(s), self-blame (i.e., feeling responsible for the anomaly and/or feeling responsible for a bad decision regarding the anomaly), and coping through avoidance of emotions or behavioral disengagement as opposed to using coping strategies such as acceptance and positive reframing (Kersting et al., 2007; Korenromp et al., 2009; Maguire et al., 2015). Positive reframing has additionally been found to be associated with post-traumatic growth (Lafarge, Mitchell, & Fox, 2013, 2016). Although grief typically subsided by one year post-termination for most parents, certain experiences such as anniversary dates (e.g., due date, date of termination), seeing other pregnant women, hearing announcements of pregnancies and birth, or a subsequent pregnancy triggered feelings of grief for some women, even at one year after the loss (Maguire et al., 2015).

Providing Emotional Support to Parents Making Decisions after Learning of a Fetal Anomaly

Medical personnel: The front line of support for parents learning of a fetal abnormality are the medical personnel treating them. While providing clear, comprehensive, and balanced information is seen as key by medical professionals (Lafarge, Mitchell, Breeze, & Fox, 2017; Skotko, 2005), the emotional impact that doctors, nurses, sonographers, and genetic counselors have on these distressed parents may often be underestimated by the medical providers themselves. It has been this author's experience that patients' appreciation for a kind word or sympathetic shoulder to cry on is recollected even years after a loss. Couples choosing pregnancy termination need practical help making arrangements for the termination in a timely manner. All of the following have been reported as valued by patients both before and after undergoing a TOPFA: attentive listening, nonjudgmental and understandable communication, prompt referral to specialists for diagnostic confirmation and long-term prognoses, sensitive scheduling of appointments (when a physician has sufficient time and fewer pregnant patients are in the office), creating and collecting mementos for parents (and keeping them available should parents initially not wish to take them home, as many do later change their minds), continuity of care, and staying in touch after decisions have been made including scheduling follow-up appointments to allow parents to express ongoing emotions, ask questions, and give medical personnel the opportunity to inform parents of the long-term course of grief and healing.

Parents who choose to continue a pregnancy when the fetus has an anomaly compatible with life need to be able to maintain hope for their child's life trajectory. Parents describe considerable uncertainty regarding their child's development after delivery (Bernhardt et al., 2014). Medical personnel need to reinforce the activities parents are likely to be able to engage in with their child rather than what they won't be able to do. Parents need to be contacted periodically to assess ongoing needs and creation of a care plan for the baby after birth should be discussed. Connecting parents with other families raising a child with a similar disorder may be appreciated. If it is deemed appropriate, information regarding options for adoptive or foster care placement of the baby can be provided (Sheets et al., 2011). For parents continuing a non-viable pregnancy, reassurance that medical personnel will continue to be available to support them throughout the duration of the pregnancy and birth, as well as afterward, can provide comfort to parents who may fear being abandoned by others who they believe did not support their decision. Referral to resources for perinatal palliative or hospice care should also be provided.

Mental health professionals: High rates of distress among parents after undergoing a TOPFA suggest a potential need for counseling, but, at present, there is no evidence-based guide for the preferred or most effective type of counseling for this unique loss. There is no evidence for the effectiveness of universal intervention as preventative treatment for grief (Wittouck, Van Autreve, De Jaegere, Portzky, & van Heeringen, 2011). Medication alone is not effective for complicated grief, either, although adding medication to an effective cognitive behavioral treatment (CBT) may alleviate comorbid depressive or PTSD symptoms for patients with complicated grief (Shear et al., 2016).

The grief after the loss of a baby after a termination due to fetal abnormality is particularly challenging to parents: many never see their baby (e.g., if termination by D&E or parents choose not to see a delivered intact baby), there are few if any recollections of the unborn baby and few concrete memories shared with others, and especially because of the role parents played in making a decision to end the pregnancy. Preoccupation with the circumstances of the death (e.g., repeatedly questioning of whether the baby felt any pain) and hypervigilance to the threats of what now feels like an unsafe world are common among these traumatically bereaved parents. Because of the similarities of some symptoms of PTSD and complicated grief (e.g., avoidance, intrusions, and maladaptive appraisals [American Psychiatric Association, 2013]) and the multiple ways in which trauma, grief, and depression interface in many parents after a TOPFA, distinguishing between them may be difficult in clinical practice.

This author has been influenced by two approaches to complicated grief and PTSD in her work with individuals/couples who have undergone a TOPFA.[1] The cognitive behavioral model (Boelen, Van Den Hout, & Van De Bout, 2006; Shear, 2015) explains the occurrence and perceptions of complicated grief as being due to:

- insufficient integration of the loss – treated through creating a meaningful and coherent narrative about the loss;
- negative global beliefs about the self, world, and future, along with catastrophic misinterpretations of grief symptoms – treated by challenging negative beliefs and catastrophic misinterpretations through cognitive restructuring;
- both anxious avoidance of cognitive and overt reminders of the loss and depressive avoidance of social cues and recreational activities through behavioral withdrawal – treated by having patients gradually confront avoided aspects of loss (e.g., places, objects, memories) through exposure techniques and helping patients set new life goals and re-engage in meaningful activities.

The cognitive processing therapy (CPT) model of PTSD as applied to bereavement conceptualizes the maintenance of PTSD symptoms as a result of intrusions caused by avoidance, arousal caused by incomplete and faulty processing of the experience, along with inaccurate thoughts, beliefs, and assumptions about the traumatic experience, and behavioral avoidance (Resick, Monson, & Chard, 2008). Unlike the emotional processing theory of PTSD which similarly posits that recovery comes from emotional processing but explains engagement with the trauma-related thoughts and feelings as leading to healing through habituation to fear (Foa, Keane, Friedman, & Cohen, 2009; Foa, Steketee, & Rothbaum, 1989), the CPT model focuses more on the content of cognitions and the impact of distorted cognitions on emotions and behaviors, positing healing through affective expression which brings about affective changes in the trauma memory rather than through fear reduction through exposure (Resik et al., 2008). The goals of CPT for traumatic bereavement are to help the patient:

- Eliminate any stuck points, i.e., problematic cognitions that are blocking their recovery. (Contrary to avoidance found in classic PTSD, some bereaved individuals ruminate and are reluctant to let go of images in their minds for fears of further losing the loved one, i.e., forgetting);
- Develop balanced and productive beliefs about the event, self, others, and the world;
- Eventually focus on the life of the person who died, not just the way he/she died. Unable to do this, parents after a TOPFA may need to focus on in utero memories of pregnancy and remember the likely pain and life challenges their child would have faced.

The author's psychotherapeutic treatment of these parents has been guided by the integration of treatment research for both grief and trauma. Combining elements of Shear's treatment for complicated grief and Resick's treatment for traumatic PTSD has proved useful in this author's approach to treating those experiencing long-term emotional distress after a TOPFA. The two approaches overlap quite a bit. Trauma-focused cognitive-behavioral interventions including psychoeducation, imaginal exposure to reduce avoidance, anxiety, arousal, and distress associated with remembering the trauma, anxiety management, and cognitive reframing techniques to address distorted beliefs and thought patterns that perpetuate PTSD symptoms have been found to reduce symptoms of acute stress and PTSD (Bisson & Andrews, 2007; Foa et al., 2009; Mendes, Mello, Ventura, Passarela, & Mari, 2008; Powers, Halpern, Ferenschak, Gillihan, & Foa, 2010; Resick, Nishith, Weaver, Astin, & Feuer, 2002), as well as complicated grief (Shear, Frank, Houch, & Reynolds, 2005). Adding elements relevant to the traumatic loss experienced by this particular population, i.e., guilt, self-blaming, feeling betrayed by one's body, and G-d, is also important.

Early Phase of Psychotherapeutic Support

The shock and distress of this type of pregnancy loss often results in parents seeking psychological support within a matter of weeks after undergoing a TOPFA. Many are at a loss as to how they are supposed to feel and how they "should" be grieving. Others are worried about how they will react with the passage of time.

This author highly recommends seeing both members of a couple after a TOPFA, especially for the initial session. This allows the clinician to support and validate their common loss and determine how they are coping as a couple. Therapeutic goals within one to two months post-TOPFA include the following:

Establish a therapeutic alliance. Create a trusting relationship through empathy, develop a nonjudgmental attitude, support the parents for the difficult decision they made, listen carefully to parental language (e.g., term they use to refer to their baby), help parents to contain the intensity of their emotions in the first session, show understanding and respect for the variability in patterns of grieving and coping, and be sensitive to culturally diverse approaches to grief.

Ensure patient's safety and stability. Assess patterns of sleep, eating, and ability to care for other children, if present (and help arrange for support if necessary). Assess for suicidality (note many patients express a passive wish to die after the trauma (McCoyd, 2007), but this can be differentiated from an actual suicidal threat). Provide suggestions for self-care, as needed. Determine prior or concurrent trauma and stressors to determine if more intensive care is needed at present. Help parents recognize the tendency toward hindsight bias, i.e., knowing now how much they are hurting and incorrectly concluding from this that they made the wrong decision. Help patients contextualize their decision-making process, reviewing information they had at the time, the extent of their research to obtain that information, what they were thinking and feeling at the time, and how challenging it is to make these decisions with uncertainty, in the absence of clear and decisive information about the extent of likely impairment and the wide spectrum of severity possible. Help patients recognize they are likely feeling sadness for the abnormal baby and the difficult decision they confronted rather than for the actual decision they made, no matter how painful it remains.

Provide a safe environment for parents to share their experience, helping to contain intense emotionality, at present. Validate the significance of their loss and right to grieve. Demonstrate willingness to witness the full experience from learning of a problem, decision-making to terminate, and decisions made thereafter. Offering soothing, affect containment techniques can help reduce emotional overwhelm and avoid premature termination at this early stage of psychotherapeutic intervention. Later, having parents share tangible mementos may help them process the reality of their loss and validate its significance to them. Be aware that parents are quite observant of your reaction to any photographs, being fearful of any negative reaction to their baby's appearance. Note and comment positively on intact features, if possible (e.g., sweet mouth, perfectly formed fingers).

Assess how couple is coping to identify those at risk. Is support available from family and friends? Are the partners able to express feelings and provide support to each other? Have either used self-destructive behaviors to avoid emotional pain?

Psychoeducation. Provide normative information regarding the traumatic grieving process (i.e., symptoms, adaptation, recovery), and common gender differences. Address common patient reactions to typically increased feelings of sadness as initial emotional shock wears off. Reinforce this as progress in the grieving process rather than a step backward, and that grief may last many months or more. Inform patients of symptoms of major depression, PTSD, and complicated grief that may indicate a need for additional psychological help. Introduce the dual process model of adaptive coping (Stroebe & Schut, 1995) which posits normal grief oscillating between a focus on loss (the sad emotions) and a restoration focus (creating plans to meet future-valued life goals and engage in pleasurable activities). This validates the patient's need to re-establish some balance in their lives and reduces guilt that women, especially, may experience for any glimpse of calm or happiness they may feel. After the first month, the author encourages couples to set aside time on a daily basis to think about their losses (the baby, their future dreams, their plans for parenthood, etc.), setting some time boundaries of approximately 20–30 minutes, to ensure they are not avoiding all thoughts and feelings about their experience, but also not getting stuck in these memories and unable to return to the present. Coping techniques (e.g., cognitive restructuring, grounding techniques) can also be introduced. Prepare patients for loss of the strong support they may have received from others immediately after the loss, as this may dissipate with time while their grief may remain quite intense (Geerinck-Vercammen & Kahai, 2003).

Offer practical help for the following. Couple relationship – Inform about different intensities of grief expressed and variations in ways of coping, possible different needs for communication and physical intimacy.

Return to work – Manage expectations and provide suggestions for how to make the re-entry easier (e.g., initially return for only half of the week; suggest a colleague notify others of the reason you prefer others be told for your absence as well as your wishes regarding expressions of sympathy, e.g., keep them brief or not at all; if your door is closed please don't enter); walk into work with a compassionate colleague to ease the re-entry process; help parents accept they will not initially function at peak levels of capability as focus and concentration may be impaired.

Follow-up medical visits – If not offered by the obstetrician, suggest patients ask to be seen when fewer pregnant women are in the office. Help patients accept they may experience intense emotion in the presence of the doctor. Help them create a list of questions they may have for their doctor.

Negotiating the social environment – Identify a range of social supports so as not to overtax the spouse. Help patients develop realistic expectations of others, i.e., some will be supportive, others may not be. Some may have no prior experience with traumatic loss and may minimize their loss or incorrectly assume parents will recover quickly and immediately start trying to conceive again. Their loss may also evoke intense feelings of fear and vulnerability in others of childbearing age. Decisions to protect oneself from interactions with others that the patient does not find comforting should be respected. Anger and disappointment in others may be somewhat softened by gently helping patients acknowledge that before their loss they may not have understood what others in this situation were feeling. If patients experience others pushing them to move on before they feel ready, explain that society, in general, doesn't acknowledge the normal long-term nature of grief. Helping parents who believe their sorrow is the only way to remember and respect their deceased child discover other ways to remember and honor their baby which may be beneficial.

Needs of surviving children – Educate parents about the acute sensitivity of children to their parents' emotional state, as well as children's natural tendency for self-blame (thus indicating the need to tell children that you are not sad about anything they have done). Children, depending on their age, may also have their own need to grieve the loss of a sibling. Most parents, however, if they do choose to tell the child of the death of the baby, choose not to inform them of the termination decision (France, Hunt, Ziebland, & Wyke, 2013). Parents need to assure children of their continued attention to meeting their child's need for security and safety through their actions, but if unavailable for this others trusted by the child(ren) need to be available to them.

Teach self-soothing techniques –Techniques such as diaphragmatic breathing, grounding techniques, and distress tolerance can help patients struggling with intense emotions. Try to keep parents from taking their total attention away from their grief, however.

Provide relevant resources – books, reputable online resources, local support groups for experiencing a TOPFA (as parents often feel as though they do not fit in a spontaneous pregnancy loss group and may feel guilty for their expression of grief for a decision they made in such a group).

Facilitate rituals – In all likelihood, some may have already been completed. Plan for the "firsts" by raising awareness of future anniversary dates that may trigger emotions (e.g., due date, anniversary of date of loss, holidays especially Mother's and Father's Day). Share ideas of how others have marked these dates and honored their baby.

For many patients, this may be sufficient intervention at this juncture. Follow-up calls are often appreciated along with the reminder of the continued availability of the mental health professional for consultation or support, if needed.

Middle Phase of Psychotherapeutic Support (Beyond Approximately Two Months Post-Loss)

The role of the mental health professional at this point in time is to help guide patients through the aftermath of their traumatic event, help them effectively manage their emotional distress, and facilitate the development of a "new normal," i.e., a new understanding of the world, their beliefs, and their goals.

There is a good deal of symptom overlap between PTSD and prolonged grief after a TOPFA. Both can involve intrusive thoughts, emotions, and sensory experiences, a tendency to avoid thoughts and feelings about the experience, guilt, and feelings of isolation as well as being stuck in the grief. The author has addressed these symptoms through imaginal reliving, in vivo exposure, and CPT as these treatment modalities have shown promise in reducing the intensity of both grief and PTSD symptoms (Resick & Schnicke, 1993; Shear, Frank, Houck, & Reynolds, 2005). Stroebe and Schut's (1999) dual-process model of bereavement is also useful in helping patients alternate between a focus on their loss and, at other times, a focus on activities that can help them restore their emotional reserves.

This author has found the following goals useful for patients who are approximately two months or more post-TOPFA:

Offer treatment rationale. Explain that symptoms being experienced (e.g., intrusions, numbing, hyperarousal, behavioral avoidance) are common reactions to traumatic events and may be contributing to symptom maintenance. Treatment will involve fully processing their traumatic loss and reviewing their maintaining factors. An analogy this therapist has found useful for patients has been suggested by Ehlers and Clark (2000). It involves comparing the trauma memory to a cupboard in which many objects have been quickly thrown in such that they are quite disorganized with items falling out at unpredictable times and making it impossible to fully close the cupboard door. Organizing the cupboard entails looking at each thing and putting it into its place. Only by doing this can the cupboard door be closed and remain so. The therapist then explains that the patient's re-experiencing symptoms are isolated, unintegrated memory fragments that are being unintentionally triggered by various situational cues that resemble some aspect of the traumatic event and result in the individual experiencing them as if they were happening in the "here and now.". The patient's symptoms are being maintained by unhelpful cognitive (e.g., thought suppression) and behavioral (e.g., avoidance) strategies as well as by cognitive distortions. The mental health professional will introduce the patient to the use and benefits of exposure, the relationship between thoughts and emotions, the importance of meaning and attributions the patient has attached to the traumatic events experienced, and build the patient's internal and interpersonal resources.

Assess the patient's resources, coping skills, and attachment history. These are relevant to the client's ability to cope with both their loss experience and the therapy for traumatic bereavement. Techniques of distress tolerance and emotional regulation will be introduced to help individuals learn to tolerate and modulate their affect as well as self-sooth after the emotionally challenging therapeutic exercises are completed (Linehan, 1993).

Focus on loss. Exposure to traumatic memories in a safe environment has been found to be effective in treating both PTSD (Foa, Keane, Friedman, & Cohen, 2009; Resick & Schnicke, 1993) and complicated grief (Boelen, deKeijser, van den Hout, & van den Bout, 2007; Shear et al., 2005; Wittouck et al., 2011). Avoidance of thinking about painful memories precludes the client from fully integrating their trauma narrative in an organized, coherent manner (Ehlers & Clark, 2000). The author has found that incorporating suggestions involving prolonged exposure from Resick and Schnicke's (1993) CPT for trauma is useful. Patients are asked to write (preferably by hand) an *Impact Statement* (a full account of their trauma experience from learning of a fetal anomaly through the termination procedure and after, including remembering the trauma with all sensory and emotional memories that they have and the impact of the event on them (e.g., answering questions about why they believe it happened to them and what effect it has had on them regarding their beliefs about themselves, others, and the world)). Alternatively, they may be asked to audio-record an *Imaginal Revisiting* of the trauma in session (Shear et al., 2005). Imaginal revisiting entails reliving the trauma in their mind's eye, making the image as realistic as possible, by including sensory details, thoughts, and feelings, along with what was happening to the extent they can handle. The patient is asked to describe, verbally, the reliving of the trauma in the first person and in the present tense. The therapist assists patients staying in their memories by asking questions such as,

> What do you see?, How does that feel?, Where do you feel that?, What is going through your mind as this is happening?, What were you thinking right before you made your decision?, What information did you actually have at this time of the decision?

Patients are encouraged to experience their emotions as fully as possible to allow the affective element of their stored trauma memory to undergo revision and lessen the distress level over repeated exposures.

Help normalize the patient's desire to avoid this difficult aspect of therapy while emphasizing its empirical effectiveness in reducing long-term distress. Reinforcing the patient's capacity to experience intense emotions without losing their sanity or being permanently paralyzed by this can help them regain feelings of control over their emotions. This exercise is likely to need repeating with the therapist encouraging the client to include additional sensory and emotional details to promote progress. Self-soothing techniques may be used before and after the exposure but both the patient and the therapist are to avoid their use during the exposure experience itself so as not to reinforce avoidance of the emotional experience.

Patients are asked to read or listen to their account of the experience in session. The therapist can periodically ask the patient to assess their level of distress to help determine "stuck points" or "hot spots" (i.e., distorted appraisals or interpretations that result in unrealistic beliefs about themselves or others) that are associated with particularly strong levels of distress that are likely precluding effective processing of the trauma. They are asked to read or listen to the account daily between sessions, as well, during the time they have set aside to focus on their loss. When thoughts of their loss occur outside of these circumscribed, time-bounded periods, they are advised to change their focus to something else, putting these thoughts on the backburner until their chosen time to concentrate on the loss. This stimulus control procedure can help patients regain some sense of control over intrusive thoughts and reduce emotional overwhelm.

Patients are asked to re-write their impact statement or re-record their revisiting experience throughout therapy as the nature of the trauma memory changes during the course of therapy. If patients are avoiding specific situations, a hierarchy of these situations can be created with the intention of encouraging gradual in vivo exposure.

Cognitive restructuring and reappraisal. Whereas fear has been found to be more responsive to exposure techniques, the self-blame and guilt that patients commonly feel after a TOPFA may respond better to cognitive reappraisal techniques (Rothbaum, Meadows, Resick, & Foy, 2000) and help patients re-build their shattered assumptions about themselves and the world.

The process of cognitive restructuring helps patients actively incorporate updated information, i.e., what they know now that they didn't know at the time of their decisions, including their current intense emotional distress. Socratic questioning on the part of the therapist is used to help patients challenge their often distorted cognitions, especially those of self-blame, hindsight bias, and guilt. For example, therapists can challenge patients by asking: what is the evidence for/against this belief, would the evidence you are presenting stand up in a court of law, are you thinking in all-or-nothing terms, are your judgments based on feelings rather than facts, what would you say to a good friend in the same circumstances if they were thinking this way?

- Addressing feelings of guilt. CPT has been found effective in reducing trauma-related guilt (Nishith, Nixon, & Resick, 2005). Parents often express self-doubt regarding their decision and whether they are grieving properly, have a right to grieve their baby, or are wallowing in their grief and making others uncomfortable. They need help to discover that they had no good options in their situation, made a decision most appropriate for their circumstances, or chose what to them felt like the least bad decision, and now they would be suffering regardless of the choice they made.

  Reassurance that there is no one right or wrong way to grieve can comfort parents. Helping them discover ways to remember their unborn child beyond intense sadness and tears can help parents, especially mothers, to recognize that if her pain diminishes with time, she has other ways to maintain her attachment to her baby.

  Culpability in having been instrumental in making the decision to end the desired pregnancy often significantly contributes to guilt and may compromise the grieving process. Guilt may also be experienced if parents felt relief in having prevented the birth of a severely disabled child. Gently point out that when both having the baby and not having the baby felt wrong and parents are responsible to make a decision, guilt may be inevitable.

  A frequently heard and very painful lament from mothers is, "I killed my baby," which violates their belief that parents are supposed to protect their children. Rather than trying to remove guilt feelings too quickly, mental health professionals (MHPs) should, rather, try to determine their cause (e.g., a personal value violated, denial of feelings of helplessness, a belief that bad outcomes should be punished) and help patients accept their feelings. If the feelings persist, however, the MHP can try to help the patients transform their guilt to regret (e.g., "While I did make the decision to end my baby's life, I wish I would have had the option to allow the baby to lead a full life without ongoing physical pain, suffering, or a life-limiting condition. But I did not."). Help patients recognize their intent (to protect vs. harm), the positive aims their decision served, and evidence that they have to the contrary of this overgeneralized belief that they are a murderer. This will help them form a more balanced view of what they did and who they are. It is the experience of this author that, with time, most patients come to recognize that although they did make a decision to end the life of their baby, the decision was made from love based on their assessment of the quality of life the baby would have and the impact this would have on their family. This can lead patients to accept that without intention to do harm, blame is not appropriate. Other sources of parental guilt can include feelings of ambivalence about the pregnancy that are normal but are misinterpreted, having wished the baby had died on his/her own, feeling relief immediately after making the decision or the termination was completed, and guilt and shame that one's body failed to create a healthy baby.

Unrealistic standards to which parents often hold themselves can be altered by acknowledging that we do not always have the control we desire. Having made a termination decision, patients often lose trust in themselves and question whether they can be good parents to a healthy child. Recognizing that US culture tends to believe that "good" mothers don't have "bad" babies (Ladd-Taylor & Umansky, 1998) helps parents see the emotional bind which they confronted. Referral to an open-minded and compassionate clergy person also helps some patients with their feelings of guilt. Suggesting parents write a supportive letter to a hypothetical friend in the same circumstances, reflecting on their feelings of guilt, challenging their automatic thinking patterns, and correcting unrealistic assumptions they are holding can help foster their developing a new perspective on their pregnancy loss and its circumstances. Creating a therapeutic ritual with patients to help them say good-bye to guilt (e.g., casting pieces of paper with various sources of the parent's guilt written on them either into the ocean or into the universe in a helium balloon) may also assist in reducing guilt. If guilt cannot be released, however, parents may need to learn to accept and live with this guilt, but with compassion for having been in a no-win situation rather than with ongoing self-punishment.

- There are other faulty beliefs for which cognitive reappraisal can be used. Examples include:

"If I follow the rules (e.g., take folic acid, avoid alcohol and sushi), nothing bad will happen to me." Help patients recognize that this "just world belief" is a probability statement not an absolute so it can be transformed into a more realistic, accurate belief such as "If I follow the rules (i.e., taking reasonable precautions), I reduce my risk of something bad happening, but cannot completely eliminate all risks." This belief, along with self-blame, often reflects patients' attempts to control everything, something which we all learn is not possible.

"It wouldn't hurt this much if I made the right decision." This is an example of emotional reasoning. Our emotions are not a good barometer of the rightness or wrongness of a decision, as even wise decisions can result in pain. Help patients recognize it is the existence of the anomaly in their baby that is causing the emotional pain, and they are likely to experience emotional pain whether they terminated the pregnancy or had a baby who was forced to cope with medical and social challenges (McCoyd, 2007).

"I will never (or should never) feel happiness again." Gently guide parents through Socratic questions to conclude that the length or intensity of their suffering does not constitute proof of love, remembrance, or attachment to their baby. Reassure them that they will always remember their baby. This experience of loss and a fulfilled life with compassion for self and others, some of it learned through this experience, may be the best tribute they can offer to their baby. Encourage patients to allow themselves brief periods of happy moments (even just five minutes) and gradually add to this.

"I couldn't handle this again." After a traumatic experience, individuals become more anxious about other potentially frightening and catastrophic events. This anxious state often creates hypervigilance which results in their being more likely to perceive perils or interpret ambiguous situations as threatening (Mogg & Bradley, 1992). While guarantees of safety are not possible, patients can learn they don't have to behave as if a repetition of this same situation has a high probability, unless they learn through additional genetic testing that they are carriers of a genetic disease (in which case they may need to undergo additional procedures or testing in a subsequent pregnancy). Asking patients if they actually know of anyone who has improbably bad luck all or much of the time or having the catastrophizing patient predict the worst, best, and most likely outcome may help them put some of their fears in perspective.

Focus on restoration. Gradually and periodically return focus to the patient's life goals, the couple relationship, and social relationships. Reinforce the patient's reincorporation of previously pleasurable and mastery activities using activity scheduling. A restorative focus will hopefully contribute to rebuilding patient resilience. Suggest they increase their exercise level to the level allowed by their obstetrician or reproductive endocrinologist. Reintroducing social activities is likely to present patients with decisions about attending baby- and child-centered events. Patients should be encouraged to do what feels right to them and recognize that others will be available to share their friend or family member's joyful events now. If they choose to attend, help them mitigate the situation (e.g., come late, leave early, help prepare food in the kitchen, develop an exit strategy in advance) and not berate themselves if they become emotional while at the event.

• Update impact of event or imaginal revisiting. Have patients re-write and update their impact statement or re-record imaginal revisiting the trauma at the end of this phase of treatment. Note changes in how they think about the traumatic loss, what they believe now about themselves, others, and the world. As with any other therapeutic issue, there is no one-size-fits-all therapy for those who have experienced a TOPFA. Individual differences in symptom presentation suggest the importance of applying therapeutic protocols flexibly so as to best incorporate the individual patient's needs, values, resources, experiences, and social and cultural backgrounds.

Late Phase of Psychotherapeutic Support and Working with Patients during a Subsequent Pregnancy

While some patients may have processed their loss at this point in time, others who are of advanced age and/or have used assisted reproductive technology to conceive their pregnancy can feel a tremendous sense of urgency to conceive as soon as possible. Not yet having had time to effectively process their traumatic loss can leave them feeling numb or too emotionally raw to navigate the multitude of conflicted emotions, for example, anxiety, sadness, fear, and hope, likely to arise in a subsequent pregnancy.

The following goals of the MHP for this phase of psychotherapeutic intervention include:

Preparing for the future and implementing future goals. Identify future goals that reflect the patient's values and needs. Delineate concrete strategies to work to reach these goals. This can help patients regain a sense of purpose as they reinvest in their lives and readjust to a new normal. Demonstrate the therapist's confidence in the patient's ability to recover from their loss, having them imagine themselves in one to two years from now, and asking them what might have happened in the interim that has resulted in a de-intensifying of their feelings of grief?

If patients wish to conceive another baby, prepare them that a future pregnancy will be informed by their prior loss as they now realize that a pregnancy is a hope, not a guarantee, and they need to recognize that they are likely to feel differently in a subsequent pregnancy as a result. They need to be prepared to experience a range of emotions that are likely to be triggered in a new pregnancy (Forray, Mayes, Magriples, & Epperson, 2009; Hamama, Rauch, Sperlich, Defever, Seng, & Fainman, 2010; Turton et al., 2009). Parents will need to be informed of their specific risks, if any, in a subsequent pregnancy, as well as the unknown risks, albeit small, that any pregnancy faces. Healthcare professionals need to provide additional time during appointments for these patients to address their fears and conflicted feelings, and offer nonjudgmental support. Medical providers also need to be aware of the tendency for mothers to demonstrate emotional cushioning in a subsequent pregnancy (Cote'-Arsenault & Donato, 2011) in which they may wish to delay announcement of the pregnancy and preparations for parenting, and try to avoid emotional attachment to the baby. Expecting the worst is another way women try to protect themselves, reflecting the erroneous belief, this author has found, that they will hurt less this way if the pregnancy does not work out. Although anxiety in a subsequent pregnancy is fully understandable, accurate information and cognitive reappraisals of parents' unrealistic predictions of danger can be beneficial in building a willingness to tolerate the uncertainty that comes with every pregnancy, an important therapeutic goal in light of the data on the impact on infants exposed to prenatal maternal distress (Kinsella & Monk, 2009).

Prepare patients for the upsurge of negative feelings around milestones and anniversary dates (e.g., due date, date of baby's death, holidays). Help them predict other situations likely to re-trigger a resurgence of emotions (e.g., being asked in a subsequent pregnancy if this is their first baby). Help prepare parents for the resurgence of memories of a prior loss that are often triggered by the subsequent birth of a healthy child. Help them to differentiate their healthy new baby from memories of their deceased baby, create positive ways to remember their loss, and honor both their past and present babies and themselves.

Parents may also need help to prepare for parenting after a TOPFA. They need to re-build trust in their ability to be competent and loving parents and create realistic expectations of themselves as parents to avoid a compensatory need to be a perfect parent or be overprotective of their children.

Finding meaning in the loss experience. Making sense of the event, finding benefit in the experience, and identity reconstruction all play a role in finding meaning after a loss (Davis et al., 1998). Finding meaning, however, takes time. Recognizing not only what was lost but also what was gained often results in a new appreciation of one's life and the people in it (Neimeyer, Burke, Mackay, & van Dyke Stringer, 2010). It requires an individual exploration and should not be forced on patients, however, nor should patients feel a sense of failure if they do not find meaning in the loss, as a significant subset of individuals do not search for meaning yet have ultimately been found to adjust well to loss (Wortman, 2004). Some patients also experience post-traumatic growth, i.e., a return beyond their baseline level of functioning to a sense of new possibilities in life, enhanced interpersonal relationships, and increased empathy for others (Lafarge, Mitchell, & Fox, 2017).

Ending treatment. Review progress with the patient(s). Consolidate and reinforce treatment gains, strengths, and coping skills acquired that can be used to face future life issues, crises, or losses. Discuss the possibility of relapse and differentiate between a lapse (a partial return to an earlier period of emotional difficulty) and a relapse (fully returning to the beginning of the individual's grief process) to help overcome frustration and maintain motivation to overcome obstacles. Discuss feelings engendered by ending treatment. Recognize that new life events may re-trigger memories and feelings about their loss. Offer follow-up appointments, as needed.

Support for Parents Choosing to Continue a Pregnancy with a Fetal Abnormality

Communicating the news of a fetal anomaly is a complex process, typically requiring repetition, clarification, and additional comprehensive and balanced information from a multidisciplinary team offering multiple resources (Sheets et al., 2011). This allows parents to make a decision regarding the pregnancy that is most appropriate to their circumstances. Ongoing care is needed to help support parents as they cope with the anxiety and uncertainty of the pregnancy. The type of support patients need depends on whether the fetal anomaly is viable or non-viable.

If a pregnancy with a diagnosed fetal anomaly is viable, parents' greatest early needs are for information about the anomaly, how the patient and baby can be medically treated, and the prognosis and likely ability of the child to function in various domains. Referral to specialists for this information as well as to discuss a post-delivery plan is necessary. Women continuing a pregnancy with a viable anomaly have been found to navigate through various stages of distress (Titapant & Chuenwattana, 2014). Initially, there is a stage of intense negative psychological reactions where women react to the loss of the ideal child they had imagined having and may experience impairment in their sense of self-worth. A healing stage typically follows in which distress declines and women use strategies of minimizing or discrediting the bad news to re-build hope, often choosing not to reveal the anomaly to others and reducing the amount of information they seek out regarding the abnormality. Finally, in the third stage as women near their due date, intense psychological reactions may re-emerge as parents begin to worry about the uncertainty of their baby's future and how they will manage the baby's birth and thereafter. Parents need help in planning for the practical obstetrical and birth needs, as well as learning about possible emotional reactions to expect. Information about resources and services available in their geographic area as well as nationally is very helpful.

It has been suggested that society as a whole may overemphasize a disability over the remaining abilities of any individual and believe a certain level of health is required to live a good or acceptable quality of life. Disabled individuals dispute this as they perceive themselves as healthy, having a good life, and able to thrive even in the midst of a generally unwelcoming society (Asch, 1999). Favorable research on living with a disability, and its positive impact on parents, siblings, and disabled individuals themselves (Skotko, Levine, & Goldstein, 2011a, 2011b, 2011c) may also help parents recast hope for their child's and their own future. Mental health professionals working with parents receiving a diagnosis of a fetal anomaly would do well to explore their own beliefs and emotional reactions toward various disabilities to ensure they have an open mind and non-judgmental attitude toward parents choosing to continue such a pregnancy.

After the birth of a child with a medical problem or disability, parents, especially mothers, typically become stronger, with reduced fear and apprehension (Guiliani et al., 2014). It may take most mothers 6–12 months, however, to fully process their infant's health issues and disability after which they typically become staunch advocates for their child and his/her needs (Wright, 2002). Multi-disciplinary support, both medical and psychological, can be offered to parents as they face the ongoing challenges of raising a child with a disability.

For those parents who choose to continue a pregnancy that is incompatible with life until a natural prenatal or postnatal demise of the baby, involvement with the healthcare team in decision-making and creating an advanced care birth plan can result in the most positive birth experience possible under these circumstances and allow patients to feel empowered in their role as parents (English & Hessler, 2013). The introduction of perinatal palliative care has given parents assistance in making meaningful plans for their baby's birth and life closure, addressing the physical, social, spiritual, and practical issues of the family, often including siblings and grandparents. In this way, parents and close family have the opportunity to create memories of the baby (Caitlin, 2005), memories they may cherish as they will have so few available to them. While the extant literature is still limited, research thus far reports that parents typically have a positive reaction to the emotional outcome offered through perinatal palliative care (Breeze, Lees, Kumar, Missfelder-Lobos, & Murdoch, 2007; Calhoun, Napolitano, Terry, Bussey, & Hoeldtke, 2003).

Conclusions

Neither the decision to terminate a pregnancy due to fetal anomaly nor the decision to continue the pregnancy is a decision taken lightly by most parents. Coming to terms with these decisions may require both time and emotional support. These non-normative losses can certainly alter a patient's world view. Interventions that promote acceptance and reframing may assist parents in creating new narratives of their experience. Efforts to reduce the stigma of abortion as well as provide additional support and resources for both parents who choose to interrupt their pregnancy or continue the pregnancy after a diagnosis of fetal anomaly may help build greater support for these parents and lessen the intensity of their grief responses, as disenfranchised losses that are neither socially sanctioned nor publically shared result in their lack of validation by others which can intensify parents' emotional responses. Further research is needed into the most beneficial short- and long-term support for patients coping with a diagnosis of fetal abnormalities. Sensitive medical and psychological caregivers can help parents process their loss, integrate it into their identity, and restructure their world view so that despite the difficulty of the experience, our patients can rebuild hope and eventually find the strength to re-engage and re-build a meaningful life.

Note

1 The following psychotherapeutic approach to treatment has been adapted from Chapter 14, Helping Patients Cope with Their Decisions, by J.P. Galst, in J.P. Galst & M.S. Verp (Eds), *Prenatal and Preimplantation Diagnosis: The Burden of Choice* (pp. 287–321). New York: Springer.

References

ACOG practice bulletin #77. (2007). Screening for fetal chromosomal abnormalities. *Obstetrics and Gynecology*; *109*: 217–227.

American Psychiatric Association. DSM-5. (2003). *Diagnostic and Statistical Manual of Mental Health Disorders*. 5th ed. Arlington, VA: American Psychiatric Association.

Barry, L.C., Kasl, S.V., & Prigerson, H.G. (2002). Psychiatric disorders among bereaved persons: The role of perceived circumstances of death and preparedness for death. *American Journal of Geriatric Psychiatry*; *10*(4): 447–457.

Bernhardt, B.A., Soucier, D., Hanson, K., Savage, M.S., Jackson, L., & Wapner, R.J. (2013). Women's experience receiving abnormal prenatal chromosomal microarray testing results. *Genetics in Medicine*; *15*(2): 139–145. doi: 10.1038/gim.2012.113

Biggs, M.S., Upadhyay, U.D., McCulloch, C.E. & Foster, D.G. (2016). Women's mental health and well-being 5 years after receiving or being denied an abortion. A prospective, longitudinal cohort study. *JAMA Psychiatry*, doi: 10.1001/jamaPSYCHIATRY.2016.3478. Downloaded from http://jamanetwork.com on 12/16/2016

Bisson, J., & Andrew, M. (2007). Psychological treatment of post-traumatic stress disorder (PTSD). *Cochrane Database of Systematic Reviews*; *18*(3): CD003388.

Boelen, P.A., deKeijser, J., van den Hout, M.A., & van den Bout, J. (2007). Treatment of complicated grief: A comparison between cognitive-behavioral therapy and supportive counseling. *Journal of Consulting and Clinical Psychology*; *75*(2): 277–284.

Boelen, P.A., Van Den Hout, M., & Van De Bout, J. (2006). A cognitive-behavioral conceptualization of complicated grief. *Clinical Psychology Science and Practice*; *13*: 109–128. doi: 10.1111/j.1468-2850.2006.00013

Breeze, A.C.G., Lees, C.C., Kumar, A., Missfelder-Lobos, H.H., & Murdoch, E.M. (2007). Palliative care for prenatally diagnosed lethal fetal abnormality. *Archives of Disease in Childhood- Fetal and Neonatal Ed*; *92*(1): F56–8. doi: 10.113i6/adc.2005.092122

Caitlin, A. (2005). Thinking outside the box: Prenatal care and the call for a prenatal advance directive. *Journal of Perinatal and Neonatal Nursing*; *19*(2): 169–176.

Calhoun, B.C., Napolitano, P., Terry, M., Bussey, C., & Hoeldtke, N.J. (2003). Perinatal hospice. Comprehensive care for the family of the fetus with a lethal condition. *Journal of Reproductive Medicine*; *48*(5): 343–348.

Choi, H., Van Riper, M., & Thoyre, S. (2012). Decision making following a prenatal diagnosis of Down syndrome: An integrative review. *Journal of Midwifery and Women's Health*; *57*(2): 156–164.

Cope, H., Garrett, M.E., Gregory, S., & Ashley-Koch, A. (2015). Pregnancy continuation and organizational religious activity following prenatal diagnosis of a lethal fetal defect are associated with improved psychological outcome. *Prenatal Diagnosis*; *35*: 761–768. doi: 10.1002/pd.4603

Cote'-Arsenault, D., & Donato, K. (2011). Emotional cushioning in pregnancy after perinatal loss. *Journal of Reproductive and Infant Psychology*; *29*(1): 81–92. doi: 10.1080/02646838.2010.513115

Davies, V., Gledhill, J., McFadyen, A., Whitlow, B., & Economides, D. (2005). Psychological outcome in women undergoing termination of pregnancy for ultrasound-detected fetal anomaly in the first and second trimesters: A pilot study. *Ultrasound in Obstetrics and Gynecology*; *25*(4): 389–392.

Doka, K.J., & Martin, J. (2010). *Grieving beyond Gender: Understanding the Ways Men and Women Mourn*. New York: Routledge.

Ehlers, A., & Clark, D.M. (2000). A cognitive model of posttraumatic stress disorder. *Behaviour Research and Therapy*; *38*: 319–345.

English, N.K., & Hessler, K.L. (2013). Prenatal birth planning for families of the imperiled newborn. *Journal of Obstetric, and Gynecologic Neonatal Nursing*; *42*(3): 390–399. doi: 10.111/1552-6909.12031

Foa, E.B., Keane, T.M., Friedman, M.J., & Cohen, J.A. (Eds.). (2009). *Effective Treatments for PTSD, Second Edition*. New York: Guilford.

Foa, E.G., Steketee, G., & Rothbaum, B.O. (1989). Behavioral/cognitive conceptualizations of post-traumatic stress disorder. *Behavior Therapy*; *20*(2): 155–176. doi: 10.1016/S0005-7894(89)80067-X

Forray, A., Mayes, L.C., Magriples, U., & Epperson, C.N. (2009). Prevalence of post-traumatic stress disorder in pregnant women with prior pregnancy complications. *Journal of Maternal Fetal Neonatal Medicine*; *22*(6): 522–527. doi: 10.1080/14767050902801686

France, E.F., Hunt, K., Ziebland, S., & Wyke, S. (2013). What parents say about disclosing the end of their pregnancy due to fetal abnormality. *Midwifery*; *29*: 24–32.

Galst, J.P. (2015). Helping patients cope with their decisions. In J.P. Galst & M.S. Verp (Eds.). *Prenatal and preimplantation diagnosis: The burden of choice* (pp. 287–321). New York: Springer.

Geerinck-Vercammen, C.R., & Kahai, H.H. (2003). Coping with termination of pregnancy for fetal abnormality in a supportive environment. *Prenatal Diagnosis*; *23*(7): 543–548.

Georgsson-Ohman, S., Sissel, S., Waldenstrom, U, Grunewald, C., & Olin-Lauritzen, S. (2006). Pregnant women's responses to information about an increased risk of carrying a baby with Down syndrome. *Birth*; *33*(1): 64–73.

Giuliani, R., Tripani, A., Pellizzoni, S., Clarici, A., Lonciari, I., D'Ottavio, G., et al. (2014). Pregnancy and postpartum following a prenatal diagnosis of fetal thoracoabdominal malformation: The parental perspective. *Journal of Pediatric Surgery*; *49*(2): 353–358. doi: 10.1016/j.jpedsurg.2013.07.025

Hamama, L., Rauch, S.A., Sperlich, M., Defever, E., & Seng, J.S. (2010). Previous experience of spontaneous or elective abortion and risk for posttraumatic stress and depression during subsequent pregnancy. *Depression and Anxiety*; *27*(8): 699–707. doi: 10.1002/da.20714

Hamamy, H.A., & Dahoun, S. (2004). Parental decisions following the prenatal diagnosis of sex chromosome abnormalities. *European Journal or Obstetrics and Gynecology and Reproductive Bioiogyl*; *116*(1): 58–62.

Hickerton, C.L., Aitken, M.A., Hodgson, J., & Delatycki, M.B. (2012). "*Did you find that out in time?*": New life trajectories of parents who choose to continue a pregnancy where a genetic disorder is diagnosed or likely. *American Journal of Medical Genetics Part A*; *158A*: 373–383. doi: 10.1001/ajmg.a.34399

Hoyert, D.L., Mathews, T.J., Menacker, F., Strobino, D.M., & Guyer, B. (2006). Annual summary of vital statistics: 2004. *Pediatrics*; *117*(1): 168–183. doi: 10.1542/peds.2005-2587

Jeon, K.C., Chen, L.S., & Goodson, P. (2012). Decision to abort after a prenatal diagnosis of sex chromosome abnormality: A systematic review of the literature. *Genetics in Medicine*; *14*(1): 27–38.

Johnson, C.Y., Honein, M.A., Flanders, W.D., Howards, P.P., Oakley Jr., G.P., & Rasmussen, S. (2012). Pregnancy termination following prenatal diagnosis of anencephaly or spina bifida: A systematic review of the literature. *Birth Defects Research Part A: Clinical and Molecular Teratology*; *94*(11): 857–863.

Kaasen, A., Helbig, A., Malt, U.F., Naes, T., Skari, H., & Haugen, G.N. (2013). Paternal psychological response after ultrasonographic detection of structural fetal anomalies with a comparison to maternal response: A cohort study. *BMC Pregnancy and Childbirth*; *13*: 147. doi: 10.1186/1471-239313-147

Kersting, A., Kroker, K., Steinhard, J., Ludorff, K., Wesselmann, U., Ohrmann, P. et al. (2007). Complicated grief after traumatic loss: A 14-month follow up study. *European Archives of Psychiatry and Clinical Neuroscience*; *257*(8): 437–443.

Kinsella, M.T., & Monk, C. (2009). Impact of maternal stress, depression and anxiety on fetal neurobehavioral development. *Clinical Obstetrics and Gynecology*; *52*(3): 425–440. doi: 10.10971GRF.060

Kleinveld, J.H., Ten Kate, L.P., van den Berg, M., van Vugt, J.M., & Timmermans, D.R. (2009). Does informed decision making influence psychological outcomes after receiving a positive screening outcome? *Prenatal Diagnosis*; *29*(3): 271–273. doi: 10.1002/pd.2186

Korenromp, P.M., Christiaens, G.C., & van den Bout, J. (2005a). Long-term psychological consequences of pregnancy termination for fetal abnormality: A cross-sectional study. *Prenatal Diagnosis*; *25*: 253–260.

Korenromp, M.J., Page-Christiaens, G.C.M.L., van den Bout, J., Mulder, E.J.H., Hunfeld, J.A.M., Bilardo, C.M. et al. (2005b). Psychological consequences of termination of pregnancy for fetal anomaly: Similarities and differences between partners. *Prenatal Diagnosis*; *25*(13): 1226–1233.

Korenromp, M.J., Page-Christiaens, G.C., van den Bout, J., Mulder, E.J., Hunfeld, J.A., Potters, C.M. et al. (2007). A prospective study on parental coping 4 months after termination of pregnancy for fetal anomalies. *Prenatal Diagnosis*; *27*(8): 709–716.

Korenromp, M.J., Page-Christiaens, G.C., van den Bout, J., Mulder, E.J., & Visser, G.H. (2009). Adjustment to termination of pregnancy for fetal anomaly: A longitudinal study of women at 4, 8, and 16 months. *American Journal of Obstetrics and Gynecology*; *201*(2): 160.e1–7. doi: 10.1016/j.ajog.2009.04.007

Ladd-Taylor, M., & Umansky, L. (1998). *Bad Mothers: The Politics of Blame in Twentieth Century America*. New York: New York University Press.

Lafarge, C. (2016). Women's experience of coping with termination of pregnancy for fetal abnormality: Coping strategies, perinatal grief and posttraumatic growth. Post-doctoral thesis, University of West London. Downloaded 1/15/17 at http://repository.uwl.ac.uk/id/eprint/1769.

Lafarge, C., Mitchell, K., Breeze, A.C.G., & Fox, P. (2017). Pregnancy termination for fetal abnormality: Are health professionals' perceptions of women's coping congruent with women's accounts? *BMC Pregnancy and Childbirth*; *17*: 60. doi: 10.1186/s12884-017-1238-3

Lafarge, C., Mitchell, K., & Fox, P. (2013). Perinatal grief following a termination of pregnancy for fetal abnormality: The impact of coping strategies. *Prenatal Diagnosis*; *33*(12): 1173–1182. doi: 10.1002/pd.4218

Lafarge, C., Mitchell, K., & Fox, P. (2017). Posttraumatic growth following pregnancy termination for fetal abnormality: The predictive role of coping strategies and perinatal grief. *Anxiety, Stress, & Coping*; *12*(1): 1–15. doi: 10.1080/10615806.2016.1278433

Lawson, K.L. (2003). Perceptions of deservedness of social aid as a function of prenatal diagnostic testing. *Journal of Applied Psychology*; *33*: 76–90.

Linehan, M.M. (1993). *Skills Training Manual for Treating Borderline Personality Disorder*. New York: Guilford.

Locock, L., & Alexander, J. (2006). 'Just a bystander'? Men's place in the process of fetal screening and diagnosis. *Social Science and Medicine*; *62*(6): 1349–1359.

Lou, S., Nielsen, C.P., Hvidman, L., Petersen, O.B., & Risor, M.B. (2016). Coping with worry while waiting for diagnostic results: A qualitative study of the experiences of pregnant couples following a high-risk prenatal screening result. *BMC Pregnancy and Childbirth*; *16*: 321–328. doi: 10.1186/s12884-016-1114-6

Maguire, M., Light, A., Kuppermann, M., Dalton, V.K., Steinauer, J.E., & Kerns, J. (2015). Grief after second-trimester termination for fetal anomaly: A qualitative study. *Contraception*; *91*: 234–239. doi: 10.1016/j.contraception.2014.11.015

Mansfield, C., Hopfer, S., & Marteau, T.M. (1999). Termination rates after prenatal diagnosis of Down syndrome, spina bifida, anencephaly, and Turner and Klinefelter syndromes: A systematic literature review. *Prenatal Diagnosis*; *19*(9): 808–812.

McCoyd, J.L. (2007). Pregnancy interrupted: Loss of a desired pregnancy after diagnosis of fetal anomaly. *Journal of Psychosomatic Obstetrics and Gynaecology*; *28*(1): 37–48.

McCoyd, J.L. (2013). Preparation for prenatal decision-making: A baseline of knowledge and reflection in women participating in prenatal screening. *Journal of Psychosomatic Obstetrics and Gynaecology*; *34*: 3–8.

Mendes, D.D., Mello, M.F., Ventura, P., Passarela, C.M., & Mari, J. (2008). A systematic review on the effectiveness of cognitive behavioral therapy for posttraumatic stress disorder. *International Journal of Psychiatry in Medicine*; *38*(3): 241–259.

Mezei, G., Pepp, C., Toth, P.E., Beke, A., & Papp, Z. (2004). Factors influencing parental decision making in prenatal diagnosis of sex chromosome aneuploidy. *Obstetrics and Gynecology*; *104*: 94–101.

Mogg, K., & Bradley, B.P. (1992). Selective attention and anxiety: A cognitive-motivational perspective. In T. Dalgeish & M.J. Power (Eds.). *Handbook of cognition and emotion* (pp. 145–170). Chichester, UK: John Wiley & Sons.

Natoli, J.L., Ackerman, D.L., McDermott, S., & Edwards, J.G. (2012). Prenatal diagnosis of Down syndrome: A systematic review of termination rates (1995–2011). *Prenatal Diagnosis*; *32*(2): 142–153.

Neimeyer, R.A., Burke, L.A., Mackay, M.M., & van Dyke Stringer, J.G. (2010). Grief therapy and the reconstruction of meaning: From principles to practice. *Journal of Contemporary Psychotherapy*; *40*: 73–83. doi: 10.1007/sl0879-009-9135

Nishith, P., Nixon, R.D., & Resick, P.A. (2005). Resolution of trauma-related guilt following treatment of PTSD in female rape victims: A result of cognitive processing therapy targeting comorbid depression? *Journal of Affective Disorders*; *86*(2–3): 259–265.

Powers, M.B., Halpern, J.M., Ferenschak, M.P., Gillihan, S.J., & Foa, E.B. (2010). A meta-analytic review of prolonged exposure for posttraumatic stress disorder. *Clinical Psychology*; *30*(6): 635–642. doi: 10.1016/j.cpr.2010.04.007

Redlinger-Grosse, K., Bernhardt, B., Berg, K., Muenke, M., & Biesecker, B.B. (2002). The decision to continue: The experiences and needs of parents who receive a prenatal diagnosis of holoprosencephaly. *American Journal of Medical Genetics*; *112*: 369–378. doi: 10.1002/1jmg.10657

Resick, P.A., Monson, C.M., & Chard, K.M. (2008). *Cognitive Processing Therapy: Veteran/military Version*. Washington, DC: Department of Veterans' Affairs.

Resick, P.A., Nishith, P., Weaver, T.L., Astin, M.C., & Feuer, C.A. (2002). A comparison of cognitive-processing therapy and prolonged exposure and a waiting condition for the treatment of chronic posttraumatic stress disorder in female rape victims. *Journal of Consulting and Clinical Psychology*; 70: 867–879.

Resick, P.A., & Schnicke, M.K. (1993). *Cognitive Processing Therapy for Rape Victims*. Newbury Park, CA: SAGE.

Rothbaum, B.O., Meadows, E.A., Resick, P., & Foy, D.W. (2000). Cognitive-behavioral therapy. In E.B. Foa, T.M. Keane, & M.J. Friedman (Eds.). *Effective treatment for PTSD: Practice guidelines from the International Society for Traumatic Stress Studies* (pp. 60–83). New York: Guilford.

Sandelowski, M., & Barroso, J. (2005). The travesty of choosing after positive prenatal diagnosis. *Journal of Obstetrical and Gynecological Neonatal Nursing*; 34(3): 307–318.

Schechtman, K.B., Gray, D.L., Baty, J.D., & Rothman, S.M. (2002). Decision-making for termination of pregnancies for fetal anomalies: Analysis of 53,000 pregnancies. *Obstetrics and Gynecology*; 99(2): 216–222.

Shear, M.K. (2015). Complicated grief. *New England Journal of Medicine*; 372: 153–160.

Shear, K., Frank, E., Houck, P.R., & Reynolds, C.F. 3rd. (2005). Treatment of complicated grief: A randomized controlled trial. *Journal of the American Medical Association*; 293(21): 2601–2608.

Shear, M.K., Reynolds, C.F. III, Simon, M., Zisook, S., Wang, Y., Mauro, C., et al. (2016). Optimizing treatment of complicated grief: A randomized clinical trial. *Journal of the American Medical Association Psychiatry*; 73: 685–694. doi:10.1001/jamapsychiatry.2016.0892

Sheets, K.B., Crissman, B.G., Feist, C.D., Sell, S.L., Johnson, L.R., Donahue, K.C., et al. (2011). Practice guidelines for communicating a prenatal or postnatal diagnosis of Down syndrome: Recommendations of the national society of genetic counselors. *Journal of Genetic Counseling*; 20(5): 432–441. doi: 10.1007/s10897-011-9375-8

Skotko, B.G. (2005). Prenatally diagnosed down syndrome: Mothers who continued their pregnancies evaluate their health care providers. *American Journal of Obstetrics and Gynecology*; 192: 670–677.

Skotko, B.G., Levine, S.P., & Goldstein, R. (2011a). Having a son or daughter with down syndrome: Perspectives from mothers and fathers. *American Journal of Medical Genettics A*; 155A(10): 2335–2347. doi: 10.1002/ajmg.a.34293

Skotko, B.G., Levine, S.P., & Goldstein, R. (2011b). Having a brother or sister with Down syndrome: Perspective from siblings. *American Journal of Medical Genetics A*; 155A(10): 2348–2359. doi: 10.1002/ajmg.a.34228

Skotko, B.G., Levine, S.P., & Goldstein, R. (2011c). Self-perceptions from people with Down syndrome. *American Journal of Medical Genetics A*; 155A(10): 2360–2369. doi: 10.1002/ajmg.a.34235

Stroebe, M., & Schut, H. (1999). The dual process model of coping with bereavement: Rationale and description. *Death Studies*; 23: 197–224.

Titapant, V., & Chuenwattana, P. (2014). Psychological effects of fetal diagnoses of non-lethal congenital anomalies on the experience of pregnant women during the remainder of their pregnancy. *Journal of Obstetrical and Gynaecological Research*; Sept 26. doi: 10.1111/jcog.12504 [E pub ahead of print].

Turton, P., Hughes, P., Evans, C.D.H., & Fainman, D. (2001). Incidence, correlates and predictors of posttraumatic stress disorder in the pregnancy after stillbirth. *British Journal of Psychiatry*; 178: 556–560. doi: 10.1192/bjp.178.6.556

Viaux-Savelon, S., Dommergues, M., Rosenblum, O., Bodeau, N., Aidane, E., Philippon, O., et al. (2012). Prenatal ultrasound screening: False positive soft markers may alter maternal representations and mother-infant interaction. *Plos-ONE*; 7(1): e30935. doi: 10.1371/journal.pone.0030935

White-van Mourik, M.C.A., Connor, J.M., & Fersguson-Smith, M.A. (1992). The psychosocial sequelae of a second trimester termination of pregnancy for fetal anomaly. *Prenatal Diagnosis*; 12(3): 189–204.

Wittouck, C., Van Autreve, S., De Jaegere, E., Portzky, G., & van Heeringen, K. (2011). The prevention and treatment of complicated grief: A meta-analysis. *Clinical Psychology Review*; 31: 69–78. doi: 10.1016/j.cpr.2010.09.005

Wool, C. Systematic review of the literature: Parental outcomes after diagnosis of fetal anomaly. (2011). *Advances in Neonatal Care*; 11(3): 182–192.

Wortman, C.B. (2004). Posttraumatic growth: Progress and problems. *Psychological Inquiry*; 15: 81–90.

Wright, J. (2002). Transcendence: Phenomenological perspective of the mother's experience of having a child with a disability. (Doctoral dissertation, Widener University, 2002). *Dissertation Abstracts International*: 63–12B.

6

Miscarriage and Pregnancy Loss

Natalène Séjourné and Nelly Goutaudier

Current Scientific Knowledge

While contraceptive methods and medically assisted procreation have led to a better control of human reproduction, the course of pregnancy cannot be totally controlled. Despite medical progress, interruption of pregnancy is still quite common. Moreover, while late miscarriages and fetal deaths in utero are unusual, miscarriages or early termination of pregnancy are more frequent with prevalence rates ranging from 12% to 24% of pregnancies (Carter et al., 2007; Larsen, Christiansen, Kolte, & Macklon, 2013). Pregnancy loss is a difficult experience to cope with for future parents and, while quite common, being confronted to miscarriage appears to be a traumatic event for women. Indeed, even if abortion is very early and occurs when pregnancy is not yet visible, many women experience it as a loss of a future baby and have to mourn projects related to the baby-to-be. Thus, miscarriage might clearly be a difficult experience to cope with and, in addition to loss-related grief, many women develop anxiety and depressive symptoms. Surprisingly, despite their frequency and their psychological impact on women, miscarriages remain quite taboo and spontaneous abortions receive less attention compared with late fetal death. As such losses can impact well-being, and lead to psychopathological symptoms and feelings of loneliness, it appears of prime importance to focus on prevention and treatment that might be implemented to help women to cope with such event.

Miscarriages and Pregnancy Loss: Definition and Characteristics

Types of Miscarriage and Pregnancy Loss

While many definitions currently exist (see section: Pregnancy Loss Depending on the Countries: An Overview), miscarriage is considered as the expulsion (from the maternal organism) of an embryo or fetus before 22 weeks of gestation (Delabaere et al., 2014). Beyond this threshold, the fetus is considered as viable, and, as the fetus always dies in the uterus and is not expelled, it is referred to as stillbirth or intrauterine fetal death (Regan, 2001). Miscarriage is different from ectopic pregnancy in which the fetus is developing outside the uterus. This particular pregnancy is more risky for mothers, and requires more care than miscarriage. Even if the 20–22 weeks' gestation threshold was proposed – as many definitions currently exist – most of recent studies often use the 24-week threshold corresponding to clinical reality (Mandelbrot, 2003).

Miscarriage is a common condition, with rates as high as one in four pregnancies (Murphy, 1998). Studies have reported rates ranging from 15% to 20% depending on studies (Lok & Neugebauer, 2007; Ogden & Maker, 2004; Shelley Healy, & Grover, 2005). As early pregnancy loss is sometimes not detected, prevalence rates might be higher (Garcia-Enguidanos, Calle, Valero, Luna, & Dominguez-Rojas, 2002; Garel & Legrand, 2005; Maconochie, Doyle, Prior, & Simmons, 2007; Regan, 2001; Regan & Rai, 2000). Nevertheless, new techniques to diagnose pregnancy using hormonal dosing now allow one to detect miscarriages that would have been missed before – leading some authors to speculate higher rates up to 32% (Wang et al., 2003; Zinaman, O'Connor, Clegg, Selevan, & Brown, 1996). While Hemminki and Forssas (1999) have reported that 4% of women experienced more than one miscarriage, recurring miscarriage might only be considered if women had three consecutive miscarriages. Considering this definition, this type of miscarriage is relatively rare and only affects 0.5–1% of pregnancies (Exalto, 2005). It is important to note that miscarriage occurs differently depending on women. Some have bleeding as a warning sign of pregnancy loss (in most of the cases, they are not dangerous for women's health) while others have no warning signs and discover the termination of pregnancy during a routine ultrasound.

It is important to note that the majority of miscarriages are early. They occur before 12 weeks' gestation and do not affect more than 1–2% of pregnancies after this period (Regan & Rai, 2000). Intrauterine fetal deaths are even more uncommon with a worldwide prevalence of 2% of pregnancies (Quibel, et al., 2014). Moreover, the rate of stillbirth in high-income countries is between 1.3 and 8.8 per 1,000 births (Alderdice, 2017).

Box 6.1 Pregnancy Loss Depending on the Countries: An Overview

Changes in definitions of pregnancy losses and differences between countries sometimes make data difficult to compare. As Lee and Rowlands (2015) point out, legal definitions that distinguish miscarriage from stillbirth are different depending on the countries with, for instance, a threshold at 20 weeks of pregnancy in Australia and 24 weeks in the United Kingdom. The results also depend on the fact that we consider in priority the weight of the fetus less than or greater than 500 grams or the gestational age (Lawn et al., 2016).

In accordance with the WHO recommendations, the French legislation has changed the viability threshold from 28 to 22 weeks' gestation. Thus, from 22 weeks' gestation, or a weight greater than 500 grams, a child can be considered as "alive" and viable and receive a birth or death certificate. Considering this threshold, if the child is stillborn, a death certificated is delivered and funerals are possible (Garel & Legrand, 2005). Thus, this change in definition has led to an increase of stillbirth rate in France after 2002 (Serfaty, 2014).

In France, perinatal bereavement is defined as the process following the loss of a child between 22 weeks' gestation and the first seven days of life (Dayan, 1999). However, many authors emphasized that this restrictive definition may mask the psychic mechanisms developed in earlier pregnancy losses such as miscarriage or abortion and include them in perinatal losses (Dayan, 1999; Hanus, 2001; Leon, 1995; Wallerstedt & Higgins, 1996).

Several authors have highlighted the need to refine the definitions and terminologies of perinatal losses (Delabaere et al., 2014; Kolte et al., 2015) and in particular the term of abortion which is charged emotionally for the patients who prefer the term of miscarriage (Silver, Branch, Goldenberg, Iams, & Klebanoff, 2011).

Despite these scientific and methodological differences, it is also important to highlight the social and cultural differences related to pregnancy loss. Thus, the rate of stillbirth was 18.4 per 1,000 total births in 2015 (Lawn et al., 2016), and Alderdice (2017) states that this differs considerably from one country to another and that the vast majority of stillbirths occur in low- and middle-income countries. Moreover, the social consequences of stillbirth are not the same for all women, especially in low- and middle-income countries where women can be blamed for the loss of the unborn child and can then be excluded from the village, forced to divorce or abused (Burden et al., 2016; Heazell et al., 2016).

Perinatal Bereavement

Bereavement corresponds to the painful work of accepting loss (Bacqué, 1997). Bowlby (1984) describes four phases of bereavement that an individual experiences when confronted to the loss of a loved one. The numbing phase usually lasts from a few hours to a week and is characterized by a state of shock and difficulties accepting the new. The languishing phase is characterized by an awareness of the reality of loss and also by nostalgia, intense distress, and anger. Finally, the disorganization and despair phase is a necessary step for the loss to be recognized and for the re-organization phase to be started.

Generally, perinatal bereavement is well recognized and is related to the bereavement of a loved one. According to Bowlby (1984), despite the recent bond between parents and the baby, the pattern of reactions is quite similar to the one developed by individuals who have lost a spouse. Nevertheless, it was not until the 1980s that miscarriage was considered as a source of bereavement and that its effects were studied in terms of grief, anxiety, depression, stress, shame, and guilt (Frost, Bradley, Levitas, Smith, & Garcia, 2007). Indeed, the suffering experienced after an early perinatal loss suggests bereavement related to fetal (Dayan, 1999; Thomas, 1995) or a neonatal death (Leppert & Pahlka, 1984; Stirtzinger, Robinson, Stewart, & Ralevski, 1999).

During pregnancy, the child is a fantasy and the mother-to-be has a representation of her baby that is very different from its biological reality (Bydlowski, 2002; Flis-Trèves, 2004). The development of the fetus in the mother's fantasy does not always follow the physiological rhythm (Marinopoulos, 2005) and pregnant women often dream of a baby who does not correspond to the embryogenic fetus (Bydlowski). Early emotional investment, daydreams, and imaginary life about the upcoming child make the involuntary pregnancy loss a painful experience. Even though pregnancy is early, the baby may already be extremely present in the parents' life (Robinson, Baker, & Nackerud, 1999). The loss of an unborn child also symbolizes the loss of a new stage of life, or a dream (Kowalski, 1990). Although there is no relationship with the baby, this loss symbolizes the loss of strong emotional investment for parents (Oppenheim, 2002) and thus results in feeling of emptiness (Toedter, Lasker, & Aldaheff, 1988).

In addition, the evolution of Western societies and the advances in medicine have led to many changes in childbearing and have consequences regarding conception. It has also led to changes regarding the place of the baby-to-be and the significance of the loss (Flis-Trèves, 2004; Marino-poulos, 2005). As Medicine focuses on the very beginning of life, an early personalization of the fetus has thus occurred (Flis-Trèves, 2004). Ultrasound now allows a three- or four-dimensional view of the unborn baby and alters the perception of future parents. This image which is particularly difficult to forget for future parents confronted with the interruption of pregnancy.

Using interviews conducted on women who have experienced miscarriage, several authors have found that women are going through the same phases of bereavement described by Bowlby (Conway, 1995; Leppert & Pahlka, 1984). Pregnancy loss occurs on several levels. It is a real loss, with the loss of the embryo or the fetus, and also symbolic one, as it threatens the realization of the desire to have a child and the social status of being a mother (Flis-Trèves, 2004; Garel & Legrand, 2005). Moreover, given the feeling of omnipotence experienced by women during pregnancy, miscarriage can be experienced as a failure (Garel & Legrand). Perinatal bereavement can also be complicated by parents' sense of responsibility. The younger the baby, the more responsible the parents feel for their health and development, making grief more painful and source of guilt (Hanus, 2001).

Specificities of bereavement following miscarriage have to be acknowledged (Frost et al., 2007; Lok & Neugebauer, 2007; Rousseau, 1988). The absence of a person to bury and physical memories make it particularly difficult to cope with (Brier, 1999). According to Frydman (1997), bereavement without body is even more difficult as no representation exists, excluding a ceremony and possibilities of recollection. In addition, as early spontaneous abortion does not allow any registration, miscarriage is characterized by a lack of evidence (Roegiers, 2003) and a social "non-existence" (Bacqué, 1997).

Stirtzinger and Robinson (1989) emphasize the importance of bereavement and explain that suffering after a miscarriage is not a pathological reaction but rather a normal response to a significant loss. Rousseau (1988) suggests different psychological mechanisms that might lead grief to become pathological: absence of conscious grief or "denial", ambivalence and chronicity due to the persistence of anger. The period of psychological disturbance, the complexity of perinatal bereavement, the failure to recognize the importance of this loss, and the impossibility of elaboration can lead to a maintenance of sadness and thus cause personal and family difficulties (Bacqué, 1997; Lok & Neugebauer, 2007; Stirtzinger & Robinson, 1989).

Well-Being and Health

Miscarriage has clearly an impact on general health and well-being. Thus, six weeks after miscarriage, women reported more somatic symptoms than those who were pregnant (Thapar & Thapar, 1992). Warsop, Ismail, and Iliffe (2004) assessed well-being and psychological health in a female sample of 63 women after miscarriage and found that, using the General Health Questionnaire-30, 43% were considered as psychopathological "cases" immediately after the announcement of miscarriage and more than one-third (37%) were still considered as cases six weeks later. Janssen, Cuisinier, Hoogduin, and Graauw (1996) observed that six months after the termination of pregnancy, women (n = 227) had higher scores of depression, anxiety, and somatization than those who had given birth to an alive baby (n = 213). Garel et al. (1992) noted that three months after miscarriage, many women reported sleep disturbances, medical consultations for psychological difficulties, and use of medication (anxiolytics sleeping pills, antidepressants) vitamins or supplements. The use of sleeping pills was almost three times higher than in women with no history of miscarriage (29% vs. 11%).

Miscarriage, Pregnancy Loss, and Psychopathology

The experience of miscarriage is characterized by emptiness and guilt (Adolfsson et al., 2004), and women might experience several feelings and/or psychological conditions such as devastation, grief, trauma, dysphoria, fear, and injustice (Abboud & Liamputtong, 2003; Brier, 1999; Garel et al., 1992). The impact of miscarriage has been extensively studied in terms of psychopathology, and numerous studies have assessed grief, depressive, anxiety, or posttraumatic stress symptoms that may be developed as a result of spontaneous abortion. While the impact of a miscarriage can persist over an extended period of time (Klier, Geller, & Ritsher, 2002; Robinson, Stirtzinger, Stewart, & Ralevski., 1994), it seems that the intensity of emotional pain decreases over time (Cuisinier, Kuijpers, Hoogduin, Graauw, & Janssen, 1996; Janssen, Cuisinier, Graauw, & Hoogduin, 1997; Madden, 1994). Thus, one year after the loss, mental health of women who experienced perinatal loss is similar to those of women who gave birth to an alive baby (Janssen et al., 1996). Swanson,

Connor, Jolley, Pettinado, and Wang (2007) have reported a decrease in distress during the first six weeks following miscarriage but not beyond, suggesting a six-week crisis period.

Depression and Depressive Symptoms

Friedman and Gath (1989) were among the first to investigate psychiatric consequences of miscarriage and found that 48% of women reported depressive disorders assessed with the Present State Examination, which is four times more than women from community samples. As a result of miscarriage, 20–55% of women develop depressive symptoms (Lok & Neugebauer, 2007). Such symptoms usually develop during the first month and resolve during the following year (Carter et al., 2007). In China, a longitudinal study comparing 280 women who had miscarried with 150 non-pregnant women showed that women who experienced miscarriages had higher scores on General Health Questionnaire and Beck Depression Inventory than non-pregnant women. Nevertheless, differences were no longer significant at one year after the loss (Lok, Yip, Lee, Sahota, & Chung, 2010). It is important to note that hormonal postpartum fluctuations, associated with the vulnerability of developing depression, and hormonal changes after miscarriage may also increase the risk of depression (Carter et al.).

Experiencing one or more miscarriages would have a long-term negative impact on mental health and such impact has been found in several countries with no significant cultural differences. Indeed, women with a history of miscarriage are more likely to develop depressive symptoms and depression than others (Toffol, Koponen, & Partonen, 2013). Several authors reported that in the first days or weeks following the loss, the average score of depression is higher in women who experienced miscarriages than in women from community samples (Beutel, Rainer, von Rad, & Weiner, 1995; Broen, Moum, Bödtker, & Ekeberg, 2006; Robinson et al., 1994; Thapar & Thapar, 1992). Neugebauer et al. (1992b) reported that 15 days after their miscarriage, of the 282 women who completed questionnaires, 36.2% scored higher on the Center for Epidemiologic Studies Depression Scale Revised (CES-D). Two weeks after miscarriage, the proportion of women with significant depressive symptoms was 3.4 times higher compared to pregnant women and 4.3 times higher than among women from community samples (Neugebauer et al., 1992a). Women who experienced miscarriages still scored higher on the CES-D at two months following miscarriage than women from community samples (Neugebauer, 2003). Stirtzinger et al. (1999) reported that one year after miscarriage, 50% of the 119 women who completed questionnaires had a critical score on the CES-D. In developing countries (Bangladesh), a higher rate of depression has been found in women after perinatal loss compared to women who have given birth to an alive child (Gausia et al., 2011). A study conducted in Sri Lanka compared the risk of developing depression in a sample of 137 mothers who experienced miscarriage 6–10 weeks before the completion of questionnaires and in 137 pregnant women without a history of miscarriage in the past 12 months. The risk of developing depression was twice higher in women with a history of miscarriage, but this difference was no longer significant while taking into account age and weeks' gestation (Kulathilaka, Hanwella, & de Silva, 2016).

In France, an exploration of depressive symptoms from clinical interviews showed that two days after miscarriage, 43% of women showed an intense depressive reaction and three months later, 51% of women presented full criteria for depression according to the DSM-III (Garel et al., 1992). Six months after experiencing miscarriage, Neugebauer et al. (1997) found a prevalence of 10.9% in women who had a miscarriage ($n = 229$) vs. 4.3% in women from a community sample ($n = 230$). A prevalence of 5.2% of minor depression was found among women who had a miscarriage while only 1% of women from a community sample reported such symptoms (Klier, Geller, & Neugebauer, 2000). Regarding fetal death, the risk of depression was four times higher in women nine months after stillbirth or in women whose infant die within 28 days of life, compared with women who gave birth to an alive child (Gold, Leon, Boggs, & Sen, 2016).

Anxiety Symptomatology and Anxiety and Related Disorders

Anxiety is a common reaction with 20–40% of women reporting anxiety symptoms after miscarriage (Athey & Spielvogel, 2000; Lok & Neugebauer, 2007). Anxiety appears to develop immediately after miscarriage, decrease over the following six months, and return to its initial level one year later (Carter et al., 2007). As for depressive symptoms, women have higher scores of anxiety than women from community samples (Broen, Moum, Bödtker, & Ekeberg, 2006). After recurrent miscarriage (two or more), Roswell, Jongman, Kilby, Kirchmeier, and Orford (2001) observed that out of 37 women, 48.6% had an important anxiety score (> 11) five weeks after the loss, 29.7% ten weeks later, and 27% after sixteen weeks.

While anxiety symptoms have been widely assessed, few studies have focused on the prevalence of anxiety disorders. Using the Diagnostic Interview Schedule, Geller, Klier, and Neugebauer (2001) focused on such disorders among a sample of 229 women who experienced miscarriage and compared prevalence rates with 230 women from a community sample. Six months after miscarriage, the incidence of an anxiety episode (recurrent or not) such as panic disorder or phobic disorder was not significantly different between groups. However, women who had a miscarriage were significantly more likely to develop an obsessive-compulsive disorder. While the tendency of women to develop a panic disorder after pregnancy loss observed by Geller et al. was not significantly higher than community sample, Carter et al. (2007) noted that, clinically, it is not uncommon to observe women developing panic attacks after miscarriage. A recent study found that women who experienced perinatal loss (between 20 weeks' gestation and one month of life) had more characteristics of anxiety disorders than those who gave birth to a child nine months after the loss, especially for generalized anxiety disorder (GAD) and social phobia, which were twice as common among bereaved women (Gold, Boggs, Muzik, & Sen, 2014).

Anxiety and Depressive Symptoms: The Common Response

Many studies have been conducted on both anxiety and depressive symptoms using the Hospital Anxiety and Depression Scale (HADS). Paton, Wood, Bor, and Nitsun (1999) reported that, at four to six weeks following miscarriage, among the 38 women who completed questionnaires, 35% had an important symptomatology regarding anxiety and 9% reported high depressive symptoms. Walker and Davidson (2001) reported an average anxiety score of 7.6 at three weeks and three months after miscarriage ($n = 40$). Nikcevic et al. (1998a) assessed anxiety and depressive symptomatology in a sample of 204 women who experienced miscarriages.[1] Clinically anxiety and depression (HADS> 8) were observed in 45% and 15% of women respectively. Considering scores above 11, the percentages were 23% and 3%.

Prettyman et al. (1993) found that among 65 women, one week after miscarriage, 41% had a significant anxiety score and 22% had depression (score> 11). At six weeks, the percentage of anxiety cases decreased (18%) and increased at 12 weeks (32%), while the percentage of cases of depression decreased over time (8% and 6% respectively). Two years later, there was no significant difference, with 26% of women scoring above a threshold score of 11 for anxiety and none for depression (Cordle & Prettyman, 1994).

Grief and Bereavement

Grief following miscarriage is frequent with a prevalence rate of 40% in women developing such reaction (Athey & Spielvogel, 2000; Lok & Neugebauer, 2007). The main symptoms include sadness, nostalgia for the lost child, desire to talk about loss, and the search for an explanation (Lok & Neugebauer). Sadness is widely experienced with 67% of women reporting having felt very sad three weeks after the loss and 40% two to four months later (Conway & Russel, 2000). A study reported that of the 300 women who had a miscarriage, only 4% had no grief response, while the majority (75%) reported decrease of grief during the following month and 21% of women reported an unresolved reaction one month after the loss (Turner et al., 1991). Nikcevic et al. (1998a) reported that in a sample of 204 women who experienced miscarriage, the average grief score on the Expanded Texas Inventory of Grief (TGI; see "Operational Guidelines" for details on scales) was comparable to the one reported by individuals who lost a loved one. Beutel, Rainer, von Rad, and Weiner (1995) focused on distinguishing bereavement and depressive responses in a sample of 125 women who had experienced a miscarriage. For instance, 20% of women reported a bereavement reaction and sadness, grief for their loss, and desire to talk about it, and look for support and comfort. Depressive reactions affected 12% of women who also reported discouragement, irritability, ruminations, agitation, and high level of anxiety, with physical complaints and sleep disorders. Finally, 20% of women reported mixed reaction of grief and depression.

Complicated Grief: From Normal to Pathological Reactions

Complicated grief (CG) reactions after pregnancy loss are important to focus on as it differs from grief in many aspects. Unlike the expected grief following lost, CG is defined as prolonged and abnormal and involved excessive grieving, and preoccupying thought about the lost one (Wittouck, Van Autreve, De Jaegere, Portzky, & van Heeringen, 2011). CG symptoms last for at least one month after six months of bereavement (Shear et al., 2011). While CG is an unusual grief response, only occurring in 6–18% of bereaved individuals (Kersting, Brähler, Glaesmer, & Wagner, 2011; Prigerson et al., 2009), it is more common following child loss (Keesee, Currier, & Neimeyer, 2011). Such grief has been shown to be associated with lower quality of life, significant sleep disruption, somatic symptoms, and suicidal ideation (Latham, & Prigerson, 2004; Marques et al., 2013; Silverman et al., 2000). While depression, anxiety, and PTSD symptoms are commonly reported in women who have experienced a perinatal bereavement, a lack of empirical data remains on CG in perinatally bereaved women as well as its associated features. Nevertheless, CG following perinatal loss might be developed as a result of an intense feeling of "not having been able to take care of the baby", and intense ruminations (Frost & Condon, 1996). As in other grief reactions, a history of trauma and lack of perceived social support might lead women to develop CG (Black, Wright, & Limbo, 2015). A recent study has shown a prevalence of 12.4% in women suffering from CG following perinatal lost (McSpedden, Mullan, Sharpe, Breen, & Lobb, 2017).

Posttraumatic Stress Disorder Symptoms

Most women considered miscarriage as a very stressful event (Robinson et al., 1994; Stirtzinger et al., 1999). Wojnar, Swanson, and Adolfsson (2011) highlighted the importance of the loss of control which is of prime importance in the experience of miscarriage. Indeed, during a miscarriage, women have to face challenges and events that are beyond their control. In addition, it is important to note that 35% of women still felt pregnant one month after miscarriage (Friedman & Gath, 1989), and, two years following the loss, 68% were still upset when thinking about miscarriage (Cordle & Prettyman, 1994). Miscarriage is an unexpected event that can involve sudden pain, bleeding, hospitalization, and operation and thus constitute a physically traumatic event. Several authors have reported that miscarriage can lead to posttraumatic stress disorder (PTSD) (Born et al., 2006; Lee & Slade, 1996a; Tedstone & Tarrier, 2003). Based on interviews, Bowles et al. (2000) estimate about 10% of acute stress disorders and 1% of PTSD due to miscarriage.

In Norway, Broen et al. (2004) compared the psychological impact of miscarriage and voluntary termination of pregnancy. Ten days after the event, 47.5% of women who had a miscarriage reached the threshold score on the Impact of Event Scale compared to 30% in women who had an abortion. However, two years after the event, this percentage was 2.6 for women who experienced miscarriage, compared with 18.1% for women who had an abortion. Ten weeks after recurrent miscarriage (two or more), Roswell et al. (2001) found that the mean score on the IES for intrusion and avoidance was similar to individual showing stress. In England, Walker and Davidson (2001) showed that three weeks after discovering miscarriage during an ultrasound, in a sample of 40 women, 15% met the DSM-IV criteria for acute stress disorder and 35% met six of the seven criteria (structured clinical interview for dissociative disorders (SCID-D)). The mean score on the IES was 32.4 (intrusion 16.6 and avoidance 14.3) three weeks after miscarriage and 26.8 (intrusion 14.2 and avoidance 12.6) three months later. One study found that in a sample of women who had a miscarriage or an ectopic pregnancy, 28% met criteria for PTSD at one month after the loss and 38% at three months (Farren et al., 2016). In the Netherlands, Engelhard, van den Hout, and Arntz (2001) assessed PTSD symptoms among 113 women who experienced pregnancy loss. One month after the loss, the prevalence was 25% and the severity of symptoms was similar to the one observed in other trauma populations. This prevalence was 7% four months after the miscarriage. A large study comparing women who had experienced late pregnancy lost (stillbirth or infant death under 28 days of life) and live-birth mothers found that nine months after the loss, women who lost a baby were seven times more likely to develop PTSD than women who gave birth to an alive child (Gold, Leon, Boggs, & Sen, 2016).

Absence of Identified Cause and Feelings of Guilt

Early and sporadic miscarriage is a natural physiological process during which a pregnancy with an abnormality is interrupted. As Exalto (2005) highlighted, an important selection occurs before and immediately after implantation. As a consequence, 30% of pregnancy will be ended during the pre-implantation period, 30% after implantation (loss of pre-clinical pregnancy), 10% during the clinical period (miscarriage), and only 30% will result in childbirth. Egg chromosomal abnormalities are one of the most frequent causes of early miscarriages and are found in at least 50% of spontaneous abortions (Goddijn & Leschot, 2000; Stirrat, 1990). Early termination of pregnancy can also be caused by hormonal infection or disorder, while uterine malformations are the cause of late miscarriages (Lansac et al., 2000). Nevertheless it is important to note that the cause of a miscarriage is not always known (Garel & Legrand, 2005; Regan, 2001) and that 15–20% of spontaneous abortions remain unprovoked (Lansac et al., 2000).

The lack of medical explanation is particularly difficult for women (Séjourné, Callahan, & Chabrol, 2011) and many women feel guilty and look for possible causes of their miscarriage (Séjourné, et al.). The search for meaning is central when a person has to cope with a stressful event. The fundamental beliefs about the self, others, and the world have been changed and many people will try to find "why such an event has happened" (Janoff-Bulman, 1992). Accepting the loss is particularly important in facilitating the grieving process (Parkes & Weiss, 1983). This search for meaning is very common in early pregnancy loss (Maker & Ogden, 2003; Nikčević et al., 1998; Simmons, Singh, Maconochie, Doyle, & Green, 2006) and is generally associated with more psychological distress (Jind, 2003; Nikčević & Nicolaides, 2014). Women's roles regarding the cause of their miscarriage seem to be related to their reactions. Several studies have suggested that women who felt responsible for miscarriage had more intense emotional distress than others (James & Kristiansen, 1995; Robinson et al., 1994; Stirtzinger, et al., 1999). Warsop et al. (2004) showed that women who had a "personalized" explanation questioned activities that they considered as negative were more likely to develop disturbance in well-being than those who had physical explanations. Likewise, women who attributed their miscarriage to a medical problem were less anxious than others (Tunaley, Slade, & Duncan, 1993). Although knowing the cause of miscarriage does not seem to have a positive impact on the evolution of women's mood (Nikcevic, Kuczmierczyk, Tunkel, & Nicolaides, 2000; Roswell et al., 2001), Nikcevic, Tunkel, and Nicolaides (1999a) found that women for whom the cause of miscarriage was identified reported less self-accusations than others. Looking for a cause was reported to have a negative impact, as the level of anxiety among women who did not have an explanation remained high, whereas it declined for those who knew the cause (Nikcevic, 2003). Providing medical information seems to help women to find meaning in the pregnancy loss (Nikčević & Nicolaides, 2014).

Impact on Family and Personal Life

Interruption of pregnancy affects not only the mother but also the entire family. Having children at the time of pregnancy loss might have a positive impact on the way miscarriage is experienced or, on the contrary, a negative once (Thomas, 1995). Children's reactions following the termination of their mother's pregnancy have been widely documented (Cain, Erickson, Fast, & Vaughan, 1964; Rousseau, 1995). Some children are too young to understand but may be affected by change in their parents' behaviors and show signs of discomfort. O'Leary and Gaziano (2011) focused on consequences of a perinatal loss for siblings. Children are confronted to two losses and have to mourn their little brother or sister and also mourn their parents as the parents they used to be before the loss. Indeed, parents might be overwhelmed by their own grief and do not realize their children's sadness. Children might then play a special role by filling their parents' need for love and overprotection (Garel & Legrand, 2005).

Miscarriage can have long-term consequences on women's relationships. Some may feel fragile and vulnerable while others may be more distant and less sensitive (Garel & Legrand, 2005). Stirtzinger et al. (1999) found that 16.5% of women reported difficulties with their spouses and 28.9% with their families three months after the miscarriage, and 8.4% and 19% a year later. While the majority of women were supported by their spouses and friends, Conway (1995) argued that they did not feel encouraged to talk about their miscarriage by the community (neighbors, colleagues, etc.). Flis-Trèves (2004) mentions the silence surrounding miscarriages. Indeed, women's feelings of failure and guilt are often misunderstood and minimized.

Many authors have shown the differences between men and women that might play a role in couple's issues. Thus, if the death of their child results in a special bond, parent's reactions differ in duration, in intensity, in parental attachment, and in the way to cope with loss (Wallerstedt & Higgins, 1996). According to Beutel, Willner, Deckardt, Von Rad, and Weiner (1996), 75% of women reported that their spouse was sympathetic immediately after the loss but not necessarily afterward, while 14% of spouses did not talk about the event. If some men internalize their grief in order not to become a burden for their spouse, others, frustrated at being unable to arrange things, become irritable (Herz, 1984). Swanson, Karmali, Powell, and Pulvermakher (2003) found that miscarriage affected interpersonal and sexual relationships. Thus, one year after the event, women reported being more distant socially (32%) or sexually (39%) and 26% of women said they were closer. In a Portuguese study, Serrano and Lima (2006) found that while the couple relationships were not affected by recurrent miscarriages, there were some changes in sexual relationship. Of the 294 women who had a miscarriage, 16.5% reported difficulties with their spouses following the loss (Stirtzinger et al., 1999). According to the study by Defrain, Millspaugh, and Xie (1996), while 61% of the 193 respondents reported that their couple was stronger due to miscarriage, 11% observed a deterioration in marital life, and 1.5% divorced. Another study found that 12% of couples broke up as a result of pregnancy loss (Aerde, 2001). Marital difficulties, especially because of the differences in the way of experiencing grief, have also been reported as a result of stillbirth (Burden et al., 2016). A review and meta-analysis (Burden et al.) underline that stillbirth can lead to social isolation as some bereaved parents will avoid activities leading them to be in contact with babies or with elements reminding them of the loss of their unborn child.

What about Men?

Most of research works have been conducted on women sample and the experience of men has been largely ignored (Murphy, 1998; Puddifoot & Johnson, 1999). While fathers' reactions were mentioned in one study in 1964 (Cain et al., 1964), they were not fully studied until 1976 (Rousseau, 1995). A literature review found that only four studies focusing on depressive symptomatology in a male sample after a miscarriage were conducted. One month after pregnancy loss, 5–17% of men were suffering from depressive symptoms and this prevalence decreased afterward (Lewis & Azar, 2015). In their comparative study conducted on 56 couples, Beutel et al. (1996) found that 10% of men and 29% of women had a high depression score. One month after miscarriage, Cumming et al. (2007) observed a prevalence of clinical anxiety (> 11) in 28.3% of women and in 12.4% of men and high depression score was found in 10% of women and 4% of men. Immediately after the miscarriage, 43.4% of the male sample had high GHQ-12 scores. These scores decreased significantly during the first three months. While lower scores were found compared to women, some men might reported scores suggesting psychological distress (Kong, Chung, Lai, & Lok, 2010). Johnson and Baker (2004) have shown that, in men samples, miscarriage is often associated with short-term negative emotional outcomes.

Despite role change in the family, men believe that they are expected to be emotionally strong and capable of coping with their feelings (Kimble, 1991; McGreal, Evans, & Burrows, 1997). Nevertheless, several qualitative studies have shown the suffering of men after miscarriage (Lacroix, Got, Callahan, & Séjourné, 2016; McCreight, 2004). Indeed, even if the unborn child may seem unreal to men given the lack of physical reality (DiMarco, Menke, & McNamara, 2001), fathers attachment would develop before birth (McGreal et al., 1997). As a consequence, they would experience an amount of grief that is comparable to the one reported by women (Kohn & Moffitt, 1992). However, the majority of participants from McCreight's study (2004) reported that their grief had been neglected by society, generating negative affects such as anger or despair. According to a phenomenological study conducted on five participants (Murphy, 1998), the first emotions reported by men, such as shock or skepticism, then lead to anger, suffering, frustration, guilt, or relief and solitude. Several qualitative studies have shown that negative affects are frequently related with the presence of shock or sideration during the announcement of the termination of pregnancy and a feeling of emptiness following the loss (Lacroix et al., 2016; McCreight, 2004; Murphy, 1998). In a qualitative study, Murphy highlighted feelings of sadness and loss evoked by men that add to the difficulty of seeing their spouse suffer. Most of men recognize that their spouses have more intense feelings and identify their primary role as support (Lacroix et al.; Miron & Chapman, 1994). Many men would feel the need to suppress their emotions in order to support their spouses (Lacroix et al.; Miron & Chapman; Murphy) and some men would find it especially difficult to be unable to support their spouse as they would like to (Lacroix et al., 2016). According to Mouras and Brun (2003), it is the repression of the feminine dimension of paternity and the identification of men with social roles that would lead them to internally live the grief. While Fréchette (1997) reported that this attitude is aimed at supporting their wives and being a contributing figure, a lack of communication in the couple is a factor of vulnerability (Schaap et al., 1997).

Several studies have focused on coping strategies developed by spouses to cope with the termination of pregnancy (Armstrong, 2001; DeVille, Reilly & Callahan, 2012; Johnson & Baker, 2004;

Kersting & Wagner, 2012; Murphy, 1998) and highlighted some differences between men and women (Kerstin & Wagner). While women use problem-oriented strategies with a search for increased social support (Stinson, Lasker, Lohman, & Toedter, 1992), men would seek less social support (Johnson & Baker, 2004). Men tend to avoid conversation and look for distraction rather than talking about loss (Beutel et al., 1996). They also tend to intellectualize (Lang, Gottlieb, & Amsel, 1996), internalize, and deny their grief (Kersting et al., 2004). However, some men would seek activities that would allow them to think about the situation and their occupations would then be considered as coping strategies and not as a flight (Armstrong, 2001). A number of men seem to hide their feelings (Kimble, 1991; Lacroix et al., 2016; McGreal et al., 1997). Rinehart and Kiselica (2010) highlighted that hiding or avoiding emotions is not an indicator of absence of grief. According to these authors, men are encouraged to do so by society and individuals around them, and it is appears of prime importance for health professionals to consider men's needs following miscarriage.

As in women, a great variability in the emotions and reactions can be observed (Abboud & Liamputtong, 2003; Lacroix et al., 2016; Séjourné, Chabrol, & Callahan, 2009) and some men, picturing themselves becoming a father at the time of birth, report not feeling concerned by miscarriage which might be considered as a defense mechanisms such as repression or suppression. While not always intentional, hiding some indicators of grief would lead to a misjudgment of their own experiences (McCreight, 2004). Jaoul et al. (2013) highlighted that a number of men experiencing recurrent miscarriages would have particularly defensive personality profiles showing a restriction of affects that might be a factor of additional suffering for their spouse and/or themselves. It seems that men are more likely to develop chronic sadness when they do not receive enough support and understanding (Lasker & Toedter, 1991) and that not expressing grief openly would lead to negative symptoms (McCarthy, 2002). It is therefore important to encourage men to share their emotions and to talk about their experiences. Given the needs expressed by men (Khan, Drudy, Sheehan, Harrison, & Geary, 2004), it appears necessary to include spouses in support interventions following a miscarriage (DiMarco et al., 2001; Jaoul et al., 2013).

Subsequent Pregnancy: A Particular Step

Pregnancy loss is a major event that can have an impact on the experience of the subsequent pregnancy as well as on the parental attitudes toward the child to come (Lamb, 2002). Pregnancy following stillbirth is particularly difficult for parents who experience a wide range of emotions such as depressive symptoms but also panic, anxiety, or optimism. Parents also mention their inability to experience the normal excitement of pregnancy and can isolate themselves and stay away from other parents (Burden et al., 2016). The delay between miscarriage and new pregnancy is particularly important. Rousseau (1988) mentions the problem of "the replacement child" and the fact that when the pregnancy occurs quickly after the loss, it can disturb the bereavement of the lost child and be experienced as the continuity of the previous pregnancy. Carter et al. (2007) emphasized that while health professionals often recommend a period of six months, women seem to choose to get pregnant when they feel ready. Thus, the majority of women are pregnant again within one year of miscarriage (Klier et al., 2005). Cordle and Prettyman (1994) observed that two years after their miscarriage, 80% of the 50 women interviewed had once again become pregnant. However, 16% decided not to become pregnant. Garel et al. (1994) also observed that 18 months after their miscarriage, some women did not want to become pregnant nor had ambivalent feelings related to health problems or fear of another failure. The sadness and depression caused by miscarriage make it difficult for women to consider pregnancy immediately after the loss (Garel & Legrand, 2005). Nevertheless, it is important to note that a positive impact of a new pregnancy was also demonstrated. Franche and Bulow (1999a) observed that women who were pregnant again after perinatal loss had less grief and coping difficulties than others. However, the persistence of grief indicated that the grieving process was not disturbed by a new pregnancy. Carter et al. (2007) emphasize the importance of treating depression before a new pregnancy and the need for specific support.

The experience of pregnancy after a miscarriage is of prime importance and several authors have highlighted the importance of anxiety (Côté-Arsenault, Hill, & Mahlangu, 1999; Geller, Kerns, & Klier, 2004). Indeed, parents are then confronted with mixed feelings of hope and worry about pregnancy (DeBackere, Hill, & Kavanaugh, 2008). A qualitative study has shown that while pregnant women with a history of one or more miscarriages try to distance themselves from their new pregnancy, they also focus on symptoms related to pregnancy and seek information about their pregnancy. The well-being of the baby and their ability to cope with another loss appear to be one of the most important concern (Côté-Arsenault, Bidlack, & Humm, 2001). Pregnant women after perinatal loss have higher scores of anxiety, depression, and grief than those without a history of pregnancy loss (Gaudet, Séjourné, Camborieux, Rodgers, & Chabrol, 2010). Likewise, couples with a history of perinatal loss report significantly more depressive symptoms and pregnancy-related anxiety than others (Franche & Mikail, 1999). One study found that during pregnancy following stillbirth, among the 66 women who participated, 59 reported that stillbirth was a traumatic event and 21% met full criteria for PTSD during the third trimester of pregnancy and 4% a year after the birth of their healthy baby (Turton, Hughes, Evans, & Fainman, 2001). A qualitative study found that fathers also expressed anxiety during pregnancy as a result of perinatal loss (Armstrong, 2001). Moreover, women who experienced neonatal loss had more grief than those who experienced miscarriage or intrauterine death during the subsequent pregnancy (Hutti, Armstrong, & Myers, 2013).

The impact of loss seems to extend beyond pregnancy as women with a history of miscarriage are more likely to develop depression at one month postpartum than women without antecedent (Bicking, Kinsey, Baptiste-Roberts, Zhu, & Kjerulff, 2015). If the negative impact of stillbirth on quality of life was not reported in all studies, recent research emphasizes that stillbirth can significantly alter self-esteem, identity, the relationship to life and death, or the feeling of parental control over pregnancy, parenting, and child-rearing (Heazell et al., 2016). The number of miscarriages and utero fetal death significantly predict depressive and anxiety symptoms during the subsequent pregnancy and this association was reported to persist after the birth of a healthy child (Robertson Blackmore et al., 2011). Tsartsara and Johnson (2006) found that while pregnancy-related anxiety was higher during the first trimester of pregnancy, there was no difference in prenatal attachment. In addition, during the third trimester of pregnancy there was no significant difference in anxiety but attachment had considerably increased for all women. However, a Jordanian study showed that grief was negatively correlated with attachment to the child born after perinatal loss (Al-Maharma, Abujaradeh, Mahmoud, & Jarrad, 2016). More than half of pregnant women after perinatal loss would develop an emotional cushioning mechanism to deal with anxiety and doubt associated with this new pregnancy and to avoid the prenatal bonding given the fear of another loss (Côté-Arsenault & Donato, 2011).

Certain dates are particularly important during the subsequent pregnancy (Côté-Arsenault & Mahlangu, 1999) and the fear of repetition disappears or decreases after the anniversary of miscarriage (Garel & Legrand, 2005). During a pregnancy following a perinatal loss, ultrasound is particularly important and can be a reminder of traumatic memories. It is especially important for parents to be prepared for this reminder process (O'Leary, 2005). Geller et al. (2004) evidenced that while it is totally common for women with a history of perinatal loss to be more anxious about the possibility of another loss, the subsequent pregnancy does not necessarily lead to psychopathological outcomes.

Box 6.2 Focus on Medical Termination of Pregnancy (MTP)

While new investigative techniques, such as ultrasound or amniocentesis, can confirm the "normality" of the fetus and allow the continuation of gestation without worry, it can lead to the diagnosis of a fetal abnormality, impacting the parental couples' projects. Confronted to the anomaly of their child, whether or not allowing life, parents may decide to interrupt the course of pregnancy at any stage. They will no longer have to consider the life of the child but its death, and will be confronted with the bereavement of a human being that they have never seen, but desired and invested. MTP is considered as a trauma as the brutality of the drama can lead to a state of shock (Kersting et al., 2004). Many studies have been conducted on depressive and anxiety symptoms following MTP. While some authors have reported that only 10% of women would develop severe and persistent psychological disorders (Zolese & Blacker, 1992), others reported higher prevalence rates. Thus, based on a qualitative study, Rousseau and Fierens (1994) found that a quarter of women reported pathological mourning, and many reported disruptions in their relationships with their children and partner. Likewise, Connor, Ferguson-Smith, and White-van Mourik (1992) found that two years after the MTP, 20% of women still reported crying, sad mood, and irritability. Hunfeld, Wladimiroff, and Passchier (1997) detected 38% of clinically significant distress four years after the interruption. For Legros (2001), their pain and thoughts would be the only reminder of the existence of their child and would allow them to preserve a bond. Risk of complicated grief (CG) is especially high after termination of a pregnancy due to fetal abnormality (Kersting & Wagner, 2012).

While showing the difficult experience of MTP, interviews also reveal the importance for women to feel like being mothers and to be considered as such. Thus, between the announcement and the medical intervention, the pregnancy is reinvested and is pleasantly lived (Gaudet, Séjourné, Allard, & Chabrol, 2008).

Operational Guidelines

Support and Care Following Perinatal Loss

Historically, perinatal loss was not considered as a significant loss. The dead baby was immediately taken away from the parents and medication was given to the mother in order to soothe her pain. The WHO recommends to help parents facing the reality by confronting the loss. Currently, the usual practice in hospitals and maternity wards aims to promote better recovery after loss. Thus, multidisciplinary teams provide support and assistance to plan the period after hospitalization (Bennett, Litz, Sarnoff Lee, & Muguen, 2005). It is usual to facilitate the grieving process by encouraging parents to have direct contacts with the dead baby, such as seeing or holding it, and memories are sometimes offered to parents such as a picture, a lock of hair, or a foot print. Assistance may also be provided by a chaplain or social worker to deal with the grieving process or to organize the funeral (Bennett et al.). Discussion groups can sometimes be proposed as well as a follow-up by a counselor or a psychologist.

Hughes, Turton, Hopper, and Evans (2002) compared anxiety, depressive, and PTSD symptoms in pregnant women as a result of perinatal loss based on whether or not they chose to see and/or to hold the baby. The results suggest that in a sample of 65 women, those who did not see or hold their baby in the arms had few symptoms than others during the subsequent pregnancy. Gauthier (1993) find a significant correlation between depressive symptoms and the lack of visualization and physical contact with the dead baby. This meeting allows parents to face the reality of the event (Bacqué, 1995; Rousseau, 1988), to perceive the baby as real, and to constitute and collect memories of its existence (Bennett et al., 2005). After an abortion, the encounter with the child and the rituals in the mourning process seem particularly important (Gaudet et al., 2008). Frydman (1997) emphasizes the importance of rituals and accompaniment in the symbolic elaboration. Given their structuring dimension, all these concrete or symbolic steps have been able to help the majority of mothers in the elaboration of grief (Mouras, 2003). However, their absence following a medical termination of pregnancy has been reported to be a risk factor for emotional instability and anxiety and depressive symptomatology (Payne, Kravitz, Notman, & Anderson, 1976).

Bennett et al. (2005) reported that these experiences may also force parents to confront intense feelings of sadness, grief, and/or shock in a potentially premature way, which may be non-therapeutic. Thus, standardized applications of perinatal bereavement management may disrupt an individual's or a couple's adaptation (Bennett et al.). However, it is important to note that the potential consequences of loss require some vigilance or intervention. Hughes and Riches (2003) suggest the need to take into account the cultural and social contexts of loss when taking care of bereaved parents. These differences may explain the variations in responses to usual care. Indeed, while, in some cultures, seeing the dead baby and having certain rituals may be therapeutic, in other cultures, seeing or touching the baby may be associated with beliefs, superstitions, or negative meanings.

For Bennett et al. (2005), following the announcement of a perinatal loss, meeting the couples before birth for allowing them to talk about the shock, fear, and surprise associated with the loss of their fetus, could be beneficial. It is also an opportunity to anticipate childbirth and its aftermath, including whether parents will want to see, hold, and/or name the child. After childbirth, focusing on the parents' experience related to these decisions is important, as well as mentioning practical aspects such as funerals, how to announce the news to the loved ones and possible siblings. Depending on the couple's characteristics (psychiatric history, coping mechanisms), psycho-education can be provided as well as recommendations on what the couple may have to face during the following weeks and months following the loss. Information on how to find support, both formal and informal, can also be addressed and telephone follow-up may be considered.

Scales for Screening

For assessing distress following the termination of pregnancy, some scales might be used. While psychopathology following miscarriage has been widely assessed using scales used in clinical practice and psychological research to measure depressive, anxiety symptoms, or traumatic responses, other scales specific to loss, bereavement, and grief can be used.

The Perinatal Grief Scale (Potvin, Lasker, & Toedter, 1989; Toedter, Lasker, & Janssen, 2001) is based on the different dimensions of grief mentioned in the literature. It assesses grief, coping difficulties and despair through 33 items. While this scale has been used in many studies, the use of certain terms is not necessarily appropriate following premature loss of pregnancy.

The Impact of Miscarriage Scale (Swanson, 1999a) consists of 24 items divided into four factors (devastating event, loss of a baby, personal meaning, and isolation).

The Perinatal Grief Intensity Scale (Hutti, dePacheco, & Smith, 1998) is based on a theoretical model and a qualitative study and allows us to study factors that might influence the intensity of grief using 14 items. This questionnaire is specific to loss during early pregnancy and allows us to evaluate the meaning of loss and the intensity of grief.

The Texas Grief Inventory Adjusted for Miscarriage (Nikcevic, Snijders, & Nicolaides, 1999b) is a modified version of the Texas Grief Inventory (Zisook, Devaul, & Click, 1982), adapted for miscarriage and including 17 items. Three sub-scales can be used to measure grief, feelings of grief, and perceived miscarriage. The authors emphasize the neutrality of the language of the tool and the fact that it measures both universal aspects of the experience of mourning and others typical of this loss.

Satisfaction and Relationships with Caregiver

It is important to note that care following miscarriage might vary depending on the type of loss. Indeed, while some women have to experience curettage or aspiration as outpatients, others take a medication to induce the expulsion. Nevertheless, the type of care does not seem to have any impact on women's psychological distress (Neugebauer et al., 1992b; Nielsen, Hahlin, Möller, & Granberg, 1996), on satisfaction (Kong et al., 2013) or on the intensity of depressive and/or anxiety symptoms (Neugebauer et al., 1997; Walker & Davidson, 2001). Adolfsson, Berterö, and Larsson (2006) found that women whose miscarriage was found during an ultrasound experienced more grief than others. As a result of perinatal loss, women are hospitalized in ambulatory care or in a gynecology or maternity ward. Maternal hospitalization may be difficult to cope with, as women have to be confronted with their pregnancy (Cecil, 1994). While several authors have highlighted that some women are satisfied with care provided by the medical staff (Lasker & Toedter, 1994; Paton et al., 1999), some women report lack of emotional support and sensitivity (Cuisinier et al., 1993; Lasker & Toedter, 1991; Paton et al., 1999). One Australian qualitative study showed that lack of information, insensitive comments, and lack of empathy during hospitalization are the most negative aspects of women's experience following miscarriages (Rowlands & Lee, 2010b). Some authors observed that while women needed to talk about it, the medical staff did not question them much about how they experienced miscarriages (Conway & Russel, 2000; Conway, 1995). The need for follow-up, more information, and specific responses regarding the implications of miscarriage are often warranted by women (Cecil, 1994; Wong, Crawford, Gask, & Grinyer, 2003). According to Brier (1999), given the anger and disappointment, women feel and need to get rid of these feelings, and some of them may perceive the medical staff as insensitive. In addition, medical staff have to deal with their own feelings and disappointments and thus have a negative attitude such as aggressiveness or avoidance (Brier; Rousseau, 2001). Corbet-Owen and Kruger (2001) suggest that medical staff are often more sensitive to physical symptoms than emotional concerns, and that listening to women can be difficult. In addition, it is important to note that while caregivers recognize the importance of post-miscarriage support, they do not necessarily perceive themselves as competent enough to support them (Prettyman & Cordle, 1992; Wong et al., 2003).

Given the frequency of miscarriages, there may be a significant gap between the experience of women and daily practice of medical staff (Cecil, 1994; Garel & Legrand, 2005; Rousseau, 1995; Simmons et al., 2006). Although miscarriage standardization exists, it may be perceived by patients as a lack of empathy (Wong et al., 2003). A Chinese study found that medical staff were not always aware of the psychological impact of miscarriage and considered it as less important than postpartum depression while patients going to hospital for an ultrasound estimated that women may be seriously psychologically affected by miscarriage (Kong, Lok, Lam, Yip, & Chung, 2010). Prettyman et al. (1993) noted that women who experienced miscarriage are less satisfied with the care received than those who experienced a later pregnancy loss. One of the difficulties experienced by women following their miscarriage may be related to the loss of the prenatal care status. Despite the lack of action, several authors insist on the importance of physicians to dedicate time to help these patients (Frydman, 1997; Rongières-Bertrand, 1997). Brown (1991) highlighted the emotional, cognitive, and instrumental elements that the medical staff can provide to help parents to cope with perinatal loss. Corbet-Owen and Kruger (2001) emphasized the need for women to see their thoughts and feelings validated by the medical staff. The role of caregivers is also to help couples to recognize, understand, and cope with their partner's grief (Corbet-Owen, 2003). An Australian longitudinal study of 998 women following miscarriage revealed that satisfaction with primary care was associated with higher mental health scores (Rowlands & Lee, 2010a).

Need for Intervention

According to studies focusing on women's need, more than 90% of women would like support for their miscarriage (Nikcevic et al., 1998a, Séjourné, Callahan, & Chabrol, 2010a). Moreover, more than one-third of women would consider emotional support (Nikcevic et al., 1998a) or psychological support (Garel et al., 1992; Séjourné, et al., 2010a) as very useful to cope with miscarriage. Women would also report a lack of information about pregnancy loss and difficulties in managing emotions related to pregnancy loss (Séjourné, et al., 2010a). Despite women's need for support, only a few seek for professional care. For instance, few women attended support group (Tunaley et al., 1993) or engaged themselves in an association for sharing experiences with women who have been through the same experience (Nikcevic et al., 1998a) and seeking help from a clinical psychologist or a psychiatrist is not that common (Garel & Legrand, 2005; Séjourné et al., 2010a).

Nevertheless, given the traumatic impact of the event, the usefulness of specific support after a miscarriage is widely documented in the literature (Lee & Slade, 1996b). In the perspective of a subsequent pregnancy, it is particularly important to evaluate bereavement (Wallerstedt, Lilley, & Baldwin, 2003) and difficulties experienced by each couple such as the reminiscences of prior losses (Touvenot, 2004). Molénat (2001) highlighted the need for prevention in the perinatal field. In this preventive approach, Dollander and de Tychey (2000, 2002) suggested that psychological support should be provided immediately after the event and not as a result of the first complications. Such approach would help to avoid the development of rigid defenses, and would allow one to prevent feelings of loneliness from developing. It would also help in establishing empathy and promoting the symbolization of loss. Garel and Legrand (2005) emphasized that it is not about dramatizing the situation or "psychiatrizing" it, but simply about "offering an opportunity to women who want to be heard" (177). Rousseau (1995) explained that the help that should be provided following miscarriage would have to "make women aware of the reality of the loss, express emotions, especially guilt (which is important to make rid of), and to reassure the couple on its subsequent fertility".

Support Interventions: What We Can Offer

It is now acknowledged that specific support interventions have to be developed. Leppert and Pahlka (1984) reported that couples who attended two psychological sessions and a telephone follow-up were able to express their feelings and felt relieved to see their feelings normalized. Carrera et al. (1998) demonstrated the effectiveness of a one-year psychological follow-up on the intensity of depressive symptomatology following perinatal loss.

Regarding miscarriage, two studies conducted in the United Kingdom evaluated the effectiveness of a specialized clinic. Findings showed a positive impact of a consultation with a specialist, addressing causes of abortion and another one with a caregiver (psychologist or midwife) managing emotional distress on well-being. Roswell et al. (2001) conducted a follow-up study on 37 women after recurrent miscarriage and were unable to observe the effectiveness of the intervention given that, except for avoidance, the symptomatology had decreased before the intervention. However, Nikcevic (2003) found that the psychological morbidity of the 283 women who attended the consultation was less important than the one reported in the literature. In order to evaluate the effects of both medical and psychological intervention separately, they compared the measures of women who only had one type on consultation (psychological vs. medical) with a control group. Women who received one type of support showed less grief, guilt, and worry during the subsequent pregnancy compared with those from the control group. However, it is important to note that few controlled and randomized studies have examined the effectiveness of support to reduce the psychological morbidity of women experiencing miscarriage. Swanson (1999a) tested the effectiveness of a specific management of three sessions allowing women to discuss their experience and difficulties during the first few months following loss and such intervention appeared to have a positive impact on emotional disorders, depressive symptoms, and anger. Adolfsson, Larsson, Wijma, and Berterö (2006) compared two types of follow-up with a midwife, —three to four weeks after a miscarriage. In the structured consultation, women were encouraged to talk about their experiences and emotions, while in the "classical" follow-up, midwives asked questions about women's health and consequences of miscarriage. Four months after the miscarriage, women who received the structured consultation reported less grief that those who were asked about health and consequences.

Lee, Slade, and Lygo (1996b) focused on the effectiveness of a one session psychological debriefing on the emotional adaptation of 39 women who had experienced an early miscarriage. Four months after miscarriage, no differences were found between women who received the intervention and women from the control group regarding anxiety and depressive symptoms. In the United States, given that prior findings have suggested that such intervention might have a positive impact on depressive symptoms, Neugebauer et al. (1992a) have studied the effectiveness of a telephone support intervention. The effectiveness of telephone-based interpersonal support for women who have experienced miscarriage was tested within the last 18 weeks in a sample of women who have developed depressive symptoms. Women could then benefit, according to their wishes, from one to six sessions conducted by a psychologist and focusing on psycho-education of depression and interpersonal difficulties. Findings were promising as such intervention decreased depressive symptoms. Lok and Neugebauer (2007) have tested the effectiveness of follow-up by a nurse (support and educational component) immediately and two weeks after miscarriage in 280 randomized women. Although fewer women in the support group showed psychological distress three months after miscarriage, the difference was not significant. Swanson, Chen, Graham, Wojnar, and Petras (2009) compared several types of care for couples suffering from depressive symptoms and grief following miscarriage and three nursing sessions appeared the most efficient. Johnson and Langford (2010) tested the effectiveness of a supportive intervention among 40 women with early pregnancy loss. Women who received the intervention had less despair than those who received the usual care. Côté-Arsenault, Krowchuk, Schwartz, and McCoy (2014) tested the feasibility and acceptability of an intervention based on several components: home visits, "pregnancy journal", and learning tasks aiming to reduce anxiety resulting from perinatal loss. Such intervention appeared to be useful for women.

A preliminary study has also demonstrated the efficacy of individual cognitive behavioral therapy (CBT) to reduce anxiety and depression in women with recurrent miscarriages (Nakano, Akechi, Furukawa, & Sugiura-Ogasawara, 2013). A randomized controlled trial demonstrated the effectiveness of appropriate interpersonal psychotherapy for major depressive disorders following perinatal loss (Johnson et al., 2016).

Interpersonal Psycho-Therapy (IPT) Following Miscarriage

It is now acknowledged that cognitive behavioral therapy (CBT) and interpersonal psycho-therapy (IPT) (see Cuijpers, Donker, Weissman, Ravitz, & Cristea, 2016; Karyotaki et al., 2017; for meta-analytic reviews) are two of the most efficient empirically based psychotherapeutic interventions for mood disorders. For the last decades, a growing attention has been paid to IPT. Even though different types of IPT currently exist, IPT has been reported to be a time-limited treatment (acutely, 12–16 weeks) divided into three phases: a beginning (one to three sessions) phase, a middle phase, and an end phase (three sessions). Considering the high prevalence of depressive disorders following miscarriage, a recent pilot study has tested the efficacy of such treatment on major depressive disorder (MDD) following miscarriage (Johnson et al., 2016). IPT consisted in group sessions divided into several sessions focusing on four topics: (1) the emotions related to grief, (2) understanding what happened, (3) grieving with others, and (4) holding the memory and moving forward. Findings showed that IPT was feasible and an acceptable treatment for MDD following miscarriage. IPT was reported to reduce depressive and PTSD symptoms.

The Internet: A New Way to Help Women?

Interestingly, the Internet provided new opportunities to obtain information and provide support following perinatal loss. Indeed, using the Internet as a source of information is quite common and it has been shown that medical staff would encourage women to use the Internet appropriately to secure information (Geller, Psaros, & Kerns, 2006).

Some women use the Internet to seek support but also to engage in grieving. Using the Internet is particularly efficient as users engage in collective work of emotions (Davidson & Letherby, 2014). Given that many women use the Internet discussion forums following their miscarriage, and that it leads to a strong sense of community and support (Capitulo, 2004), this approach seems to be particularly interesting (Séjourné, Callahan, & Chabrol, 2010a). It is important to note that, for the last decades, such groups have increased and a recent search using Google revealed that more than 33,000 groups related to health currently exist (Gold, Boggs, Mugisha, & Palladino, 2012). A recent study found that women participating or consulting the Internet forums were more affected by depressive, grief anxiety symptoms higher than those who did not consult the forums, suggesting that these women might use the Internet for seeking support (Séjourné et al., 2016).

What a Brief and Early Support Intervention Looks Like[2]

Psychological interviews incorporated components based on basic psychotherapeutic processes and specific components from CBT. Empathetic listening has to be used to promote the expression of emotions, particularly regarding sadness and guilt that can occur after a miscarriage and that are not always recognized and accepted by women. The educational component is based not only on information regarding causes and frequency of miscarriages, but also on psychological reactions and repercussions that might happened.

Positive reinforcements and promotion of self-encouragement have to be used.

Box 6.3 Three Steps of a Psychological Intervention for Miscarriage: An Overview

Step 1: Subjective Experiences and Basic Psychoeducative Components

* Women have to be explained that an individual does not react directly to the event and that it is the subjective experience that matters. It helps to reassure women about the normality of their emotions and it also provides them with a space to freely talk.
* The frequency of miscarriages has to be discussed, as reminding women of the large number of spontaneous abortions might have a positive impact on cognitions. It can also prevent them from feeling guilty as miscarriages are frequent events and nothing can be done.
* It is important to ask questions about knowledge about miscarriages, beliefs about pregnancy, and the social representations of "what is a happy motherhood". Then, the possible causes of miscarriages are also discussed, in particular, to ensure that women are aware of them.

Step 2: Emotions, Social Environment, and CBT Components

* Guilt and difficulty of being confronted with a situation for which, sometimes, no explanation is given is also discussed. The substitution of alternative thoughts (what other cause can we imagine?) and the evaluation of the advantages and disadvantages of feeling guilty help women to distance from possible feelings of responsibility.
* Relationships with relatives have to be systematically discussed. The anticipation of the relatives' reactions allows us to better accept some difficult conversations with family members.
* Self-affirmation is also encouraged for helping them to express their feelings in a non-aggressive way. Benefits of speech and sharing of emotions have to be discussed.
* Relationships with the spouse are discussed in a specific way, as it is highlighted that different ways of living the same event might exist and that expressing emotions is of prime importance.

Step 3: Changes and Life to Come

* When women have children, the possible announcement of miscarriage and children's reactions have to be systematically discussed.
* Perception of their future life and the place given to miscarriage are discussed. Women have to be asked about changes caused by miscarriage in their current lives and then in their future lives. The possibility of a subsequent pregnancy and how to deal with it are also mentioned. These included discussing the normal nature of anxiety during the first weeks of pregnancy, the difficulty of avoiding such anxiety, and seeking solutions.

Recommendations

Regardless the type of loss, a follow-up by telephone may be of prime importance. All persons likely to meet women and couples experiencing perinatal loss should be informed of the potential psychological consequences of such loss. Being better informed can encourage caregivers' empathetic listening.

As different reactions can be observed, it is important to respect the person's progress and to consider that there is no rule regarding the duration and/or intensity of symptoms experienced. Likewise, the consequences might have long- or short-term impact. Women or couples may feel the need to talk about loss during the subsequent pregnancy which can be experienced in a particularly difficult way. Sometimes it is necessary to propose a follow-up or a session in order to discuss these fears. A single session might be enough for some parents who will easily talk about their fears and will ask questions but it is important to be available at that time. Using the time of hospitalization to start helping parents is important as once they are back home, some will not seek for care.

It is important to make sure that parents have resources and give him or her information about the signs and symptoms that should alert the person about the need for more formal help in the days or weeks to come. In addition, it is necessary to take into account men who may also be in pain. Discussing with the couple the possible reactions that might exist not only in women but also in men will allow the couple to discuss these aspects.

From a primary prevention perspective, it is necessary to listen but not being insistent, as every woman or man does not necessarily need support. When it seems necessary, professionals have to propose an appointment with a psychologist or a psychiatrist. Sometimes, women feel the need but do not dare to ask directly.

As early miscarriages are characterized by difficult recognition, it is of prime importance for caregivers to recognize loss and its consequences (Cote-Arsenault & Mahlangu, 1999; Cuisinier et al., 1993; Lasker & Toedter, 1994). Markin (2016) highlights the common errors that are made in the management of early perinatal losses. As women's relatives, women's caregivers might minimize the impact of miscarriage or assume that grief is resolved.

The announcement of miscarriage is a particularly important moment. Women and couples may be shocked during the announcement of pregnancy loss. Given this state of shock or the confusing emotional state, the couple may have difficulty understanding and processing the information; as a consequence, it is important to talk about these aspects during a subsequent consultation. Although the cause for each miscarriage might be unknown, most of them are the result of chromosomal abnormalities leading to miscarriage and these pieces of information may be useful for women. Similarly, it is important to clarify to some women who feel responsible that they could not have done anything to avoid a miscarriage.

One of the most important concerns of women who already have children is to know what they are going to tell them. It may therefore be important to address these issues. For instance, it is possible to explain to a young child using metaphors; that is, when you grow beans on cotton balls, you can see that all the beans do not grow.

A late fetal death will cause other concerns for the medical staff such as how to take care of the couples facing this event. Parents may find it very difficult to stay in the maternity ward after the birth of their dead baby and thus be confronted with tears and the sight of other babies. However, other patients may feel very overwhelmed by being moved to a gynecological or surgical department that they may interpret as no longer being considered as a mother. It is therefore important to ask the patient where she would like to be hospitalized. In the same way, the follow-up appointment should preferably take place in a different location than the one in which she lost her baby. It may be important to explain to parents that they have the opportunity to see their baby but that not all parents want to see or carry the baby and have a choice. Taking pictures or collecting other memories can be important if the parents want to have them, even in a delayed time. If seeing the baby and spending time with him/her can help creating memories and facilitating the grief process, some parents may feel fear. It is important to talk with them considering different options available. Preparing parents for the sight of the child, especially when the child is born very prematurely or has congenital anomalies, can be very useful, especially through a description or photos. For some parents, losing a baby can be the first painful experience of loss they are experiencing and it is important to reassure them by telling them that what they feel is normal. If the loss occurs in a multiple pregnancy, a special attention should be paid to parents whose feelings are particularly confused. If the psychological impact of a late loss is more easily taken into account than that of a miscarriage, medical follow-up should not be overlooked and may be more difficult for those women who are experiencing bleeding, pain, or rise of milk without having any baby.

Notes

1 Miscarriages were found during ultrasound at 20 days to 13 months (median duration of 187 days).
2 This psychological support intervention has been shown to be effective in treating anxious, depressive, and traumatic symptoms three weeks after pregnancy loss (Séjourné, Callahan, & Chabrol, 2010b).

References

Abboud, L. N., & Liamputtong, P. (2003). Pregnancy loss: What it means to women who miscarry and their partners. *Social Work in Health Care, 26*(3), 37–62.
Adolfsson, A., Berterö, C., & Larsson, P. G. (2006). Effect of a structured follow-up visit to a midwife on women with early miscarriage: A randomized study. *Acta Obstetricia et Gynecologica, 85*(3), 330–335.

Adolfsson, A., Larsson, P. G., Wijma, B., & Berterö, C. (2004). Guilt and emptiness: Women's experiences of miscarriage. *Health Care for Women International, 25*, 543–560.

Aerde, J. V. (2001). Des directives pour les professionnels de la santé qui soutiennent des familles après un décès périnatal. *Paediatrics and Child Health, 6*, 480–490.

Alderdice, F. (2017). The experience of stillbirth. *Journal of Reproductive and Infant Psychology, 35*, 105–107.

Al-Maharma, D. Y., Abujaradeh, H., Mahmoud, K. F., & Jarrad, R. A. (2016). Maternal grieving and the perception of and attachment to children born subsequent to a perinatal loss. *Infant Mental Health Journal, 37*(4), 411–423.

Armstrong, D. (2001). Exploring fathers' experiences of pregnancy after a prior perinatal loss. *MCN: The American Journal of Maternal Child Nursing, 26*(3), 147–153.

Athey, J., Spielvogel, & A. M. (2000). Risk factors and interventions for psychological sequelae in women after miscarriage. *Primary Care Update for Ob/Gyns, 7*(2), 64–69.

Bacqué, M. F. (1997). *Deuil et santé*. Paris: Odile Jacob.

Bacqué, M. F. (1995). *Le deuil à vivre*. Paris: Odile Jacob.

Bennett, S. M., Litz, B. T., Sarnoff Lee, B., & Maguen, S. (2005). The scope and impact of perinatal loss: Current status and future directions. *Professional Psychology: Research and Practice, 36*, 180–187.

Beutel, M., Willner, H., Deckardt, R., Von Rad, M., & Weiner, H. (1996). Similarities and differences in couples' grief reactions following a miscarriage: Results from a longitudinal study. *Journal Psychosomatic Research, 40*, 245–253.

Beutel, M., Rainer, D., von Rad, M., & Weiner, H. (1995). Grief and depression after miscarriage: Their separation, antecedents, and course. *Psychosomatic Medicine, 57*(6), 517–526.

Bicking Kinsey, C., Baptiste-Roberts, K., Zhu, J., & Kjerulff, K. E. (2015). Effect of previous miscarriage on depressive symptoms during subsequent pregnancy and postpartum in the first baby study. *Maternal and Child Health Journal, 19*, 391–400.

Black, B. P., Wright, P. M., & Limbo, R. (2015). *Perinatal and Pediatric Bereavement in Nursing and Other Health Professions*. New York: Springer Publishing Company.

Born, L., Soares, C. N., Phillips, S. D., Jung, M., & Steiner, M. (2006). Women and reproductive-related trauma. *Annals of New York Academy of Science, 1071*, 491–494.

Bowlby, J. (1984). *Attachement et perte III: La perte*. Paris: PUF.

Bowles, S. V., James, L. C., Solursh, D. S, Yancey, M. K., Epperly, T. D., & Folen, R. A. (2000). Acute and post-traumatic stress disorder after spontaneous abortion. *American Family Physician, 61*(6), 1689–1696.

Brier, N. (1999). Understanding and managing the emotional reactions to a miscarriage. *Obstetrics and Gynecology, 93*, 151–155.

Broen, A. N., Moum, T., Bödtker, A. S., & Ekeberg, O. (2006). Predictors of anxiety and depression following pregnancy termination: A longitudunal five-year follow-up study. *Acta Obstetricia et Gynecologica, 85*, 317–323.

Broen, A. N., Moum, T., Bödtker, A. S., & Ekeberg, O. (2004). Psychological impact on women of miscarriage versus induced abortion: A 2-year follow-up study. *Psychosomatic Medicine, 66*(2), 265–271.

Brown, Y. (1991). Perinatal death and grieving. *The Canadian Nurse, 87*(8), 26–29.

Burden, C., Bradley, S., Storey, C., Ellis, A., Heazell, A. E. P., Downe, S., Cacciatore, J., & Siassakos, D. (2016). From grief, guilt pain and stigma to hope and pride – A systematic review and metaanalysis of mixed-method research of the psychosocial impact of stillbirth. *BMC Pregnancy and Childbirth, 16*, 9.

Bydlowski, M. (2002, 2éme édition). *La dette de vie, itinéraire psychanalytique de la maternité*. Paris: PUF.

Cain, A. C., Erickson, M. E., Fast, I., & Vaughan, R. A. (1964). Children's disturbed reactions to their mother's miscarriage. *Psychosomatic Medicine, 26*(1), 58–66.

Capitulo, K. L. (2004). Perinatal grief online. *MCN: The American Journal of Maternal/Child Nursing, 29*(5), 305–311.

Carrera, L., Diez-Domingo, J., Montanana, V., Monleon Sancho, J., Minguez, J., & Monleon, J (1998). Depression in women suffering perinatal loss. *International Journal of Gynecology and Obstetrics, 62*, 149–153.

Carter, D., Misri, S., & Tomfohr, L. (2007). Psychologic aspects of early pregnancy loss. *Clinical Obstetrics and Gynecology, 50*(1), 154–165.

Cecil, R. (1994). Miscarriage: Women's views of care. *Journal of Reproductive and Infant Psychology, 12*, 21–29.

Connor, J. M, Ferguson-Smith, M. A, & White-van Mourik, M. C. A. (1992). The psychosocial sequelae of a second trimester termination of pregnancy for foetal abnormality. *Prenatal Diagnosis, 12*(3), 189–204.

Conway, K. (1995). Miscarriage experience and the role of support systems: A pilot study. *British Journal of Medical Psychology, 68*, 259–267.

Conway, K., & Russel, G. (2000). Couples' grief and experience of support in the aftermath of miscarriage. *British Journal of Medical Psychology, 73*, 531–545.

Corbet-Owen, C. (2003). Women's perceptions of partner support in the context of pregnancy loss(es). *South African Journal of Psychology, 33*(1), 19–27.

Corbet-Owen, C., & Kruger, L. M. (2001). The health system and emotional care: Validating the many meanings of spontaneous pregnancy loss. *Families, Systems and Health, 19*(4), 411–427.

Cordle, C. J., & Prettyman, R. J. (1994). A 2-year follow-up of women who have experienced early miscarriage. *Journal of Reproductive and Infant Psychology, 1*, 37–43.

Côté-Arsenault, D., Krowchuk, H., Schwartz, K., & McCoy, T. P. (2014). Evidence-based intervention with women pregnant after perinatal loss. *American Journal of Maternal Child Nursing, 39*(3), 177–186.

Côté-Arsenault, D., & Donato, K. (2011). Emotional cushioning in pregnancy after perinatal loss. *Journal of Reproductive and Infant Psychology, 29*, 81–92.

Côté-Arsenault, D., Bidlack, D., & Humm, A. (2001). Women's emotions and concerns during pregnancy following perinatal loss. *MCN, The American Journal of Maternal Child Nursing, 26*(3), 128–134.

Côté-Arsenault, D., & Mahlangu, N. (1999). Impact of perinatal loss on the subsequent pregnancy and self: Women's experiences. *Journal of Obstetric Gynecology and Neonatal Nursing, 28*(3), 274–282.

Cuijpers, P., Donker, T., Weissman, M. M., Ravitz, P., & Cristea, I. A. (2016). Interpersonal psychotherapy for mental health problems: A comprehensive meta-analysis. *American Journal of Psychiatry, 173*(7), 680–687.

Cuisinier, M. C. J., Kuijpers, J. C., Hoogduin, C. A. L., de Graauw, C. P. H. M., & Janssen, H. J. (1993). Miscarriage and stillbirth: Time since the loss, grief intensity and satisfaction with care. *European Journal of Obstetrics, Gynecology and Reproductive Biology, 52*, 163–168.

Cumming, G., Klein, S., Bolsover, D., Lee, A., Alexander, D., Maclean, M., & Jurgens, D. (2007). The emotional burden of miscarriage for women and their partners: Trajectories of anxiety and depression over 13 months. *BJOG, 114*, 1138–1145.

Dayan, J. (1999). *Psychopathologie de la périnatalité.* Paris: Masson.

Davidson, D., & Letherby, G. (2014). Griefwork online: Perinatal loss, lifecourse disruption and online support. *Human Fertility, 17*(3), 214–217.

DeBackere, K. J., Hill, P. D., & Kavanaugh, K. L. (2008). The parental experience of pregnancy after perinatal loss. *Journal of Obstetric, Gynecologic, & Neonatal Nursing, 37*(5), 525–537.

Defrain, J., Millspaugh, E., & Xie, X. (1996). The psychosocial effects of miscarriage: Implications for health professionals. *Families, Systems and Health, 14*(3), 331–347.

Delabaere, A., Huchon, C., Lavoue, V., Lejeune, V., Iraola, E., Nedellec, S., … Carcopino, X. (2014). Standardisation de la terminologie des pertes de grossesse: Consensus d'experts du Collège national des gynécologues et obstétriciens français (CNGOF). *Journal de Gynécologie Obstétrique et Biologie de la Reproduction, 43*(10), 756–763.

De Ville, E., O'Reilly, A., & Callahan, S. (2012). Le rôle du conjoint dans les stratégies de coping mises en place chez les femmes lors d'une fausse couche. *Psychologie Française, 58*, 41–51.

DiMarco, M. A., Menke, E. M., & McNamara, T. (2001). Evaluating a support group for perinatal loss. *MCN: The American Journal of Maternal Child Nursing, 26*(3), 135–140.

Dollander, M., & de Tychey, C. (2002). Fragilité psychologique de l'enfant en devenir et période prénatale. *L'évolution Psychiatrique, 67*(2), 290–311.

Dollander, M., & de Tychey, C. (2000). Pertes pré et périnatales: prévenir la psychopathologie ultérieure. *Perspectives Psychiatriques, 39*(5), 383–389.

Engelhard, I. M., van den Hout, M. A., & Arntz, A. (2001). Posttraumatic stress disorder after pregnancy loss. *General Hospital Psychiatry, 23*, 62–76.

Exalto, N. (2005). Recurrent miscarriage. *International Congress Series, 1279*, 247–250.

Farren, J., Jalmbrant, M., Ameye, L., Joash, K., Mitchell-Jones, N., Tapp, S., … Bourne, T. (2016). Post-traumatic stress, anxiety and depression following miscarriage or ectopic pregnancy: A prospective cohort study. *BMJ Open, 6*(11), e011864.

Flis-Trèves, M. (2004). *Le deuil de maternité.* Paris: Calmann-lévy.

Franche, R. L., & Bulow, C. (1999a). The impact of a subsequent pregnancy on grief and emotional adjustment following a perinatal loss. *Infant Mental Health Journal, 20*(2), 175–187.

Franche, R. L., & Mikail, S. F. (1999b). The impact of perinatal loss on adjustment to subsequent pregnancy. *Social Science and Medicine, 48*, 1613–1623.

Fréchette, L. (1997). Deuil à la suite d'accidents de procréation et de décès de nourrissons. *Frontières, 9*(3), 10–14.

Friedman, T., & Gath, D. (1989). The psychiatric consequences of spontaneous abortion. *British Journal of Psychiatry, 155*, 810–813.

Frost, J., Bradley, H., Levitas, R., Smith, L., & Garcia, J. (2007). The loss of possibility: Scientisation of death and the special case of early miscarriage. *Sociology of Health and Illness, 29*(7), 1–20.

Frydman, R. (1997). Mourir avant de n'être? Aspects éthiques. Colloque GYPSY In *Mourir avant de n'être?*

Garcia-Enguidanos, A., Calle, M. E., Valero, J., Luna, S., & Dominguez-Rojas, V. (2002). Risk factors in miscarriage: A review. *European Journal of Obstetrics, Gynecology and Reproductive Biology, 102*, 111–119.

Garel, M., & Legrand, H. (2005). *L'attente et la perte du bébé à naître.* Paris: Albin Michel.

Garel, M., Blondel, B., Lelong, N., Papin, C., Bonenfant, S., & Kaminski, M. (1994). Long-term consequences of miscarriage: The depressive disorders and the following pregnancy. *Journal of Reproductive and Infant Psychology, 12*, 233–240.

Garel, M., Blondel, B., Lelong, N., Papin, C., Bonenfant, S., & Kaminski, M. (1992). Réactions dépressives après une fausse couche. *Contraception, Fertilité, Sexualité, 20*(1), 75–81.

Gaudet, C., Séjourné, N., Camborieux, L., Rodgers, R., & Chabrol, H. (2010). Pregnancy after perinatal loss: Association of grief, anxiety and attachment. *Journal of Reproductive and Infant Psychology, 28*(3), 240–251.

Gaudet, C., Séjourné, N., Allard, M. A., & Chabrol, H. (2008). Les femmes face à la douloureuse expérience de l'Interruption Médicale de Grossesse. *Gynécologie, Obstétrique, Fertilité, 36*(5), 536–542.

Gausia, K., Moran, A. C., Ali, M., Ryder, D., Fisher, C., & Koblinsky, M. (2011). Psychological and social consequences among mothers suffering from perinatal loss: Perspective from a low income country. *BMC Public Health, 11*, 451.

Gauthier, Y. (1993). *Tragédies à l'aube de la vie, répercussions sur les familles.* Paris: Bayard.

Geller, P. A., Kerns, D., & Klier, C. M. (2004). Anxiety following miscarriage and the subsequent pregnancy: A review of the literature and future directions. *Journal of Psychosomatic Research, 56*, 35–45.

Geller, P. A., Klier, C. M., & Neugebauer, R. (2001). Anxiety disorders following miscarriage. *Journal of Clinical Psychiatry, 62*(6), 432–438.

Geller, P. A., Psaros, C., & Kerns, D. (2006). Web-based resources for health care providers and women following pregnancy loss. *Journal of Obstetric, Gynecologic, & Neonatal Nursing, 35*(4), 523–532, Colloque GYPSY I, Editions Odile Jacob.

Goddijn, M., & Leschot, N. J. (2000). Genetic aspects of miscarriage. *Baillière's Clinical Obstetrics and Gynaecology, 14*(5), 855–865.

Gold, K. J., Leon, I., Boggs, M. E., & Sen, A. (2016). Depression and posttraumatic stress symptoms after perinatal loss in a population-based sample. *Journal of Women's Health, 25*(3), 263–269.

Gold, K. J., Boggs, M. E., Muzik, M., & Sen, A. (2014). Anxiety disorders and obsessive compulsive disorder 9 months after perinatal loss. *General Hospital Psychiatry, 36*, 650–654.

Heazell, A. E., Siassakos, D., Blencowe, H., Burden, C., Bhutta, Z. A., Cacciatore, J., … Mensah, O. K. (2016). Stillbirths: Economic and psychosocial consequences. *The Lancet, 387*(10018), 604–616.

Herz, E. (1984). Psychological repercussions of pregnancy loss. *Psychiatric Annals, 14*, 454–457.

Hanus, M. (2001). *Les deuils dans la vie.* Paris: Maloine.

Hemminki, H., & Forssas, E. (1999). Epidemiology of miscarriage and its relation to other reproductive events in Finland. *American Journal of Obstetrics and Gynecology, 181*, 396–401.

Hughes, P. M., & Riches, S. (2003). Psychological aspects of perinatal loss. *Current Opinion in Obstetrics and Gynecology, 15*, 107–111.

Hughes, P., Turton, P., Hopper, E., & Evans, C. D. H. (2002). Assessment of guidelines for good practice in psychosocial care of mothers after stillbirth: A cohort study. *Lancet, 360*, 114–118.

Hunfeld, J. A., Wladimiroff, J. W., & Passchier, J. (1997). Prediction and course of grief four years after perinatal loss due to congenital anomalies: A follow-up study. *British Journal of Medical Psychology, 70*, 85–91.

Hutti, M. H., Armstrong, D. S., & Myers, J. A. (2013). Evaluation of the perinatal grief intensity scale in the subsequent pregnancy after perinatal loss. *Journal of Obstetric, Gynecologic, & Neonatal Nursing, 42*(6), 697–706.

Hutti, M. H., dePacheco, M., & Smith, M. (1998). A study of miscarriage: Development and validation of the perinatal grief intensity scale. *Journal of Obstetric Gynecology and Neonatal Nursing, 27*(5), 547–555.

James, D. S., & Kristiansen, C. M. (1995). Women's reactions to miscarriage: The role of attributions, coping styles, and knowledge. *Journal of Applied Social Psychology, 25*(1), 59–76.

Janoff-Bulman, R. (1992). *Shattered Assumptions: Towards a New Psychology of Trauma.* New York, NY: Free Press.

Janssen, H., Cuisinier, M., Graauw, K., & Hoogduin, K. (1997). A prospective study of risk factors predicting grief intesity following pregnancy loss. *Archive of General Psychiatry, 54*, 56–61.

Janssen, H., Cuisinier, M., Hoogduin, K., & Graauw, K. (1996). Controlled prospective study on the mental health of women following pregnancy loss. *American Journal of Psychiatry, 153*(2), 226–230.

Jaoul, M., Ozon, A., Marx de Fossey, I., Riazuelo, H., Molina Gomes, D., Chudzic, L., & Wainer, B. (2013). Etude des aspects psychologiques des fausses couches a répétition à l'aide d'un questionnaire de personnalité approfondi: le MMPI-2. *Gynécologie Obstétrique & Fertilité, 41*, 297–304.

Jind, L. (2003). Parents' adjustment to late abortion, stillbirth or infant death: The role of causal attributions. *Scandinavian Journal of Psychology, 44*, 383–394.

Johnson, J. E., Price, A. B., Kao, J. C., Stout, R., Gobin, R. L., & Zlotnick, C. (2016). Interpersonal psychotherapy (IPT) for major depression following perinatal loss: A pilot randomized controlled trial. *Archives of Women's Mental Health, 19*(5), 845–859.

Johnson, O., & Langford, R. W. (2010). Proof of life: A protocol for pregnant women who experience pre-20-week perinatal loss. *Critical Care Nursing Quarterly, 33*(3), 204–211.

Johnson, M. P., & Baker, S. R. (2004). Implication of coping repertoire as predictor of men's stress, anxiety and depression following pregnancy, childbirth and miscarriage: A longitudinal study. *Journal of Psychosomatic Obstetrics and Gynecology, 25*, 87–98.

Karyotaki, E., Riper, H., Twisk, J., Hoogendoorn, A., Kleiboer, A., Mira, A., … Andersson, G. (2017). Efficacy of self-guided internet-based cognitive behavioral therapy in the treatment of depressive symptoms: A meta-analysis of individual participant data. *JAMA Psychiatry, 74*(4), 351–359.

Kersting, A., Brähler, E., Glaesmer, H., & Wagner, B. (2011). Prevalence of complicated grief in a representative population-based sample. *Journal of Affective Disorders, 131*(1), 339–343.

Kersting, A., Reutemann, M., Ohrmann, P., Baez, E., Klockenbusch, W., Lanczik, M., & Arolt, V. (2004). Grief after termination of pregnancy due to fetal malformation. *Journal of Psychosomatic, Obstetric and Gynaecololy, 25*(2), 163–169.

Kersting, A., & Wagner, B. (2012). Complicated grief after perinatal loss. *Dialogues in Clinical Neurosciences, 14*, 187–194.

Keesee, N. J., Currier, J. M., & Neimeyer, R. A. (2008). Predictors of grief following the death of one's child: The contribution of finding meaning. *Journal of Clinical Psychology, 64*(10), 1145–1163.

Kimble, D. (1991). Neonatal death: A descriptive study of fathers' experiences. *Neonatal Network, 9*, 45–50.

Khan, R. A., Drudy, L., Sheehan, J., Harrison, R. F., & Geary, M. (2004). Early pregnancy loss: How do men feel? *Irish Medical Journal, 97*(7), 217–218.

Klier, C. M., Geller, P. A., & Ritsher, J. B. (2002). Affective disorders in the aftermath of miscarriage: A comprehensive review. *Archives of Women's Mental Health, 5*, 129–149.

Klier, C. M., Geller, P. A., & Neugebauer, R. (2000). Minor depressive disorder in the context of miscarriage. *Journal of Affective Disorders, 59*(1), 13–21.

Kohn, I., & Moffitt, P. L. (1992). *Pregnancy Loss. A Silent Sorrow.* London: Headway, Hodder and Stoughton.

Kolte, A. M., Bernardi, L. A., Christiansen, O. B., Quenby, S., Farquharson, R. G., Goddijn, M., & Stephenson, M. D. (2015). Terminology for pregnancy loss prior to viability: A consensus statement from the ESHRE early pregnancy special interest group. *Human Reproduction, 30*: 495–498.

Kong, G., Lok, I., Yui, A., Hui, A., Lai, B., & Chung, T. (2013). Clinical and psychological impact after surgical, medical or expectant management of first-trimester miscarriage – A randomised controlled trial. *Australian and New Zealand Journal of Obstetrics and Gynaecology, 53*, 170–177.

Kong, G., Chung, T., Lai, B., & Lok, I. (2010). Gender comparison of psychological reaction after miscarriage-a 1-year longitudinal study. *BJOG, 117*, 1211–1219.

Kong, G., Lok, I., Lam, P., Yip, A., & Chung, T. (2010). Conflicting perceptions between health care professionals and patients on the psychological morbidity following miscarriage. *Australian and New Zealand Journal of Obstetrics and Gynaecology, 50*, 562–567.

Kowalski, K. (1990). No happy ending: Pregnancy loss and bereavement. *NAACOG's Clinical Issues in Perinatal and Women's Health Nursing, 2*(3), 368–380.

Kulathilaka, S., Hanwella, R., & de Silva, V. A. (2016). Depressive disorder and grief following spontaneous abortion. *BMC Psychiatry, 16*, 100.

Lacroix, P., Got, F., Callahan, S., & Séjourné, N. (2016). La fausse couche: du côté des hommes. *Psychologie Française, 6*(3), 207–217.

Lamb, E. H. (2002). The impact of previous perinatal loss on subsequent pregnancy and parenting. *The Journal of Perinatal Education, 11*(2), 33–40.

Lang, A., Gottlieb, L. N., & Amsel, R. (1996). Predictor of husbands' and wives' grief reactions following infant death: The role of marital intimacy. *Death Studies, 20*, 33–57.

Lansac, J., Berger, C., & Magnin, G. (2000). *Obstétrique.* Paris: Masson, collection pour le praticien.

Larsen, E. C., Christiansen, O. B., Kolte, A. M., & Macklon, N. (2013). New insights into mechanisms behind miscarriage. *BMC Medicine, 11*(1), 154.

Lasker, J. N., & Toedter, L. J. (1991). Acute versus chronic grief: The case for pregnancy loss. *American Journal of Orthopsychiatry, 61*, 510–522.

Lasker, J. N., & Toedter, L. J. (1994). Satisfaction with hospital care and interventions after pregnancy loss. *Death Studies, 18*, 41–64.

Latham, A. E., & Prigerson, H. G. (2004). Suicidality and bereavement: Complicated grief as psychiatric disorder presenting greatest risk for suicidality. *Suicide and Life-Threatening Behavior, 34*(4), 350–362.

Lawn, J. F., Blencowe, H., Waiswa, P., Amouzou, A., Mathers, C., Hogan, D., ... Cousens, S. (2016). The Lancet ending preventable stillbirths series study group with the Lancet stillirth epidemiology investigator group. Stillbirths: Rates, risk factors and acceleration towards 2030. *Lancet, 387*(10018), 587–603.

Lee, L., McKenzie-McHarg, K., & Horsch, A. (2017). The impact of miscarriage and stillbirth on maternal–fetal relationships: An integrative review. *Journal of Reproductive and Infant Psychology, 35*(1), 32–52.

Lee, C., & Slade, P. (1996a). Miscarriage as a traumatic event: A review of the literature and new implications for intervention. *Journal of Psychosomatic Research, 40*(3), 235–244.

Lee, C., Slade, P., & Lygo, V. (1996b). The influence of psychological debriefing on emotional adaptation in women following early miscarriage: A preliminary study. *British Journal of Medical Psychology, 69*, 47–58.

Lee, C., & Rowlands, I. J. (2015). When mixed methods produce mixed results: Integrating disparate findings about miscarriage and women's wellbeing. *British Journal of Health Psychology, 20*, 36–44.

Legros, J. P. (2001). Arrêt de vies in utero ou l'errance des fœtus, un possible deuil. *Etudes sur la mort, 119*, 63–75.

Leon, I. G. (1995). Conceptualisation psychanalytique de la perte d'un enfant en période périnatale. *Devenir, 7*(1), 9–30.

Leppert, P. C., & Pahlka, B. S. (1984). Grieving characteristics after spontaneous abortion: A managment approach. *Obstetrics and Gynecology, 64*(1), 119–122.

Lewis, J., & Azar, R. (2015). Depressive symptoms in men post-miscarriage. *Journal of Men's Health, 11*(5), 8–13.

Lok, I. H., Yip, A. S., Lee, D. T., Sahota, D., & Chung, T. K. (2010). A 1-year longitudinal study of psychological morbidity after miscarriage. *Fertility and Sterility, 93*(6), 1966–1975.

Lok, I. H., & Neugebauer, R. (2007). Psychological Morbidity following miscarriage. *Best Practice and Research Clinical Obstetrics and Gynaecology, 21*(2), 229–247.

Maconochie, L., Doyle, P., Prior, S., & Simmons, R. (2007). Risk factors for first trimester miscarriage – Results of a UK-population-based case-control study. *BJOG, 114*, 170–186.

Madden, M. E. (1994). The variety of emotional reactions to miscarriage. *Women and Health, 21*(2/3), 85–104.

Maker, C., & Ogden, J. (2003). The miscarriage experience: More than just a trigger to psychology morbidity? *Psychology and Health, 18*(3), 403–415.

Mandelbrot, L. (2003). Avortements spontanés tardifs. In Cabrol, D., Pons, J. C., Goffinet, F. *Traité d'obstétrique*. Paris: Flammarion Médecine-Sciences.

Marinopoulos, S. (2005). *Dans l'intime des mères*. Paris: Fayard.

Markin, R. D. (2016). What clinicians miss about miscarriages: Clinical errors in the treatment of early term perinatal loss. *Psychotherapy, 53*, 347–353.

Marques, L., Bui, E., LeBlanc, N., Porter, E., Robinaugh, D., Dryman, M. T., ... Simon, N. (2013). Complicated grief symptoms in anxiety disorders: Prevalence and associated impairment. *Depression and Anxiety, 30*(12), 1211–1216.

McCarthy, M. (2002). *Gender differences in reactions to perinatal loss: A qualitative study of couples*. Unpublished doctoral dissertation, California School of Professional Psychology, San Diego.

McCreight, B. S. (2004). A grief ignored: Narratives of pregnancy loss from a male perspective. *Sociology of Health and Illness, 26*(3), 326–350.

McGreal, D., Evans, B. J., & Burrows, G. D. (1997). Gender differencies in coping following loss of a child through miscarriage or stillbirth: A pilot study. *Stress Medicine, 13*(3), 159–165.

McSpedden, M., Mullan, B., Sharpe, L., Breen, L. J., & Lobb, E. A. (2017). The presence and predictors of complicated grief symptoms in perinatally bereaved mothers from a bereavement support organization. *Death Studies, 41*(2), 112–117.

Miron, J., & Chapman, J. S. (1994). Supporting: Men's experiences with the event of their partner's miscarriage. *Canadian Journal of Nursing Research, 26*(2), 61–72.

Molénat, F. (2001). *Naissances: pour une éthique de la prévention*. Ramonville Saint-Agne: Erès.

Mouras, M. J. (2003). La périnatalité: repères théoriques et cliniques. *Paris, 6*, 39–42.

Murphy, F. A. (1998). The experience of early miscarriage from a male perspective. *Journal of Clinical Nursing, 7*, 325–332.

Nakano, Y., Akechi, T., Furukawa, T., & Sugiura-Ogasawara, M. (2013). Cognitive behavior therapy for psychological distress in patients with recurrent miscarriage. *Psychology Research and Behavior Management, 6*, 37–43.

Neugebauer, R. (2003). Depressive symptoms at two months after miscarriage: Interpreting study findings from an epidemiological versus clinical perspective. *Depression and Anxiety, 17*, 152–161.

Neugebauer, R., Kline, J., Shrout, P., Skodol, A., O'Connor, P., Geller, P., Stein, Z., & Susser, M. (1997). Major depressive disorder in the 6 months after miscarriage. *JAMA, 277*(5), 383–338.

Neugebauer, R., Kline, J., O'Connor, P., Shrout, P., Johnson, J., Skodol, A., Wicks, J., & Susser, M. (1992a). Depressive symptoms in women in the six months after miscarriage. *American Journal of Obstetrics and Gynecology, 166*, 104–109.

Neugebauer, R., Kline, J., O'Connor, P., Shrout, P., Johnson, J., Skodol, A., Wicks, J., & Susser, M. (1992b). Determinants of depressive symptoms in the early weeks after miscarriage. *American Journal of Public Health, 82*(10), 1332–1339.

Nielsen, S., Hahlin, M., Möller, A., & Granberg, S. (1996). Bereavement, grieving and psychological morbidity after first trimester spontaneous abortion: Comparing expectant management with surgical evacuation. *Human Reproduction, 11*(8), 1767–1770.

Nikčević, A. V., & Nicolaides, K. H. (2014). Search for meaning, finding meaning and adjustment in women following miscarriage: *A Longitudinal Study. Psychology & Health, 29*, 50–63.

Nikcevic, A. V. (2003). Development and evaluation of a miscarriage follow-up clinic. *Journal of Reproductive and Infant Psychology, 21*(3), 207–217.

Nikcevic, A. V., Kuczmierczyk, A. R., Tunkel, S. A., & Nicolaides, K. H. (2000). Distress after miscarriage: Relation to the knowledge of the cause of pregnancy loss and coping style. *Journal of Reproductive and Infant Psychology, 18*(4), 339–343.

Nikcevic, A. V., Tunkel, S. A., Kuczmierczyk, A. R., & Nicolaides, K. H. (1999a). Investigation of the cause of miscarriage and its influence on women's psychological distress. *British Journal of Obstetrics and Gynaecology, 106*, 808–813.

Nikcevic, A. V., Snijders, R., & Nicolaides, K. H. (1999b). Some psychometric properties of the Texas Grief Inventory adjusted for miscarriage. *British Journal of Medical Psychology, 72*, 171–178.

Nikcevic, A. V., Tunkel, S. A., & Nicolaides, K. H. (1998a). Psychological outcomes following missed abortions and provision of follow-up care. *Ultrasound Obstetric and Gynecology, 11*, 123–128.

Ogden, J., & Maker, C. (2004). Expectant or surgical management of miscarriage: A qualitative study. *BJOG, 111*, 463–467.

O'Leary, J. M., & Gaziano, C. (2011). Sibling Grief after Perinatal Loss. *Journal of Prenatal and Perinatal Psychology and Health, 25*(3), 173–193.

O'Leary, J. (2005). The trauma of ultrasound during a pregnancy following perinatal loss. *Journal of Loss and Trauma, 10*, 183–204.

Ouibel, T., Bultez, T., Nizard, J., Subtil, D., Huchon, C., & Rozenberg, P. (2014). Morts fœtales in utero. *Journal de Gynécologie Obstétrique et Biologie de la Reproduction, 43*, 883–907.

Oppenheim, D. (2002). *Parents en deuil: le temps reprend son cours.* Ramonville Saint-Agne: Eres.

Organisation Mondiale de la Santé. (2004). *Prise en charge des complications de la grossesse et de l'accouchement.* Imprimé en suisse. Retrieved from apps.who.int/iris/bitstream/10665/43009/1/9242545872.pdf.

Paton, F., Wood, R., Bor, R., & Nitsun, M. (1999). Grief in miscarriage patients and satisfaction with care in a London hospital. *Journal of Reproductive and Infant Psychology, 17*(3), 301–315.

Parkes, C. M., & Weiss, R. S. (1983). *Recovery from Bereavement.* London: Jason Aronson.

Payne, E. C., Kravitz, A. R., Notman, M. T., & Anderson, J. V. (1976). Outcome following therapeutic abortion. *Archives of General Psychiatry, 33*(6), 725–733.

Potvin, L., Lasker, J. N., & Toedter, J. L. (1989). Measuring grief: A short version of the Perinatal Grief Scale. *Journal of Psychopathology and Behavioral Assessment, 11*, 29–45.

Prettyman, R. J., Cordle, C. J., & Cook, G. D. (1993). A three-month follow-up of psychological morbidity after early miscarriage. *British Journal of Medical Psychology, 66*, 363–372.

Prettyman, R. J., & Cordle, C. J. (1992). Psychological aspects of miscarriage: Attitudes of the primary health care team. *British Journal of General Practitionner, 42*, 97–99.

Prigerson, H. G., Horowitz, M. J., Jacobs, S. C., Parkes, C. M., Aslan, M., Goodkin, K., … Bonanno, G. (2009). Prolonged grief disorder: Psychometric validation of criteria proposed for DSM-V and ICD-11. *PLoS Med, 6*(8), e1000121.

Puddifoot, J. E., & Johnson, M. P. (1999). Active grief, despair, and difficulty coping: Some measured characteristics of male response following their partner's miscarriage. *Journal of Reproductive and Infant Psychology, 17*(1), 89–93.

Regan, L. (2001). *Miscarriage.* Londres: Orion.

Regan, L., & Rai, R. (2000). Epidemiology and the medical causes of miscarriage. *Baillière's Clinical Obstetrics and Gynaecology, 14*(5), 839–854.

Rinehart, M. S., & Kiselica, M. S. (2010). Helping men with the trauma of miscarriage. *Psychotherapy, 47*(3), 288–295.

Robertson Blackmore, E., Côté-Arsenault, D., Tang, W., Glover, V., Evans, J., Golding, J., & O'Connor, T. G. (2011). Previous prenatal loss as a predictor of perinatal depression and anxiety. *The British Journal of Psychiatry, 198*(5), 373–378.

Robinson, M., Baker, L., & Nackerud, L. (1999). The relationship of attachment theory and perinatal loss. *Death Studies, 23,* 257–270.

Robinson, G. E., Stirtzinger, R., Stewart, D. E., & Ralevski, E. (1994). Psychological reactions in women followed for 1 year after miscarriage. *Journal of Reproductive and Infant Psychology, 12*(1), 31–36.

Roegiers, L. (2003). *La grossesse incertaine.* Paris: Presses Universitaires de France, coll. Le fil rouge.

Rongières-Bertrand, C. (1997). Les gynécologues-obstétriciens face aux grossesses arrêtées. In Frydman, R., Flis-Trèves, M. (Eds.). *Mourir avant de n'être?* Paris: Odile Jacob, pp. 57–64.

Roswell, E., Jongman, G., Kilby, M., Kirchmeier, R., & Orford, J. (2001). The psychological impact of recurrent miscarriage, and the role of counselling at a pre-pregnancy counselling clinic. *Journal of Reproductive and Infant Psychology, 19*(1), 33–45.

Rousseau, P. (2001). Le deuil périnatal et son accompagnement. In Guedeney, A., Allilaire, J.-F. (Eds.). *Interventions psychologiques en périnatalité.* Paris: Masson, pp. 133–152.

Rousseau, P. (1995). Les pertes périnatales, la famille, les soignants et la société. *Devenir, 7*(1), 31–60.

Rousseau, P. (1988). Le deuil périnatal. Psychopathologie et accompagnement. *Journal de Gynécologie Obstétrique et Biologie de la Reproduction, 17,* 285–324.

Rousseau, P., & Fierens, R.M. (1994). Evolution du deuil des mères et des familles après mort périnatale. *Journal de Gynecologie Obstetrique et Biolologie de la Reproduction, 23,* 166–174.

Rowlands, I., & Lee, C. (2010a). Adjustment after miscarriage: Predicting positive mental health trajectories among young Australian women. *Psychology, Health & Medicine, 15,* 34–49.

Rowlands, I. J., & Lee, C. (2010b). 'The silence was deafening': Social and health service support after miscarriage. *Journal of Reproductive and Infant Psychology, 28,* 274–286.

Schaap, A. H. P., Wolf, H., Bruinse, H. W., Barkhof-Van De Lande, S., & Treffers, P. E. (1997). Long-term impact of perinatal bereavement: Comparison of grief reactions after intrauterine versus neonatal death. *European Journal of Obstetrics & Gynecology and Reproductive Biology, 75*(2), 161–167.

Séjourné, N., Fagny, J., Got, F., Lacroix, P., Pauchet, C., & Combalbert, L. (2016). Internet forum following a miscarriage: A place for women in particular pain? *Journal of Reproductive and Infant Psychology, 34*(1), 28–34.

Séjourné, N., Callahan, S., & Chabrol, H. (2011). Avortement spontané et culpabilité: Une étude qualitative. *Journal de Gynécologie Obstétrique et Biologie de la Reproduction, 40,* 430–436.

Séjourné, N., Callahan, S., & Chabrol, H. (2010a). Support following miscarriage: What women want. *Journal of Reproductive and Infant Psychology, 28*(4), 403–411.

Séjourné, N., Callahan, S., & Chabrol, H. (2010b). The utility of a psychological intervention for coping with spontaneous abortion. *Journal of Reproductive and Infant Psychology, 28*(3), 287–296.

Séjourné, N., Chabrol, H., & Callahan, S. (2009). La fausse couche: une expérience difficile et singulière. *Devenir, 21*(3), 143–157.

Serrano, F., & Lima, M. L. (2006). Recurrent miscarriage: Psycological and relational consequences for couples. *Psychology and Psychotherapy: Theory, Research and Practice, 79,* 585–594.

Serfaty, A. (2014). Stillbirth in France. *The Lancet, 384,* 1672.

Shear, M. K., Simon, N., Wall, M., Zisook, S., Neimeyer, R., Duan, N., … Gorscak, B. (2011). Complicated grief and related bereavement issues for DSM-5. *Depression and Anxiety, 28*(2), 103–117.

Shelley, J. M., Healy, D., & Grover, S. (2005). A randomized trial of surgical, medical and expectant management of first trimester sponaneous miscarriage. *Australian and New Zealand Journal of Obstetrics and Gynaecology, 45,* 122–125.

Silver, R., Branch, D. W., Goldenberg, R., Iams, J. D., & Klebanoff, M. (2011). Nomenclature for pregnancy outcomes: Time for a change. *Obstetrics & Gynecology, 118,* 1402–1408.

Silverman, G. K., Jacobs, S. C., Kasl, S. V., Shear, M. K., Maciejewski, P. K., Noaghiul, F. S., & Prigerson, H. G. (2000). Quality of life impairments associated with diagnostic criteria for traumatic grief. *Psychological Medicine, 30*(4), 857–862.

Simmons, R. K., Singh, G., Maconochie, N., Doyle, P., & Green, J. (2006). Experience of miscarriage in the UK: Qualitative findings from the National Women's Health Study. *Social Science and Medicine, 63,* 1934–1946.

Stinson, K. M., Lasker, J. N., Lohman, J., & Toedter, L. J. (1992). Parent's grief following pregnancy loss: A comparison of mothers and fathers. *Family Relations, 41,* 218–223.

Stirrat, G. M. (1990). Recurrent miscarriage I: Definition and epidemiology. *The Lancet, 336,* 673–675.

Stirtzinger, R. M., Robinson, G. E., Stewart, D. E., & Ralevski, E. (1999). Parameters of grieving in spontaneous abortion. *International Journal of Psychiatry in Medicine, 29*(2), 235–249.

Stirtzinger, R., & Robinson, G. E. (1989). The psychologic effects of spontaneous abortion. *CMAJ, 140*(1), 799–805.

Swanson, K. M., Chen, H. T., Graham, C., Wojnar, D. M., & Petras, A. (2009). Resolution of depression and grief during the first year after miscarriage: A randomized controlled clinical trial of couples-focused interventions. *Journal of Women's Health, 18*, 1245–1257.

Swanson, K. M., Connor, S., Jolley, S. N., Pettinado, M., & Wang, T. J. (2007). Contexts and evolution of womens' responses to miscariage during the first year after loss. *Research in Nursing and Health, 30*, 2–16.

Swanson, K. M., Karmali, Z. A., Powell, S. H., & Pulvermakher, F. (2003). Miscarriage effects on couples' interpersonel and sexual relationships during the first year after loss: Women's perceptions. *Psychosomatic Medicine, 65*, 902–910.

Swanson, K. M. (1999a). Effects of caring, measurement, and time on miscarriage impact and women's well-being. *Nursing Research, 48*(6), 288–298.

Tedstone, J. E., & Tarrier, N. (2003). Posttraumatic stress disorder following medical illness and treatment. *Clinical Psychology Review, 23*(3), 409–448.

Thapar, A., & Thapar, A. (1992). Psychological sequelae of miscarriage: A controlled study using the general health questionnaire and the hospital anxiety and depression scale. *British Journal of General Practice, 42*, 94–96.

Thomas, J. (1995). The effects on the family of miscarriage, termination for abnormality, stillbirth and neonatal death. *Child: Care, Health and Development, 21*(6), 413–424.

Toedter, L. J., Lasker, J. N., & Alhadeff, J. M. (1988). The perinatal grief scale: Development and initial validation. *American Journal of Orthopsychiatry, 58*(3), 435.

Toffol, E., Koponen, P., & Partonen, T. (2013). Miscarriage and mental health: Results of two population-based studies. *Psychiatry Research, 205*(1–2), 151–158.

Touvenot, V. (2004). Mort périnatale et transmissions intergénérationnelles: les deuils parentaux non-résolus sont-ils un facteur de risque? In de Tychey, C. (Eds.). *La prévention des dépressions*. Paris: L'Harmattan, pp. 96–102.

Tsartsara, E., & Johnson, M. P. (2006). The impact of miscarriage on women's pregnancy-specific anxiety and feelings of prenatal maternal-fetal attachement during the course of a subsequent pregnancy; an exploratory follow-up study. *Journal of Psychosomatic Obstetrics and Gynecology, 27*(3), 173–182.

Tunaley, J. R., Slade, P., & Duncan, S. B. (1993). Cognitive processes in psychological adaptation to miscarriage: A preliminary report. *Psychology and Health, 8*, 369–381.

Turner, M. J., Flannelly, G. M., Wingfield, M., Rasmussen, M. J., Ryan, R., Cullen, S., Maguire, R., & Stronge, J. M. (1991). The miscarriage clinic: An audit of the first year. *British Journal of Obstetrics and Gynaecology, 98*, 306–308.

Turton, P., Hughes, P., Evans, C. D. H., & Fainman, D. (2001). Incidence, correlates and predictors of post-traumatic stress disorder in the pregnancy after stillbirth. *The British Journal of Psychiatry, 178*(6), 556–560.

Walker, T. M., & Davidson, K. M. (2001). A preliminary investigation of psychological distress following surgical management of early pregnancy loss detected at initial ultrasound scanning: A trauma perspective. *Journal of Reproductive and Infant Psychology, 19*(1), 7–16.

Wallerstedt, C., Lilley, M., & Baldwin, K. (2003). Interconceptional counseling after perinatal and infant loss. *JOGNN, 32*(4), 533–542.

Wallerstedt, C., & Higgins, P. (1996). Facilitating perinatal grieving between the mother and the father. *Journal of Obstetric, Gynecologic and Neonatal Nursing, 25*, 389–394.

Wang, X., Chen, C., Wang, L., Chen, D., Guang, W., & French, J. (2003). Conception, early pregnancy loss, and time to clinical pregnancy: A population-based prospective study. *Fertility and Sterility, 79*(3), 577–584.

Warsop, A., Ismail, K., & Iliffe, S. (2004). Explanatory models associated with psychological morbidity in first trimester spontaneous abortion: A generalist study in a specialist setting. *Psychology, Health and Medicine, 9*(3), 306–314.

Wittouck, C., Van Autreve, S., De Jaegere, E., Portzky, G., & van Heeringen, K. (2011). The prevention and treatment of complicated grief: A meta-analysis. *Clinical Psychology Review, 31*(1), 69–78.

Wojnar, D. M., Swanson, K. M., & Adolfsson, A. S. (2011). Confronting the inevitable: A conceptual model of miscarriage for use in clinical practice and research. *Death Studies, 35*, 536–558.

Wong, M. K. Y., Crawford, T. J., Gask, L., & Grinyer, A. (2003). A qualitative investigation into women's experiences after a miscarriage: Implications for this primary healthcare team. *British Jouranl of General Practice, 53*, 697–702.

Zinaman, M. J., O'Connor, J., Clegg, E. D., Selevan, S. G., & Brown, C. C. (1996). Estimates of human fertility and pregnancy loss. *Fertility and Sterility, 65*(3), 503–509.

Zisook, S., Devaul, R., & Click, M. A. (1982). Measuring symptoms of grief and bereavement. *American Journal of Psychiatry, 139*, 1590–1593.

Zoless, G., & Blacker, C. V. (1992). The psychological complications of therapeutic abortion. *British Journal of Psychiatry, 160*, 742–749.

7

Traumatic Childbirth
The Ever-Expanding Ripple Effects

Cheryl Tatano Beck

Traumatic Childbirth

Kounin (1970) first coined the phrase "ripple effect" to describe the positive impact teachers can have on their students. A ripple effect is "a spreading effect or series of consequences caused by a single action or event" (dictionary.com). Zinker (2013) stressed that it is important to understand small ripples since they can be the first phase in growing bigger waves. Before clinicians can identify the ripple effects of traumatic childbirth, we need to know what that initial drop in the water, the birth trauma, looks like. We first need to understand the initial event that can result in these ripples.

The reported range of prevalence rates for traumatic childbirth is 23–45%. Sawyer, Ayers, Young, Bradley, and Smith (2012) found in the United Kingdom (UK) that 23% of their total sample of 125 mothers at eight weeks postpartum perceived their childbirth to be traumatic. In Australia 45.5% of the total community sample of 866 mothers at 4–6 weeks after birth reported that they had experienced traumatic births (Alcorn, O'Donovan, Patrick, Creedy, & Devilly, 2010). While in a United States (US) study of 103 mothers four weeks postpartum, Soet, Brack, and Dilorio (2003) found that 34% of the women perceived their births to be traumatic.

What is essential for clinicians to remember is that traumatic childbirth is just like beauty: it lies in the eye of the beholder (Beck, 2004a). What obstetrical healthcare providers may view as another routine birth, mothers may perceive as traumatic. Beck (2004a) conducted a phenomenological study of mothers' experiences of birth trauma. Four themes that emerged included: (1) "To care for me: Was that too much to ask?", (2) "To communicate with me: Why was this neglected?", (3) "To provide safe care: You betrayed my trust", and (4) "The end justifies the means: At whose expense? At what price?". What was discovered was that women who perceived their births to be traumatic were systematically stripped of protective layers during childbearing. During such a vulnerable time as giving birth, women did not feel cared for. They felt abandoned, alone, and stripped of their dignity as illustrated by the following quote: "I am amazed that 3½ hours in the labor and delivery room could cause such utter destruction in my life. It was truly like being the victim of a violent crime or rape" (Beck, 2004a, p. 32). Some mothers described the care they received during their birthing process as "cold" and "mechanical". Another protective layer that women were stripped of was being communicated with by labor and delivery staff. Women often described that they felt invisible as clinicians spoke to each other as if they were not present. One mother revealed that "the attending physician was saying, 'We may have lost this bloody baby'. The hospital staff discussed my baby's possible death in front of me and argued in front of me as if I weren't there" (Beck, 2004a, p. 33).Women trusted their clinicians would provide safe care but for some mothers at times they felt they received unsafe care and they feared for both their own safety and that of their unborn child. Lastly mothers felt that once the baby was born alive and in good health, no one wanted to hear what they had gone through to give birth. Success was measured only in terms of the infant and not in terms of the mother's experience giving birth.

Dinesen noted that "all sorrows can be borne if we put them into a story" (as cited in Arendt, 1958, p. 175). Persons try to make sense of a difficult life event by putting it into narrative form (Riessman, 1993). Beck (2006a) conducted a narrative analysis with 11 mothers regarding their stories of traumatic childbirth. Burke's (1969) narrative approach provided the structure for the analysis of the birth trauma stories. His focus of analysis is on five elements of a story (act, scene, agent, agency, and purpose) which examines the relationships of these five elements with each other. These terms are paired together as ratios, such as scene:agent, and imbalances are looked for to discover where tensions occur in a story. The ratio imbalance of act:agency occurred most frequently on the verbal landscape of mothers' traumatic birth stories. Predominant in women's narratives was the How (or agency) an act was done to them during labor and delivery. Clinicians did not communicate with women concerning what was going to be done to them, such as artificially rupturing membranes. Women did not feel cared for during childbirth. The glaring absence of caring and communication during childbirth was emphasized in this narrative analysis. Women described feeling like they were raped on the delivery table with everyone watching and no one offering to help them. This narrative analysis confirmed the findings of Beck's (2004a) phenomenological study of birth trauma.

An excerpt from one mother's narrative is provided to illustrate the ratio imbalance of act:agency; the uncaring manner of the nurse as she cared for this woman who was laboring to give birth to her infant who had died in utero:

> My husband went to get the nurse. The nurse said, you have only just had the gel, you couldn't be having IT yet. I said, yes. She is about to be born. The nurse checked and the head was visible. She looked shocked and said wait. I'll have to get a dish and returned with a green kidney shaped dish. The way she held the dish and the look on her face, I knew she did not want to be in the room. My husband held the dish for her. I then gave a little push and my daughter (still in her little sack) slipped quietly in the dish. The nurse took the dish from my husband and covered my daughter with a sheet. She then walked off without saying a word about where she was going. I called to her. Where are you taking her??? (I had not even seen her properly as she was still in her sack). The nurse said, I have to take IT to the doctor. She wants to see IT. Also the nurse continued to refer to me by my last name, not my first name. I said but I want to see my daughter. She said, Why? IT'S dead. She then said I have to get someone to wash IT so IT can be examined.
>
> *(Beck, 2006a, p. 461)*

Prevalence and Risk Factors of Posttraumatic Stress Disorder Following Childbirth

Grekin and O'Hara (2014) conducted a meta-analysis of the prevalence and risk factors of post-partum posttraumatic stress disorder (PTSD). Based on 78 studies their findings were divided into studies of community samples and those of at-risk samples. For community samples the prevalence rate was 3.1% with a 95% confidence interval of 2.5–3.9%. The only variable that moderated prevalence rates in community samples was age. As age increased, the prevalence of postpartum PTSD decreased. When focusing on at-risk samples the prevalence rate was 15.7% with a 95% confidence interval of 11.1–21.7%. Regarding risk factors, the correlates were categorized into two groups depending on the strength of their association with postpartum PTSD symptoms. In community samples a large effect size was reported for the risk factor of postpartum depressive symptoms. Medium effect sizes were reported for risk factors of negative interactions with labor and delivery staff, and a history of psychopathology. When considering risk factors in at-risk samples, postpartum depressive symptoms, and maternal and infant complications had large effect sizes while a history of trauma had a medium effect.

Grekin and O'Hara's (2014) meta-analysis confirmed findings of a US national survey of 859 mothers of which 18% experienced elevated levels of posttraumatic stress symptoms following childbirth (Beck, Gable, Sakala, & Declercq, 2011). Postpartum depressive symptoms predicted that 51% of the variance in posttraumatic stress symptom scores on the Posttraumatic Stress Symptoms-Self Report (PSS-SR) adapted to make it event specific for items referring to childbirth (Ayers & Pickering, 2001).

Ayers, Bond, Bertullies, and Wijma (2016) reviewed 50 studies in their meta-analysis of risk factors for birth-related posttraumatic stress measured at least one month after birth. The following pre-birth vulnerability factors were identified: prenatal depression ($r = .51$), fear of childbirth ($r = .41$), complications during pregnancy ($r = .38$), a history of PTSD ($r = .39$), and counseling for pregnancy or birth ($r = .32$). During labor and delivery risk factors most strongly related to PTSD included negative subjective birth experiences ($r = .59$), assisted vaginal or cesarean birth ($r = .48$), lack of support from staff ($r = -.38$), and dissociation ($r = .32$). During the postpartum period poor coping and stress ($r = .30$) and co-morbid depression ($r = .60$) were associated with PTSD.

Twenty-eight studies that used a diagnostic measure of PTSD were summarized by Yildiz, Ayers, and Phillips (2016). Not only the prevalence of PTSD during the postpartum year but also the point prevalence was reported. The mean prevalence of postpartum PTSD was 4.0% (95%, CI 2.77–5.71) in community samples while in the high-risk groups it was 18.5% (95%, CI 10.6–30.38). Similar patterns in point prevalence were found in both samples. For the total sample point prevalence was 5.77% at 4–6 weeks, 1.44% at three months, and the highest (6.79%) at six months. Simpson and Catling (2016) reviewed 21 articles to understand psychological traumatic birth experiences. Risk factors identified were prior mental health disorders, obstetric emergencies, neonatal complications, and poor quality of provider interactions during childbirth.

The Ripples of Traumatic Childbirth

What are the ripple effects of traumatic childbirth? Identifying these ripples can help to prevent the growth of bigger negative consequences for mothers, such as PTSD (Figure 7.1). Beck (2015) identified the following ripples from her series of studies on traumatic childbirth: posttraumatic stress symptoms, PTSD, breastfeeding, subsequent childbirth, mother-infant interaction, partners, and obstetrical care providers.

PTSD/Posttraumatic Stress Symptoms

James (2015) reviewed nine studies of women's experiences of PTSD after traumatic childbirth. Four themes guided by the cognitive model of PTSD (Elhers & Clark, 2000) were identified: the nature of trauma memory, negative appraisal of trauma and/or its sequelae, current threat, and strategies intended to control threat/symptoms.

Mothers suffering with PTSD after birth may draw on metaphorical expressions to help explain this mental health disorder more effectively with clinicians and provide rich insight into their experiences that are not captured by medical terminology. Beck (2016) conducted a metaphor analysis to investigate the language used by women with PTSD following birth as a valuable

Traumatic Childbirth

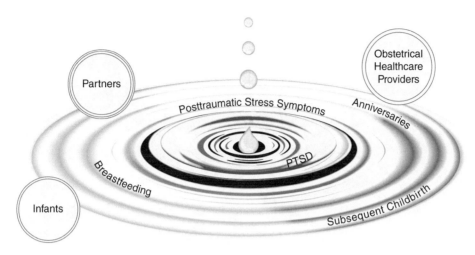

Figure 7.1   The ever-widening ripple effect of traumatic childbirth
Reprinted with permission from Beck, C.T. (2015). Middle range theory of traumatic childbirth: The ever-widening ripple effect.

source of insight. This was a qualitative secondary data analysis of a phenomenological study of PTSD due to traumatic childbirth with 38 mothers (Beck, 2004b). Nine metaphors were identified. PTSD due to childbirth is:

- A video on constant reply
- Enveloping darkness
- A dangerous ocean
- A thief in the night
- A bottomless abyss
- Suffocating layers of trauma
- A mechanical robot
- A ticking time bomb
- An invisible wall

These metaphors provide a new voice for mothers suffering with PTSD due to birth trauma and can help clinicians to identify these women so that they can get the mental health care they need and deserve.

Beck (2011) conducted a metaethnography of her six qualitative studies on traumatic childbirth and its resulting PTSD. As Figure 7.2 illustrates this synthesis revealed the far-reaching, stinging tentacles of the original trigger of birth trauma. This often invisible phenomenon to others resulted in six amplifying feedback loops. In amplifying causal looping "as consequences become continually causes and causes continually consequences, one sees either worsening or improving progressions or escalating severity" (Glaser, 2005, p. 9). Feedback is involved. When feedback lessens the impact of the original change or trigger, it is termed a balancing loop. A reinforcing loop occurs when the feedback increases the impact of a trigger.

Four of the loops in Beck's (2011) metaethnography reinforced the posttraumatic stress symptoms while two loops balanced the negative consequences by decreasing mothers' distress.

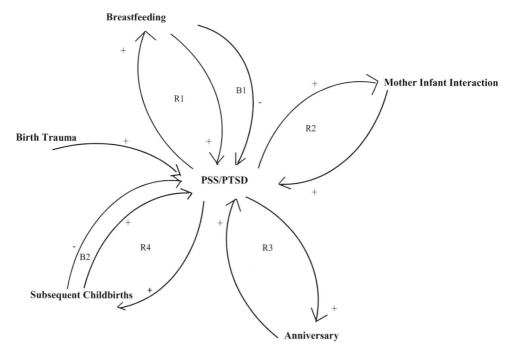

Figure 7.2 Amplifying causal loop diagram illustrating traumatic childbirth and its aftermath
Reprinted with permission from Beck, C.T. (2011). A metaethnography of traumatic childbirth and its aftermath: Amplifying causal looping. p. 307.

The impact of traumatic childbirth on mothers' breastfeeding experiences was a tale of two pathways (Beck & Watson, 2008). Reinforcing loop #1 highlights the detrimental effects posttraumatic stress symptoms can have on breastfeeding. Some women suffered with uncontrollable flashbacks when breastfeeding. Mothers shared that often they felt violated on the delivery table and so they became hypervigilant about protecting their bodies. To achieve this some mothers chose not to breastfeed in order to protect their breasts from being violated. The second path that some women chose is illustrated by balancing loop #1. Here breastfeeding helped to decrease women's posttraumatic stress symptoms as they described breastfeeding was a soothing time for them and helped them heal mentally.

Posttraumatic stress due to childbirth involved negative impacts on mother-infant interaction (reinforcing loop #2). This amplifying loop was present in all six of Beck's qualitative studies. For instance, mothers who experienced PTSD revealed that they distanced themselves from their infants who triggered their intensifying posttraumatic stress symptoms (Beck, 2004b). While breastfeeding some women felt a disturbing detachment from their infants (Beck & Watson, 2008). At the yearly anniversary of their birth trauma some mothers admitted that an emotional bond with their infants was missing (Beck, 2006b).

The third reinforcing feedback loop in Beck's (2011) metaethnography focused on the anniversary of birth trauma. This was a time of flare ups in women's posttraumatic stress symptoms. The actual day of the anniversary was especially difficult since it always was a day of celebration for everyone else but the mother since it was the child's birthday. This increased distress was also experienced in the days and weeks leading up to the child's birthday. After the anniversary day was over, mothers described that they were in a fragile state. Their invisible birth trauma wounds were reopened and raw.

Reinforcing loop #4 deals with subsequent childbirth after a previous birth trauma (Beck & Watson, 2010). During pregnancy women were filled with panic that this upcoming labor and delivery could again be traumatic. Multiple strategies were initiated to break the cycle of one traumatic birth after another, such as yoga, journaling, and self-hypnosis. Sadly for some women their worst fears came true – another traumatic birth – which re-intensified their posttraumatic stress symptoms. For other women their subsequent birth was a healing one and resulted in balancing loop #2 where their posttraumatic stress symptoms decreased. Women described feeling empowered and this brought a reverence to their birthing experience that they had longed for.

Mother-Infant Interaction and Child Development

Another ripple of traumatic childbirth extends out to mother-infant interaction. An exploratory study of the impact of posttraumatic stress symptoms after childbirth on early mother-infant interactions was conducted in Italy (Ionio & DiBlasio, 2014). Nineteen women completed the Perinatal PTSD Questionnaire (DeMier, Hynan, Harris, & Manniello, 1996) two days and two months postpartum. Their findings suggested that the number of PTSD symptoms at two months postpartum can impact early mother-infant interactions. Infants whose mothers had elevated PTSD symptoms displayed more avoidance behaviors. Mothers with PTSD symptoms were more prone to intrusive behaviors during interactions with their infants.

Webb and Ayers (2014) reviewed 14 studies which investigated the effect of depression, anxiety, and PTSD on interpretation of infant emotional expressions. Only two studies examined PTSD and those findings suggested that mothers may be more biased toward specific infant emotions leading to less sensitivity toward infants' needs. More research is needed, however, to confirm this pattern.

A prospective study of the impact of postpartum PTSD symptoms on child development at two years of age was conducted in Norway (Garthus-Niegel, Ayers, Martini, von Soest, & Eberhard-Gran, 2016). In this population-based sample ($N = 1,472$) postpartum PTSD symptoms had a small predictive relationship with poor child social emotional development at two years of age. Even after adjusting for confounding variables of mothers' depression and anxiety and infant temperament, the relationship was still significant. Boys and children who had early difficult temperament were especially susceptible to the negative impact of mothers' PTSD symptoms.

In a pilot study of 14 infants who were six months old, those whose mothers had PTSD developed poorer behavioral reactivity and emotional regulation than infants whose mothers did not have PTSD (Sanjuan et al., 2016). Infants' frontal neural activity, as measured by theta power during rest, was significantly associated with mothers' perinatal PTSD severity ($p = .004$). Sanjuan and colleagues suggested that these findings may indicate delayed cortical maturation in infants whose mothers had higher perinatal PTSD severity.

Fathers

Fathers are also included in the ripple effects of traumatic childbirth. Eight qualitative studies of fathers' experiences of complicated births that were potentially traumatic were synthesized in a metaethnography (Elmir & Schmied, 2016). Using Noblit and Hare's (1988) method four major themes were identified: (1) the unfolding crisis, (2) stripped of my role: powerless and helpless, (3) craving information, and (4) scarring the relationship. Some fathers revealed that their unresolved feelings of their partners' traumatic birth prevented them from moving on and instead led to flashbacks and nightmares.

Beck, Driscoll, and Watson (2013) conducted a qualitative study of fathers' experiences of being present at their partners' traumatic birth. The theme of helplessness was first and foremost in their descriptions of their experiences. As this father shared, "I am on an island watching my wife drown and I don't know how to swim. I not only do not know how to swim but I am drowning myself" (p. 212).

Inglis, Sharman, and Reed's (2016) sample consisted of 69 fathers who answered online questions regarding their perceptions of their partners' traumatic childbirth. Seven of these men were also interviewed. Thematic analysis revealed one global theme of Standing on the Sidelines which composed of two major themes of Witnessing the Trauma: Unknown Territory and the Aftermath: Dealing Within. Subthemes under Witnessing the Trauma included Being Unprepared, Out of Control, and Not Knowing. Under the Aftermath major themes were The Impact and Getting Past It. Lack of communication was a significant factor in these subthemes. Failure to communicate between the labor and delivery staff and the fathers exacerbated their distress.

Posttraumatic Growth in Mothers

Can there be any positive ripples of traumatic birth? Research is beginning to identify that some mothers can experience what is called posttraumatic growth which refers to the "positive psychological change experienced as a result of the struggle with highly challenging life circumstances" (Tedeschi & Calhoun, 2004, p. 1). This type of growth does not occur as a direct result of the traumatic event but rather as the result of the individual's struggle of coping or surviving their crisis. The five dimensions of posttraumatic growth include Appreciation of Life, Relating to Others, Personal Strength, New Possibilities, and Spiritual Change (Tedeschi & Calhoun, 1996). An individual does not necessarily experience growth in all five areas.

In three quantitative studies posttraumatic growth has been investigated during the postpartum period. Community samples were used. Women did not need to view their births as traumatic to be included in these studies. Sawyer and Ayers in 2009 conducted the first study on posttraumatic growth after childbirth. The Internet sample consisted of 219 women who had given birth within the previous 36 months. Women completed the Posttraumatic Growth Inventory (PTGI; Tedeschi & Calhoun, 1996). At least 50% of the sample reported at least a moderate degree of positive change following childbirth which was determined as a PTGI score of more than 62. Appreciation of Life was the posttraumatic growth dimension that received the highest endorsement (80.36%) while Spiritual Change received the least endorsement (16.44%).

A second quantitative study was conducted by Sawyer and her colleagues (2012) with a community sample of 125 women who completed the PTGI at eight weeks postpartum. A small amount of growth following childbirth, as indicated by a PTGI score of more than 41, was reported by 47.9% of the mothers. Appreciation of Life (68.1%) again was the dimension of growth most endorsed while Spiritual Change the least (22.3%). A regression analysis revealed that the strongest predictors of mothers' growth were operative birth and posttraumatic stress symptoms prenatally.

Posttraumatic growth following childbirth was examined in 193 mothers in the UK and 160 mothers in Croatia who gave birth within the last two years (Sawyer, Radoš, Ayers, & Burn, 2015). Using the PTGI (Tedeschi & Calhoun, 1996), 44% of UK mothers and 35% of Croatian mothers reported a moderate degree of positive growth after childbirth. Younger mothers in both countries reported higher levels of posttraumatic growth than older mothers.

Posttraumatic growth in mothers who perceived they had experienced a traumatic birth was examined in one qualitative study (Beck & Watson, 2016). Fifteen mothers participated in this phenomenological study via the Internet. A positive legacy of birth trauma was reported. As one participant shared, "I was broken; now I am unbreakable" (p. 268). Four themes emerged from this study: (1) opening oneself up to a new present, (2) achieving a new level of relationship nakedness, (3) fortifying spiritual mindedness, and (4) forging new paths. The first theme of Opening Oneself up to a New Present highlighted that posttraumatic growth is a process. As this woman revealed "At first, the very fabric of your being is shattered, destroyed. Nothing makes sense. The pieces do not go back together again. Rather, it is a gradual, new, very different kind of becoming" (Beck & Watson, 2016, p. 267). Struggling through their traumatic births made mothers stronger and this new strength underpinned their now different daily life. As part of their personal growth women became more empathetic and also more assertive.

The second theme focused on how mothers' relationships with others changed due to their posttraumatic growth (Beck & Watson, 2016). Communication opened up between women and their partners as the women no longer hid what they were feeling or thinking. Women felt secure enough in their relationships with their partners to be "naked" in front of them. One mother described this as achieving "relationship nakedness" (p. 268).

Fortifying spiritual mindedness, the third theme, involved a strengthening of faith. This mother explained that

> I can honestly say that overall, the most significant thing in my growth has been prayer and my personal relationship with the creator of this universe. I now believe that I was made for a purpose. Not only has He opened the right doors for me to gain healing and growth I specifically needed, but He has also given me huge insight into birth trauma which I hope to use for His glory in helping others with similar experiences.
>
> *(Beck & Watson, 2016, p. 269)*

The final theme in Beck and Watson's (2016) study of posttraumatic growth in mothers concentrated on the new paths mothers forged as they developed and achieved new professional and personal goals. Their new paths led some women to enrolling in universities to further their education while others became actively involved in volunteer work. Other women chose nursing as a new career so that they could help support women during childbirth.

Secondary Traumatic Stress in Obstetrical Healthcare Providers: Extending the Ripple Effects

For obstetrical clinicians who attend traumatic births they too can experience some ripple effects: one negative (secondary traumatic stress) and one positive (vicarious posttraumatic growth). Examples of both these ripple effects are provided by research with one type of obstetrical healthcare provider: labor and delivery nurses. Secondary traumatic stress is "the natural consequent behaviors and emotions resulting from the knowledge about a traumatizing event experienced by a significant other. This stress results from helping or wanting to help a traumatized or suffering person" (Figley, 1995, p. 10). In a mixed methods study Beck and Gable (2012) investigated the prevalence and severity of secondary traumatic stress in labor and delivery nurses and also explored the nurses' descriptions of their experiences caring for women during traumatic births. Nurses completed the Secondary Traumatic Stress Scale (STSS; Bride, Robinson, Yegidis, & Figley, 2004). With a sample of 464 labor and delivery nurses, 35% reported moderate to severe levels of secondary traumatic stress. Content analysis of the nurses' descriptions identified six themes: (1) magnifying the exposure to traumatic births, (2) struggling to maintain a professional role while with traumatized patients, (3) agonizing over what should have been, (4) mitigating the aftermath of exposure to traumatic births, (5) haunted by secondary traumatic stress symptoms, and (6) considering foregoing careers in labor and delivery to survive.

What magnified nurses' exposure to traumatic births involved four scenarios: being a new nurse, abusive births, patients whose second language was English, and adolescents as patients

(Beck & Gable, 2012). An example of how being a new nurse in labor and delivery intensified the situation is provided by the following excerpt:

> The demised infant needed to be bathed and photographed (tastefully) so that the parents had pictures of their infant to keep. It was a busy night, and I was left alone to do this. As I bathed and posed the infant for pictures, the baby was literally falling apart in my hands. It was my first experience with a term infant in this state of decomposition and it shook me to my core! I just remember feeling so alone. After photography, I wrapped the baby in blankets and after placing him in his mother's arms, I just hugged them both, and we cried together.
>
> *(p. 753)*

In the second theme of struggling to maintain a professional role, nurses echoed the incredible stress they worked under after a traumatic birth.

> The really jarring part was that I still had another patient that was in active labor and I had to maintain a positive attitude and remain upbeat when entering her room and giving her care. And that's what is expected of us nurses!
>
> *(Beck & Gable, 2012, p. 755)*

Theme 3 focused on how labor and delivery nurses often felt powerless and helpless during traumatic births. They agonized and questioned whether they had done enough to protect their patients. At times nurses felt like they had failed their patients as this quote illustrates:

> Once in the DR he (the obstetrician) checked her so roughly she was unable to push because she started screaming. I figured out that she was only 6 cm dilated and he was trying to manually dilate her with each contraction. My only clear memory is that this beautiful, intelligent, cooperative woman turned into a screaming, mindless animal under his torture. I've never felt so powerless, helpless, or useless in my life. I really feel that I failed her. She was counting on me to help her and I let that man torture her. I feel as sick to my stomach thinking about it today as I did 40 years ago when it was fresh.
>
> *(p. 756)*

In the fourth theme related to labor and delivery nurses' secondary traumatic stress, nurses described some strategies they tried to lessen the aftermath of being exposed to birth trauma (Beck & Gable, 2012). Prayer, and informal and formal debriefing are examples of these strategies. Theme 5 highlighted how labor and delivery nurses were haunted by secondary traumatic stress symptoms. This nurse shared that

> Whenever I hear a patient screaming I will flashback to a patient who had an unmedicated (not even a local) cesarean section and to the wailing of a mother when we were coding her baby in the delivery room. I feel like I will never get these sounds/images out of my head even though they occurred more than 10 years ago.
>
> *(p. 757)*

Lastly in the sixth theme labor and delivery nurses contemplated changing careers. Some nurses actually made the decision to leave labor and delivery and moved out of direct patient care to become managers. Other nurses chose to attend graduate school or go into academia. For some nurse they moved to either antepartum or postpartum units which were much less intensive care settings.

Vicarious Posttraumatic Growth in Obstetrical Healthcare Providers

Vicarious posttraumatic growth is the positive ripple effect that some labor and delivery nurses experienced. Posttraumatic growth in clinicians as a result of their work with trauma survivors is called vicarious posttraumatic growth. There are five dimensions of vicarious posttraumatic growth: Appreciation of Life, Relating to Others, Personal Strength, New Possibilities, and Spiritual Change. Beck, Eaton, and Gable (2016) examined vicarious posttraumatic growth in labor and delivery nurses who cared for women during traumatic births. The sample completed the PTGI (Tedeschi & Calhoun, 1996) in this mixed methods study. Labor and delivery nurses reported a moderate degree of vicarious posttraumatic growth. The dimension where the highest growth was reported was Appreciation of Life while New Possibilities was the dimension that reflected the least growth.

Qualitative descriptions of the labor and delivery nurses of their vicarious posttraumatic growth in Beck et al.'s (2016) mixed methods study were analyzed using content analysis. Segments of their descriptions were categorized into one of the five dimensions of vicarious posttraumatic growth. The dimension with the highest number of segments was Relating to Others while New Possibilities had the least number. Under the dimension of Relating to Others labor and delivery nurses shared how they (1) developed more compassion for patients and their families, (2) learned how amazing and inspiring their patients were, and (3) became closer with their coworkers. The following quote illustrates how awe inspiring one patient was whose baby had been born with two faces:

> The staff was horrified and did not want the mother to see the baby. I advocated for the mother who wanted to see and hold her baby. The baby only lived for a few hours but that mother did not see a horrifying thing. She saw and loved her baby. Her unconditional love spread to everyone on the unit that day. I feel so blessed to have been a part of that 'miracle'. It was a life changing event in my life because I understood the depth of a mother's love even in the face of a severely deformed baby that was dying.
>
> *(Beck et al., 2016, pp. 807–808)*

In the dimension of Personal Strength labor and delivery nurses recounted that part vicarious posttraumatic growth was their increased confidence they gained that they indeed were capable of handling difficult births. Vicarious posttraumatic growth also included spiritual changes for some nurses as their faith in God was strengthened. This nurse explained "I have always felt a higher power in our labor unit during difficult births. Like there is a guardian angel protecting the newly born. Makes me feel more spiritual" (Beck et al., 2016, p. 808).

Caring for women during traumatic births reminded labor and delivery nurses of just how precious life is and that it cannot ever be taken for granted. In this dimension of increased Appreciation of Life nurses recounted how they consciously shifted priorities in their lives as they placed an even higher value on their family, especially their children. As this nurse explained "After every traumatic birth it makes me go home and hug my family a little tighter" (p. 808). Under the New Possibilities dimension of vicarious posttraumatic growth labor and delivery nurses described some new paths in their lives that caring for women during traumatic births had led them down, such as, furthering their education, specializing in perinatal bereavement, and policy development for increased safety in childbirth.

Treatment

Eye movement desensitization and reprocessing (EMDR) therapy, cognitive behavioral therapy (CBT), and debriefing are three types of treatment available for PTSD due to childbirth.

Lapp, Agbokov, Peretti, and Ferreri (2010) reviewed studies that tested interventions for postpartum PTSD. Their conclusion was that the effectiveness of debriefing was inconclusive but that EMDR and CBT may decrease posttraumatic stress symptoms in mothers. Lapp et al. stressed, however, that randomized controlled trials are needed. Another systematic review of treatment strategies for PTSD following childbirth involved eight randomized controlled trials (Peeler, Chung, Stedmon, & Skirton, 2013). Individual and group counseling, debriefing, and expressive writing were the interventions assessed. In only three of the eight studies did the interventions result in a significant decrease in PTSD symptoms in mothers. No conclusions could be drawn because each of the three studies used a different intervention. A Cochrane review of debriefing interventions to prevent psychological trauma in mothers after childbirth was conducted by Bastos, Furuta, Small, McKenzie-McHarg, and Bick (2015). Seven trials from three countries were included and the conclusion was that high-quality evidence to inform clinical practice was not found in this review.

Healthcare providers can share with mothers struggling with posttraumatic stress that some women have reported some positive growth in their lives. We must not, however, create false hope in women that all trauma survivors will experience posttraumatic growth. Calhoun and Tedeschi (2013) suggest clinicians be "expert companions" when caring for traumatized patients. We can respect trauma survivors' struggles but at the same time we can allow the individuals to explore the potential for growth.

In their review of current issues and recommendations for future research on PTSD following childbirth, McKenzie-McHarg et al. (2015) concluded that longitudinal studies are needed to measure the prevalence and severity of PTSD plus its impact on mothers, their partners, and infants. PTSD following childbirth also needs to be integrated within maternity care pathways along with training for clinicians. Lastly they recommended alternative approaches to prepare women for labor and delivery along with testing effective interventions to decrease posttraumatic stress symptoms.

Implications for Clinical Practice

Obstetrical Healthcare Providers

To begin with clinicians need to be educated about their vulnerability to secondary traumatic stress when caring for patients who are traumatized or suffering. Continuing education programs can focus not only on secondary traumatic stress as a professional risk but also on the possibility of vicarious posttraumatic growth. These educational programs can help clinicians recognize the signs and symptoms of secondary traumatic stress in themselves and perhaps their need to seek help. An example of an already established program to prevent and treat secondary traumatic stress in healthcare providers is Gentry's (2002) Accelerated Recovery Program.

Calhoun and Tedeschi (2013) have developed an intervention to promote posttraumatic growth based on their theory. It consists of five components: psychoeducation about trauma, emotional regulation training, constructive self-disclosure, creation of new narratives with posttraumatic growth themes, and exploring new life possibilities. Holding periodic debriefing sessions for labor and delivery staff can provide valuable opportunities for self-disclosure. Writing narratives of the traumatic births that clinicians have attended can also be encouraged.

Mothers

The best way to help ensure that women will not experience a traumatic birth is for clinicians to treat all women as if they are survivors of previous trauma (Crompton, 2003). All obstetrical clinicians, not just nurses, need to practice what Highley and Mercer (1978) called for, that is, to bring reverence to caring for women during childbirth:

> Being able to assist a woman in one of the greatest tasks of her life – giving birth to and mothering a baby – is a privilege and challenge that touches every nurse who assists in her care. The challenge extends not only to the concrete physical help that the mother needs, but to the subtle consideration and attention which help her maintain her self-control and thus her self-respect.
>
> *(p. 41)*

We need to ensure that women are surrounded by protective layers of caring during childbirth. They need to feel cared for, communicated with, and respected. The glaring lack of caring of women during childbirth has been confirmed as one of the keys to the birth being viewed as traumatic. We know that prior trauma is a risk factor for women perceiving their birth as traumatic. When a multipara is admitted to labor and delivery, a careful history of her prior birthing experiences is essential. If a woman had a previous traumatic birth, she is at risk of being re-traumatized. Once known, clinicians can be alerted so that special care can be taken with this laboring woman. We need to be proactive in helping to prevent traumatic births and its resulting PTSD. Knowledge of risk factors for PTSD due to childbirth that research has uncovered, such as high levels of medical intervention, is essential so that healthcare providers are alert to these high-risk mothers. Being vigilant is critical to early signs of distress in traumatized mothers like a dazed look, being withdrawn, or experiencing dissociation. Routine assessment of mothers for posttraumatic stress symptoms using instruments such as the PSS-SR (Foa, Riggs, Dancu, & Rothbaum, 1993) is needed. Ayers and Pickering (2001) adapted the PSS-SR to make it event specific for childbirth.

Clinicians need to be alerted to the far-reaching ripple effects of traumatic birth for women: be it breastfeeding, subsequent childbirth, or its anniversary. For traumatized women, they may be in need of intensive one-on-one support as they try to initiate and sustain breastfeeding. England and Horowitz (1998) stressed that wounded women be encouraged to grieve prior traumatic births in order to lift the burden of their invisible pain. If subsequent labor and delivery has the potential to heal women, clinicians need to be aware of the effect their actions can have on women during this subsequent birth.

At anniversary time we must not fail to rescue mothers who are experiencing a flare up of their posttraumatic stress symptoms. Pediatric healthcare providers have an ideal opportunity to identify women struggling at this time when they bring their children in for annual physical exams. Further ripple effects can encompass mother-infant interactions. Clinicians need to pay close attention to this vulnerable dyad to identify if any interventions are needed.

Back in 1985 Golub and Loizzo warned that "just as a stone thrown in to water ruffles the surface in an outward direction, the feelings that arise in clinical situations generate emotional ripples of varied intensity" (p. 333). They also described how intense emotions of our patients can ripple out to all clinicians in their care. Clinicians, mothers, and their families all need to heed this warning.

References

Alcorn, K. L., O'Donovan, A., Patrick, J. C., Creedy, D., & Devilly, G. J. (2010). A prospective longitudinal study of the prevalence of post-traumatic stress disorder resulting from childbirth events. *Psychological Medicine, 40,* 1849–1859.

Arendt, H. (1958). *The human condition.* Chicago: University of Chicago Press.

Ayers, S., Bond, R., Bertullies, S., & Wijma, K. (2016). The aetiology of post-traumatic stress following childbirth: A meta-analysis and theoretical framework. *Psychological Medicine, 46,* 1121–1134.

Ayers, S., & Pickering, A. (2001). Do women get post-traumatic stress disorder as a result of childbirth? A prospective study of incidence. *Birth, 28*, 111–118.

Bastos, M. H., Furuta, M., Small, R., McKenzie-McHarg, K., & Bick, D. (2015). Debriefing interventions for the prevention of psychological trauma in women following childbirth. *Cochrane Database of Systematic Reviews, 4.* Doi: 10.1002/14651858. CD007194.pub2

Beck, C. T. (2004a). Birth trauma: In the eye of the beholder, *Nursing Research, 53*, 28–35.

Beck, C. T. (2004b). Posttraumatic stress due to childbirth: The aftermath. *Nursing Research, 53*, 216–2245.

Beck, C. T. (2006a). Pentadic cartography: Mapping birth trauma narratives. *Qualitative Health Research, 16*, 453–466.

Beck, C. T. (2006b). The anniversary of birth traumatic: Failure to rescue. *Nursing Research, 55*, 381–390.

Beck, C. T. (2011). A metaethnography of traumatic childbirth and its aftermath: Amplifying causal looping. *Qualitative Health Research, 2*, 301–311.

Beck, C. T. (2015). Middle range theory of traumatic childbirth: The ever-widening ripple effect. *Global Qualitative Nursing Research.* Doi: 10.1177/2333393615575313.

Beck, C. T. (2016). Posttraumatic stress disorder after birth: A metaphor analysis. *MCN: American Journal of Maternal Child Nursing, 41*, 76–83.

Beck, C. T., Driscoll, J. W., & Watson, S. (2013). *Traumatic childbirth.* New York: Routledge.

Beck, C. T., Eaton, C. M., & Gable, R. (2016). Vicarious Posttraumatic growth in labor and delivery nurses. *Journal of Obstetric, Gynecologic, and Neonatal Nursing, 45*, 801–812.

Beck, C. T., & Gable, R. K. (2012). Secondary traumatic stress in labor and delivery nurses: A mixed methods study. *Journal of Obstetric, Gynecologic, and Neonatal Nursing, 41*, 747–760.

Beck, C. T., Gable, R. K., Sakala, C., & Declercq, E. R. (2011). Posttraumatic stress disorder in new mothers: Results from a two-stage U.S. national survey. *Birth: Issues in Perinatal Care, 38*, 216–227.

Beck, C. T., & Watson, S. (2008). Impact of birth trauma on breast-feeding: A tale of two pathways. *Nursing Research, 57*, 228–236.

Beck, C. T., & Watson, S. (2010). Subsequent childbirth after a previous traumatic birth. *Nursing Research, 59*, 241–249.

Beck, C. T., & Watson, S. (2016). Posttraumatic growth following birth trauma: "I was broken. Now I am Unbreakable". *MCN: American Journal of Maternal Child Nursing, 41*, 264–271.

Bride, B. E., Robinson, M. M., Yegidis, B., & Figley, C. R. (2004). Development and validation of the secondary traumatic stress scale. *Research on Social Work Practice, 14*, 27–35.

Burke, K. (1969). *A grammar of motives.* Berkley: University of California Press.

Calhoun, L. G., & Tedeschi, R. G. (2013). *Posttraumatic growth in clinical practice.* New York: Routledge.

Crompton, J. (2003). Posttraumatic stress disorder and childbirth. *Childbirth Educators New Zealand Education Effects*, summer, 25–31.

DeMier, R. L., Hynan, M. T., Harris, H. B., & Manniello, R. L. (1996). Perinatal stressors as predictors of symptoms of posttraumatic stress in mothers and infants at high risk. *Journal of Perinatology, 16*, 276–280.

Elhers, A., & Clark, D. M. (2000). A cognitive model of posttraumatic stress disorder. *Behavioral Research and Therapy, 38*, 319–345.

Elmir, R., & Schmied, V. (2016). A meta-ethnography synthesis of fathers' experiences of complicated births that are potentially traumatic. *Midwifery, 32*, 6666–6674.

England, P., & Horowitz, R. (1998). *Birthing from within.* Albuquerque, NM: Partera Press.

Figley, C. R. (1995). Compassion fatigue: Toward a new understanding of the costs of caring. In B. H. Stamm (Ed.). *Secondary traumatic stress: Self-care issues for clinicians, researchers, and educators* (pp. 3–28). Luhterville, MD: Sidran Press.

Foa, E. B., Riggs, D. S., Dancu, C. V., & Rothbaum, B. O. (1993). Reliability and validity of a brief instrument for assessing posttraumatic stress disorder (PSS-SR). *Journal of Traumatic Stress, 6*, 459–473.

Garthus-Niegel, S., Ayers, S., Martini, J., von Soest, T., & Eberhard-Gran, M. (2016). The impact of postpartum post-traumatic stress disorder symptoms on child development: A population based, 2-year follow-up study. *Psychological Medicine*, Doi: 10.1017/s003329171600235x.

Gentry, J. E. (2002). Compassion fatigue: A crucible of transformation. *Journal of Trauma Practice, 1*, 37–61.

Glaser, B. G. (2005). *The grounded theory perspective III: Theoretical coding.* Valley, CA: Sociology Press.

Golub, Z. D., & Loizzo, K. (1985). The ripple effect of anger. *MCN: The American Journal of Maternal Child Nursing, 10*, 333–337.

Grekin, R., & O'Hara, M. W. (2014). Prevalence and risk factors of postpartum posttraumatic stress disorder: A meta-analysis. *Clinical Psychology Review, 34*, 389–401.

Highley, B., & Mercer, R. T. (1978). Safeguarding the laboring woman's sense of control. MCN. *The American Journal of Maternal Child Nursing, 4*, 39–41.

Inglis, C., Sharman, R., & Reed, R. (2016). Paternal mental health following perceived traumatic childbirth. *Midwifery, 41*, 125–131.

Ionio, C., & DiBlasio, P. (2014). Post-traumatic stress symptoms after childbirth and early mother-infant interactions: An exploratory study. *Journal of Reproductive and Infant Psychology, 32*, 163–181.

James, S. (2015). Women's experiences of symptoms of posttraumatic stress disorder (PTSD) after traumatic childbirth: A review and critical appraisal. *Archives of Women's Mental Health, 18*, 761–771.

Kounin, J. (1970). *Discipline and group management in classrooms*. Albany, NY: Delmar.

Lapp, L. K., Agbokov, C., Perretti, C. S., & Ferreri, F. (2010). Management of posttraumatic stress disorder after childbirth: A review. *Journal of Psychosomatic Obstetrics & Gynecology, 31*, 113–122.

McKenzie-Mcharg, K., Ayers, S., Ford, E., Horsch, A., Jomeen, J., Sayer, A., Stramrood, C., Thomson, G., & Slade, P. (2015). Posttraumatic stress disorder following childbirth: An update of current issues and recommendations for future research. *Journal of Reproductive and Infant Psychology, 33*, 219–237.

Noblit, G., & Hare, R. D. (1988). *Meta-ethnography: Synthesizing qualitative studies*. Newbury Park, CA: Sage Publications.

Peeler, S., Chung, M. C., Stedmon, J., & Skirton, H. (2013). A review assessing the current treatment strategies for postnatal psychological morbidity with a focus on post-traumatic stress disorder. *Midwifery, 29*, 377–388.

Riessman, C. K. (1993). *Narrative analysis*. Newbury Park, CA: Sage Publications.

Sanjuan, P. M., Poremba, C., Flynn, L. R., Savich, R., Annett, R. D., & Stephen, J. (2016). Association between theta power in 6-month old infants at rest and maternal posttraumatic stress disorder severity: A pilot study. *Neuroscience Letters, 630*, 120–126.

Sawyer, A., & Ayers, S. (2009). Post-traumatic growth in women after childbirth. *Psychology and Health, 24*, 457–471.

Sawyer, A., Ayers, S., Young, D., Bradley, R., & Smith, H. (2012). Posttraumatic growth after childbirth: A prospective study. *Psychology and Health, 27*, 362–377.

Sawyer, A., Radoš, S. N., Ayers, S., & Burn, E. (2015). Personal growth in the United Kingdom and Croatian women following childbirth: A preliminary study. *Journal of Reproductive and Infant Psychology, 33*, 294–307.

Simpson, M., & Catling, C. (2016). Understanding psychological traumatic birth experiences: A literature review. *Women and Birth, 29*, 203–207.

Soet, J. E., Brack, G. A., & Dilorio, C. (2003). Prevalence and predictors of women's experience of psychological trauma during childbirth. *Birth, 30*, 36–46.

Tedeschi, R., & Calhoun, L. (1996). The Posttraumatic Growth Inventory: Measuring the positive legacy of trauma. *Journal of Traumatic Stress, 9*, 455–472.

Tedeschi, R., & Calhoun, L. (2004). Posttraumatic growth: Conceptual foundations and empirical evidence. *Psychological Inquiry, 15*, 1–18.

Webb, R., & Ayers, S. (2014). Cognitive biases in processing infant emotion by women with depression, anxiety, and posttraumatic stress disorder in pregnancy or after birth: A systematic review. *Cognition and Emotion*. Doi: 10.1080/0269931.2014.977849.

Yildiz, P. D., Ayrs, S., & Phillips. L. (2016). The prevalence of posttraumatic stress disorder in pregnancy and after birth: A systematic review and meta-analysis. *Journal of Affective Disorders*. Doi: 10.1016/j.jad.2016.10.009.

Zinker, J. B. (2013). *The science of ocean waves: Ripples, tsunamis and stormy seas*. Baltimore, MD: Johns Hopkins University Press.

Part III
Postnatal Period

8

Beyond the Blues

Stress, Emotional Experiences of Women, and Intervention Methods during the Postpartum Period

Rosa Maria Quatraro and Pietro Grussu

Introduction

The postpartum period, as defined in the biomedical literature, is placed within the first six to eight weeks after childbirth—that is from the birth of the fetus and the ensuing expulsion of the placenta, to the involution of the uterus and the return to a physical condition in large part similar to the pregravid state. The involution of the reproductive system and the re-stabilization to the pre-pregnancy physiological condition are not the only events which, in the months following childbirth, characterize a woman's experience (Fahey and Shenassa, 2013).

This period, especially for first-time mothers, is characterized by the greatest personal and familial changes that a woman can experience during her lifetime. Globally, the postpartum period is seen in experiential terms as a time of enrichment when the growth of an individual is stimulated. At the same time, though, the aftermath of childbirth can also bring about conditions of emotional discomfort and stress (Bener, Gerber and Sheikh, 2012), to the point of psychopathological manifestations that are at times extreme (Paschetta et al., 2014).

Among the stressful physical elements which cannot go unmentioned are perineal pain, backache, urinary incontinence, hemorrhoids and constipation, hormonal fluctuations, the feeling of extreme fatigue and physical exhaustion, difficulty in falling asleep and sleeping, problems associated with nursing such as breast engorgement, nipple pain, mastitis, fissures and leaking breasts. At the same time, among the psychological stressors are those associated with new relational routines with one's partner and sense of belonging within the family framework, the lack of social support, preoccupations pertaining to one's own maternal role, doubts about one's ability to adequately nourish the newborn, the feeling of being unprepared to manage the growth and development of the child, the fears that some unspeakable thing might happen to the newborn child, pressures and desires associated with a return to pre-pregnancy weight, day-to-day sensitivities linked to one's body image and changes with respect to sexuality (Beck et al., 2011; Cheng and Li, 2008; Hung et al., 2011; George, 2005; Wilkins, 2006).

These situations of physical and emotional stress are made more onerous by the fact that, immediately after childbirth, the woman gives her exclusive attention to the newborn child, 24 hours per day, often without the possibility to detach herself and to rest properly. Moreover, during the postpartum period, mothers are called upon to carry out the difficult job of learning, understanding and arranging in a unique pattern the crying, the sleep and the nutritional needs of the child, together with all of the child's other behaviors.

If a woman feels uneasy about comforting or taking care of her baby, she may on occasion consider herself to be an incompetent mother (Ruchala and Halstead, 1994). At the same time, the attitude and responses that a woman gets from health professionals, from her immediate family and from her friends, as well as the responses exhibited by her child (Porter and Hsu, 2003) serve as the major validation of her feeling of adequacy—or inadequacy—in this new personal and social experience. In particular, the recognition, criticism or praise that she receives from those who surround her will also influence the expectations that a woman will have for herself as a mother, now and in the future (Hung, 2006).

An in-depth knowledge of the dynamics that characterize the perinatal period leads to an awareness that appropriate interventions of prevention and support—physical as well as emotional—are needed in order to foster a scaling down of perceived stress and a reduction of stressful life events.

The Woman and Her Transition to Motherhood: From the Relationship with the Fetus to the Relationship with the Child

A woman arrives at childbirth after a journey which lasts about ten months. During that voyage, she has had to take essential psychological and emotional strides. During pregnancy, in order to adapt psychologically and physically, the mother must, from the outset, be able to achieve a symbiotic connection with the fetus. Subsequently, with the beginning of fetal movement, she has to begin to separate herself psychologically (Soifer, 1987). At the same she must gradually develop the ability to see herself and to think of herself as "mother" so as to know how to take care of herself and her pregnancy in a time of great emotional fragility and specific physical needs. Finally, a woman must have the ability and the possibility to prepare herself psychologically for labor and delivery, in order to be able to confront the fears and fantasies inherent in childbirth (Attrill, 2002).

Generally, the feelings associated with fetal movement help the mother to carry out the task of separation as well as the task of symbiosis—two concepts that play an important role in the mother-child relationship. A good balance between these opposing forces is, in fact, one of the elements that, after childbirth, will permit the mother-child dyad to evolve together, despite the difficulty that the growth and development process brings for both mother and child.

That symbiosis is the starting point of the mother-child rapport and is the basis of an ongoing relationship that will change in intensity and characteristics with the growth and development of the child. According to Attrill (2002), the failure to achieve these goals of symbiosis and separation is a potentially predictive factor in a difficult labor and delivery, much the same as the impossibility to confront the fantasies and fears associated with childbirth, and an inappropriate emotional response to the newborn in the moments following delivery.

During the period immediately following childbirth, there is an intensification of pre-birth themes. The outcome of delivery, in particular, is a factor that can influence not only the idea that the woman has of herself as a mother, but also the strain that arises between the recovery of a mother-child symbiosis and the physical separateness confirmed by childbirth itself (Soifer, 1987, pp. 83–84).

The birth also activates the dimension of psychological separation, making the mother come into contact with an actual child who has needs and demands that she must gradually learn to comprehend and interpret. The preverbal dimension of the neonatal world, for example, requires the woman to be able to dra on her own experiences of vulnerability and fragility, but at the same time also drawn upon her most adult abilities to provide sustenance and protection to the newborn child. In that regard, Roberts (1977) identifies two new developmental tasks that the mother needs to undertake during the immediate neonatal period: the creation of an emotional bond and the formation of reciprocity.

In this phase, the mother needs to succeed in establishing an initial bond with her child and begin breastfeeding or bottle feeding (in some cases mothers do not want to, cannot or feel unable to breastfeed).

For some women, breastfeeding is a choice that follows a route with few obstacles; for others, though, it can become a critical aspect of motherhood upon which to pour preoccupations, feelings of inadequacy and a sense of guilt (Byrom, 2013; Thomson, 2015).

A woman can also find herself having to decide on which feeding method to adopt. Meeting this dilemma can be very difficult, especially when mothers are extremely ambivalent toward breastfeeding and, even after trying it, do not feel like continuing, while at the same time finding themselves unable to make a decision.

The relationship with the newborn, in some cases, is framed in terms of continuity with respect to the previous relationship with the fetus. In other cases, the woman instead experiences an evident discontinuity between the child she carried in her womb and the baby she now holds in her arms. For some, taking care of the unborn child and establishing a communicative relationship with the child do not pose particular difficulties. For others, the world of the newborn turns out to be indecipherable and uncontrollable, to the point of bringing about feelings of incompetence and inadequacy in the care of one's own child.

In this regard, it should be remembered that Winnicott (1975) spoke of primary maternal preoccupation as a "state of heightened sensitivity" which is already being developed in the final trimester of pregnancy and which permits the woman to attune herself to the needs of the newborn in an intuitive and preverbal manner (Stern, 1985). Not in all cases, however, is this attunement process straightforward and without difficulty (Tronick et al., 1998).

For some women, in fact, pregnancy ends up being charged with anxious worries, and pregnancy presents itself as a time of hardship which can be accompanied by stress and anxiety (Dayan et al., 2006; Lederman, 1990; Oates, 1989). In some cases, these emotional reactions and preoccupations are transitory (Huizing et al., 2014); in other cases, they can persist and bring dysfunctional responses on biological, cognitive-affective and relational levels into the post-partum period (Don et al., 2014). In that regard, Huizing et al. (2017) show how women with elevated levels of trait anxiety during pregnancy and with pregnancy-specific anxiety (preoccupations about the progress of the pregnancy and the health of the child) are, after the birth of the child, more at risk to have difficulty in adapting, and to experience stress associated with taking care of the baby. In particular, women who feel very worried during pregnancy have a greater probability of being worried and anxious mothers, and they are much more susceptible to typical postpartum stressors.

The First Weeks Following Delivery

With reference primarily to Western culture, upon the return home after the hospital stay, a phase begins that is new in all respects. The mother and the child seek their way of continuing the relationship that began during pregnancy. The period following childbirth is sometimes referred to as "the fourth trimester" because of the discontinuity/continuity with respect to the prenatal phase. The discontinuity comes into play because now the baby is an actual human being, with real, tangible needs that must be satisfied as they arise. Continuity is achieved in the days following delivery when the mother attributes familiar characteristics to her child and—more or less slowly—she falls in love with the newborn.

If, during pregnancy, being two people in one body gave the mother some autonomy in her movements and in the management of her day, now the woman is catapulted into a reality for which she may feel herself to be unprepared and inadequate. This particular phase is characterized, on the one hand, by the emotional and physical states of the mother and, on the other, by the impossibility of the child to gain access to the verbal and conceivable world of the mother. At first the child reaches out to the mother through cries, facial expressions, sounds (for example, during sleep, the baby produces sounds which, in the beginning, can waken the mother frequently, leading her to check on the state of her child's health) and fluids that come out of the child's body and arouse reactions of alarm or satisfaction in the mother. In this regard, we think of regurgitation and the importance of "burping" in the mother-child relationship. We think, too, of the nappy change ritual, and the "loads" that, with their odor and sound, transmit a sign to the mother of the healthy functioning of the baby's digestive system.

Mentally, the newborn is a fetus and the same being as prior to birth, propelled into a situation that is psychologically new compared to that in which the fetus lived for nine months. The child therefore needs time, continuity and care to adapt to the new reality (Vallino and Macciò, 2004). The mother is called upon to immerse herself in this neonatal world of tactile, auditory and kinesthetic sensations which differ greatly from those of the adult world and even the world of older children. The newborn asks the mother to regress, dipping into the "newborn in her", and the baby remains helpless and without bargaining power in a domain where crying is the only way to be heard when something is needed or bothersome.

In a certain sense, a mother must use her intuition to guess what her little one needs, and cannot help but put herself into the territory of trial and error. How much can a woman endure of not knowing what her child needs? For how long can she manage the process of trial and error which sometimes leads to relief for both of them, and at other times does not bring about the anticipated outcomes, or is effective only after lengthy exhausting attempts? In this continuing dance between mother and child, the inability/impossibility of relieving one's own child from discomfort, and to stop crying and upsetting himself, sometimes leads the mother to become discouraged and to lose faith in her own ability to be a good mother or, to echo Winnicott (1970), a "good enough mother".

We must also keep in mind that, in these first weeks, the mother usually reacts to the change and the emotional and hands-on workload with an emotional responsiveness which, outside of the postnatal period, would be alarming, but in this postnatal phase is often part of the normal psychological experience.

The Postpartum Period and the Ability to Adapt

In the first days following childbirth, a woman is uniquely exposed to extensive emotional turbulence. Influenced by situational aspects which can be external or internal (linked to the intimate resonances that life events have for each woman), the woman can manifest positive feelings, but negative emotions can also be exhibited. First-time mothers are especially at risk and vulnerable to the difficulties presented in the period following the birth of the child.

For example, in a qualitative study (Darvill, Skirton and Farrand, 2010) conducted on a small sample of women, the main themes that emerged were related to control, support (from mother, husband and friends who were living the same experience) and the responsibility of a new family.

Fahey and Shenessa (2013) highlight an analysis of the literature that draws attention to four factors that seem to have a significant influence on the way in which a woman will live the period immediately following childbirth:

- The ability to ask for and obtain social support;
- Self-efficacy;
- The ability to cope with the demands of the post-childbirth period;
- Realistic expectations of the post-childbirth period.

Rosa Maria Quatraro and Pietro Grussu

The Ability to Ask For and Obtain Social Support

Numerous studies have shown that social support positively affects physical and emotional health (Barrera, 1986; Razurel et al., 2011). During the postpartum period, emotional and hands-on support have a direct effect, decreasing the burden of the duties and tasks that the woman has to perform daily. Added to this, there is also indirect positive fallout: social support has, in fact, a beneficial effect on the perception of stressful life events, and improves self-esteem and the sense of self-efficacy (Cohen, 1988; Collins et al., 1993).

In the first weeks following the birth of the child, the woman often gives priority to practical hands-on support. In fact, she needs help to take care of the newborn and other children, just as she needs help with domestic chores like cooking and cleaning, so as to have time herself to eat, bathe and sleep (Negron et al., 2013).

When a woman feels that those surrounding her do not pick up on her need to be helped, the reactions are anxiety, stress and anger (Razurel et al., 2011). Moreover, the dissonance between the support that the woman expects to receive and that which she actually receives is particularly stressful (Razurel et al., 2011; Tarkka and Paunonen, 1996).

Sometimes, it is these same women who do not ask for help. This seems to be linked to the perception of being seen as ineffective in her new role—that others consider her to be a burden, that the people around her feel hurt or offended in the face of a request for help that differs from a spontaneous offer of assistance or, further, that others cannot understand what she is experiencing and therefore are not able to offer the help she needs (Negron et al., 2013).

It is important that healthcare providers keep these elements in mind to help the woman to speak about these two aspects, and also to modify her beliefs when they have no basis in reality. Conversely, when the beliefs are based on family members' real difficulty in understanding the needs of the woman and in responding to them, it is important that professionals work within a framework of acceptance of the new mother in order to activate the necessary family and social resources.

Self-Efficacy

"Self-efficacy" is defined as the ability to attain specific objectives. During the postpartum period, this ability is directly correlated with behaviors that promote well-being, and inversely correlated with stress and depression (Reece, 1992; Reece and Harkless, 1998). In particular, during the period which follows the birth of a child, self-efficacy is linked to the ability to enter into the maternal role and to feel capable of taking care of one's own child and family (Leahy-Warren et al., 2012; Mercer, 2004; Mercer and Walker, 2006).

There are three aspects which play a fundamental role in the sense of self-efficacy during the postpartum period. The first aspect is the basic performance of the tasks posed by motherhood for which multiparous mothers have a higher level of auto-efficacy (Leahy-Warren, McCarthy and Corcoran, 2011). The second is having vicarious experience because someone has demonstrated how a thing is done (Bandura, 1997), an aspect which permits a gradual increase in self-efficacy. The third aspect is the temperament of the newborn (Jones and Prinz, 2005), which is why mothers with newborns who are more difficult to console feel more incapable and tend, in the long run, to make less of an effort to console their babies, and to lose faith in their power to succeed in their objectives (Bandura, 1997; Leerkes and Crockenberg, 2002).

The Ability to Cope with the Demands of the Postpartum Period

During the postpartum period, women use different coping methods to handle the stressors they encounter. The search for social support is an example of a positive coping strategy put in place

152

by some new mothers. Often, though, to deal with the difficulties they face and with issues affecting their health, these same women use negative strategies such as avoidance or minimization (Albers, 2000; Declerq et al., 2006). This frequently leads to the mother's health concerns being overlooked, and to an inadequate response from family and carers to take charge and to help.

Realistic Expectations of the Postpartum Period

Having expectations is a natural condition and has an adaptive value. However, when expectations are based on incorrect or incomplete information and come into conflict with reality, the dissonance can be negative from an individual as well as from a relational point of view.

During the postpartum period, the dissonance between expectations and reality can be critical to the capability of the woman to cope with the difficulties that motherhood poses (Coleman, Nelson and Sundre, 1999; Lawrence, Nylen and Cobb, 2007). Women who, for example, don't feel ready to take on the post-childbirth phase, as well as those whose lived experience is worse than they had expected, have greater difficulty in adapting (Bryanton and Beck, 2010) and are at greater risk of incurring developing mental health disorders (Howell, Mora and Leventhal, 2006).

Unmet expectations with respect to one's own parenting capabilities are also associated with an inferior capacity to cope with difficulties, an increase in distress and marital dissatisfaction and a decrease in the ability to mobilize social resources (Emmanuel et al., 2011; Negron et al., 2013). Conversely, having already cared for babies or having parented, and the accuracy of information that has been received are factors associated with a greater correspondence between expectations and reality (Coleman, Nelson and Sundre, 1999; Lawrence, Nylen and Cobb, 2007). These elements therefore have a positive effect on the mother's general psychological condition.

The Maternity Blues

Definition and Description of the Condition

Within perinatal psychology and psychopathology, it was Pitt (1973) who first used the label "maternity blues" to describe a collection of psychological and psychosomatic symptoms that can occur in the period immediately after childbirth.

Globally, the term "blues" refers to the notion that the symptomatology of the woman affected by the discomfort is fundamentally characterized by a predominant low mood (Henshaw, 2003) of a transitory nature (Ferber, 2004). In fact, according to some authors (Kennerley and Gath, 1989; Newport et al., 2002), subjects with the maternity blues are characterized by the presence of mild depressive symptoms such as crying, sadness, unstable and fluctuating mood, poor concentration, irritability, anxiety, fear and disturbances of sleep and appetite. Beyond this symptomatology, the new mothers may also experience feelings of unreality and a certain detachment and disinterest toward the child (Robinson and Stewart, 1993). These women usually report feelings of "low mood" (Kennerley and Gath, 1989).

Currently, the scientific community agrees in considering the maternity blues as a collection of psychological and psychosomatic symptoms which women can exhibit in a manner that is heightened, but not pathological, in the first 10–15 days after delivery. In most mothers, the condition turns out to be transitory, and tends to resolve itself of its own accord (Grussu, 2016).

Mothers who go through a condition defined as the maternity blues during the period immediately following the birth report how much their mood differs from their usual frame of mind, and how it changes frequently, even from one day to the next. In addition, they report not only a low mood and a sense of sadness, but also an increase in their emotional sensitivity. In general, they commonly perceive that, with respect to even the recent past, they tend to react with greater intensity when presented with common situations or experiences encountered in the course of their day, and which occur in a routine life marked by new commitments and by new personal and relational responsibilities (Rondón, 2003).

Elevated levels of maternal symptomatology have been detected during the course of the first days following the birth (Kendell et al., 1981), specifically in the first four to six days (Stein, Marsh and Morton, 1981), on the fifth day (Adewuya, 2005) or in the third to eighth day following the birth of the child (O'Hara et al., 1990). Numerous studies published over the last 40 years have involved research samples from various cultural contexts. These studies have shown the frequency of maternity blues in the population of women who have just given birth to range from 8% to 84% (Harris, 1981; O'Hara et al., 1991; Oakley and Chamberlain, 1981; Tsukasaki et al., 1991).

The significant discrepancy present in the literature on the spread of the phenomenon is sustained by the absence of a shared definition and cataloguing of this disorder among scholars and researchers who take an interest in the maternal psychological condition after childbirth. This disparity is the outcome of studies that have used survey and data collection methodologies that are, in large part, doubtful in their reliability and the possibility of generalization. In fact, in-depth reviews (Beck, 1991; Henshaw, 2003) have shown how far studies on the maternity blues have taken researchers as they circumscribe, in arbitrary and diverse ways, some of the psychological manifestations of the period immediately after childbirth. For example, in numerous studies cited in the literature, some researchers have carried out an assortment of maternal symptom assessments, in a random manner and often without any discussion, taking into consideration just one day during the postpartum period. Others, however, have carried out repeated assessments for as many as seven to ten consecutive days. Additionally, many of the assessments relating to the symptomatology present in the puerpera emerge from retrospective research (Grussu, 2016).

Recently, therefore, the intent of some researchers has been not so much to identify the possible presence of maternity blues, but to shed light on the profiles and some reactive modalities that characterize the experience of the new mothers in the immediate period after birth. Others have sought to identify psychometric tools which are able to detect and highlight the broad spectrum of lived experiences and feelings that women report going through during the period following the birth of their child.

Sensitivity and the Lived Maternal Psychological Experiences in the First Days after Childbirth

In recent years, an interesting branch of research has attempted to define, in a more precise way, the symptomatological structure of maternal mood occurring in the period after childbirth. The primary approach adopted by the researchers has been to carry out frequent and repeated surveys, using psychometric tools that allow the identification of a broad spectrum of symptoms present in the immediate postpartum, as well as the variability of the symptomatological levels that a woman develops and manifests with the passing of days.

In that regard, an Italian study of the first 15 days following childbirth carried out on a group of primiparous women at low social and medical risk profiles, with normal full-term pregnancies, vaginal births and healthy babies (Grussu and Quatraro, 2013), detected the presence of a psychological symptomatology and a level of minor mood disorders as a whole. Conversely, the somatic symptomatology was shown to be intensified in the earliest postpartum days, by the presence in the women of some spikes in distress characterized by anxiety and feelings of confusion and loss. In particular, though, the new mothers with raised levels of psychological and somatic symptoms showed greater emotional distress; however, those with a reduced symptomatology reported minor mood disturbances. Additionally, primipara women who reported higher levels of emotional distress and symptoms on the first day were still reporting higher levels of psychological suffering on the 15th day. On the whole, however, the mild mood disorders reported by mothers followed a linear trend for all 15 days after delivery. The psychological and somatic symptomatology is particularly accentuated in the first days after the birth of the child and decreases significantly in the following days. Above all, it is the somatic experience of anxiety and fatigue that tends to decrease gradually. Finally, with the imminence of, and following, the postpartum discharge from hospital, there is an anxious symptomatology.

Insofar as the possibility of identifying and using specific tools for the detection of maternity blues is concerned, the research group of Mike O'Hara at the University of Iowa (Buttner et al., 2012) has developed the Daily Experiences Questionnaire (DEQ). This tool has shown itself to be particularly useful for the detection of mood variability present in postpartum women, by identification of the Positive Affect (PA) and the Negative Affect (NA).

On the one hand, the data obtained by administering this instrument suggest that, within the first week postpartum, the woman's affective structure is not significantly differentiated from that detected in the weeks prior to the birth of the child; on the other hand, the descriptors of mood status measured by the DEQ are very useful as they facilitate the capture of multiple indications that make up the factors of emotional distress typical of the maternity blues.

The DEQ has additionally been shown to be more suitable in detecting mood status immediately after delivery when compared with other tools predominantly intended to identify depressive symptomatology (Leigh and Milgrom, 2007). Taking into account that different studies have identified a significant connection between high NA or low PA of mood and postnatal depression in the immediate postpartum (Buttner, Brock and O'Hara, 2015; Fossey, Papiernik and Bydlowski, 1997; Watanabe et al., 2008), there does indeed seem to be a promising possibility of using a tool of this kind during the hospitalization related to childbirth or in the days following discharge from hospital.

The mood disorders detected at three days after the birth are the best predictor of the level of postpartum depression present at six weeks (Lane et al., 1997), while the mood disorders detected in the first two weeks after childbirth have been shown to be predictive of postnatal depression and anxiety at 12 weeks after childbirth (Reck et al., 2009).

In a recent study by Miller and his colleagues (Miller, Kroska and Grekin, 2017), it was also observed that the levels of NA and those of PA of mood detected in the days immediately following childbirth were predictive of subsequent depressive symptomatology at two and 12 weeks postpartum. The authors therefore suggest that measurement of a woman's affective condition during the hospital stay can indeed be helpful for the early identification of those at risk for postpartum depression. This method could also be used after discharge from hospital to monitor the mood of women at risk and consequently, when feasible, promptly carry out interventions that strengthen the positive factors such as social support, and mitigate the risk factors.

Healthcare providers (gynecologists, midwives, nurses, psychologists, social workers, educators, etc.) who have taken the time to listen to and speak with pregnant women, or to connect with the same women immediately after the birth will certainly be important reference points for the new mother if the symptoms suggesting maternity blues should get worse, or be prolonged beyond 10–15 days following the birth of the child. In such situations, it can be very helpful for the woman to have a positive relationship of trust with her health professional. Such relationships can be built during specialist visits during pregnancy and reinforced by health education meetings conducted before the birth of the child or undertaken immediately after birth during the hospital stay. These ties will ultimately be fruitful if the designated health professional has nurtured in the woman the ability to verbalize her mood, is committed to gathering sufficient information on aspects such as any possible psychiatric conditions of the new mother or her family, has looked into the presence—current or past—of particular life circumstances or stressful events and has acted in advance to offer helpful advice and reassurance (Rondón, 2003).

Postnatal Stress

As already mentioned, the first weeks following childbirth have come to be seen increasingly not only as a moment exclusively of happiness, but also as a period in which the woman can go through situations and conditions that are stressful on a physical, emotional and relational level. Although the reactions to transitory distress (which can include sadness, depression, fear, anxiety and helplessness) are considered normal after childbirth, it is important that a reaction to prolonged and significant stress does not become trivialized or minimized. In other words, that reaction should attract our attention (Lefkowitz, Baxt and Evans, 2010) even when the woman, or those around her, seem to think it is normal and they attribute it to the maternity blues. We know, in fact, that the maternity blues usually occur within a limited time period (the first two weeks after childbirth); therefore, it often cannot explain nor provide a sense of the complex emotional reactivity that women experience after the birth of the child.

Postpartum stress was defined by Hung (2001) as a condition of duress, or a significantly distinct negative emotional state which is present in the first six weeks after childbirth. The factors that are associated with a higher level of stress include low income, socioeconomic disadvantage, stressful life events and inadequate social and family support (Beber et al., 2013; Gausia et al., 2009; Prost et al., 2012). During this phase, women are particularly vulnerable to stress, having to confront substantial changes linked to maternal and family obligations, as well as the compelling changes that occur in the mind and the body (Zauderer, 2009): one *becomes* a mother, gradually learning how to do things, and how to act in a context of significant changes and multiple responsibilities. In that regard, Barclay and Lloyd (1996) sought to define the experiences that women face during the postpartum period in a more precise and reliable manner. These authors assert that the concept of maternal distress permits us to understand in a more thorough way the emotional experience of motherhood that women go through in contemporary society. These same authors, however, underscore the confusion present in the literature with regard to terminology used to describe maternal stress such as stress, depression, anxiety, depressive symptoms, prenatal depression, perinatal depression and postnatal depression. In reference to this critical issue, from a recent review (Rallis et al., 2014) it emerges that the most current studies have nevertheless identified the possibility that women experience a postnatal stress both overlapping and independent of postnatal depression and anxiety. It is not clear, then, whether postnatal distress is an affective condition that can occur during the postpartum period independently of depression and anxiety, or whether it instead might be a factor which, during the postnatal period, plays a critical role in the development and retention of anxiety or a depressive disorder (Figure 8.1).

A further attempt to define the concept of maternal distress in a more precise way was developed by Emmanuel and St. John (2010). For them, it is the woman's response to the transitional phase to motherhood that includes changes to her body and to her relational and social roles, as well as her reaction to the childbirth experience and its demands, and to the losses as well as the gains associated with being a new mother. According to this view, one can have a very real mental health issue as a consequence of severe and prolonged maternal stress to the point of developing a condition of depression, maladjustment, dysfunctional modalities and emotional and relational "disconnection". These authors contend that even though maternal distress can lead to emotional issues and problems of mental health which range from feeling alone and without energy to feelings of anxiety and depression, this condition does not necessarily represent just a negative experience. It can, in fact, also portray evolutionary features linked to transitional life stages. From this

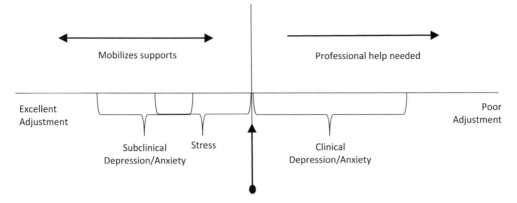

Figure 8.1 Rallis et al. (2013). The transition to motherhood: Towards a broader understanding of perinatal distress. Women and Birth 27, 68–71

perspective, the concept of maternal distress is well placed within the theory of the transitions of life developed by Meleis (Meleis et al., 2000), which shows that the transition to motherhood is not a linear action, but entails instability, confusion and distress that, in most cases, lead to a phase of recovered stability. During this period of time, in particular the mother looks for significance in events connected to motherhood, and commits to, and carries out, all those changes necessary to reach a point of greater psychological balance.

Emmanuel and St. John (2010), building on the work already carried out by Barclay and Lloyd (1996), by Rogan et al. (1997) and by Nicolson (1999), have also developed a conceptual structure of maternal distress which describes the woman's response during the transition to motherhood. For them, maternal distress is on a continuum of four categories: stress responses, adapting responses, functional and control responses, and connecting responses. The severity of the maternal distress varies from mild to severe, from low to high.

In this frame of reference, a woman with a low level of distress will experience stress, worry and restlessness in trying to adapt to her new role. Nevertheless, she will adapt to her new social status, acquire a mastery of self-care and childcare, and develop or maintain a relationship and a connection with her child, her partner, her relatives and her friends (Figure 8.2).

A woman with elevated maternal distress, however, will be unhappy, anxious and depressed. She will find it difficult to adapt to the new role of mother and to her change in social circumstances. She will feel herself to be out of control, fatigued and unable to search for and use information and resources. She will find it difficult to take care of herself and her child. Moreover, she will feel herself to be alone, disconnected and detached, and she will struggle in her relationships—with her child, her partner, and her friends and relatives.

The value of this conceptualization lies in the recognition and normalization of the feelings of distress, strain and difficulty experienced by the women in response to this transition phase, instead of labeling them, regarding them as a problem to be solved, or pathologizing them without having undertaken the necessary in-depth diagnostic analysis.

It should however be kept in mind that the stressors of the perinatal period can have negative effects on the health of the mother and the child as well as on family relationships (Glasheen, Richardson and Fabio, 2010; Meçe, 2013). Precisely for this reason, it is essential to plan for and activate specific interventions of support from the time of discharge from hospital and throughout all of the first two to three months after childbirth, with the aim of reducing postnatal stress and supporting the woman, the couple and the family during this particular phase of the life cycle.

Antecedents	Contributing factors	Attributes: Maternal distress (MD) as a continuum	Consequences
• Becoming a mother • Role changes • Body changes and functioning • Increased demands and challenges • Losses and gains • Birth experience • Changes to relationships and social context	Maternal characteristics Education Single status Age Employment status Socioeconomic status Reproductive factors Parity Unwanted pregnancy Previous perinatal loss Unplanned pregnancy Adverse childbirth experience Health and wellbeing Health status Predisposition Unhappy High or low expectations Body image Poor self-esteem & self-confidence Poor role models Functioning Readiness for childbearing Physical and social functioning ability Lifestyle Infant characteristics Excessive infant crying Baby with problems Preterm infant Relationships Partner relationships Relationships with own mother Relationships with infant and other children Social factors Social support and networks Stressful life events Domestic violence	**Low MD → High MD** Stress responses *Stress* (worry, concern mild anxiety) → *Anxiety and Depression* (Unhappy, low mood, highly anxious) Adapting responses *Adaptation* (maternal role development) → *Maladaptation* (Poor maternal role development) Function and control responses *Functional* (Coping, In control, mastery, using information and resources, energy, caring for self and infant) → *Dysfunctional* (Not coping, out of control, Inability to seek and use Information and resources, fatigue, Inability to care for self and infant) Connecting responses *Connected* (Relationships with infant, partner, relatives and friends, seeking support within the community and society) → *Disconnected* (Feeling alone, disharmony in relationships, inability to seek support)	Impact on: • Mental health status • Maternal role development • Quality of life • Ability to function • Quality of relationships • Social engagement

Figure 8.2 Emmanuel and St. John (2010). Maternal distress: A concept analysis. Journal of Advanced Studies, 66, 2104–2115

Interventions of Support during the Postpartum Period

Currently, there are diverse psychosocial and psychological interventions that are effective in the treatment of postpartum depression (Dennis and Hodnett, 2007). However, it is of great benefit to be able to act effectively in a preventative way during pregnancy and in the postnatal period, especially for those who present risk factors for the onset of postpartum depression. In that regard, in a recent meta-analytic review (Dennis and Dowswell, 2013) the authors point out that women who access psychosocial and psychological interventions are less likely to develop postpartum depression than those receiving routine treatment. Specifically, it was found that by combining three types of intervention (repeated home visits by experienced personnel, obstetric care that also included screening for postpartum depression and repeated peer calls), the risk of developing postpartum depression was reduced by 50%. This shows that supportive multifactorial interventions carried out in the initial postnatal period have proven to be effective prevention strategies.

Although psychological intervention such as cognitive-behavioral therapy shows clear evidence of efficacy in the treatment of postpartum depression (as indicated in Chapter 12), it is not yet sufficiently supported by studies that unequivocally demonstrate its validity in prevention (Dennis and Dowswell, 2013). Conversely, interpersonal therapy turns out to be a very promising method of intervention not only in therapeutic terms, but also on a preventative basis, especially in populations at risk (Dennis and Dowswell, 2013; Werner et al., 2015).

Psychosocial Interventions

In recent years, there is a more widespread awareness of the importance of having specific interventions available for the assistance and management of postnatal maternal health, including mental health. Some of these interventions have proven to be more effective, providing better postpartum stress management than the routine care provided after hospitalization (Alderdice, McNeill and Lynn, 2013; Bernard et al., 2011). Specifically, some of these psychosocial interventions, implemented in the first weeks after childbirth, have proven useful in the prevention of postpartum depression. On this question, two measures have proven to be particularly promising: home visits carried out by specialized health professionals (midwives, pediatric nurses, health assistants, psychologists) and peer-to-peer telephone support or social volunteer support (Dennis and Dowswell, 2013).

A recent review of the psychosocial interventions initiated after childbirth on an international level (Song, Kim and Ahn, 2015) identified three principal kinds of stress-reduction interventions:

1   Support programs directed toward the management of postpartum stress.
2   Educational programs that address the behaviors and characteristics of newborns.
3   Programs that foster the interaction between the mother and the newborn.

The first type of intervention is especially effective in helping the women to reduce stress. These support programs give even better results if they engage the social framework in which the mother lives by involving, for example, the husband/partner, family members, friends and experienced mothers (Cheng and Pickler, 2009; Dennis et al., 2009; Negron et al., 2013). It is therefore very important in these support interventions that healthcare professionals seek to include family members as well as support groups for mothers. Additionally, healthcare providers should not limit themselves to only suggesting support. Rather, it would be desirable to explain to the mother the importance of multi-level support, and to try to guide her toward an understanding of what expectations she has about the help she could receive and which she believes could be useful (Negron et al., 2013).

These interventions with the new mothers, conducted by skilled professionals, require not only good relational empathic skills, but also specific expertise and suitable communication and relationship training. In a review of the literature by Mercer and Walker (2006), for example, it was emphasized how interventions that foster the woman's interaction with the healthcare professional and its reciprocation have proven to be more effective than those based on information and providing instruction. Mercer (2004), like Song and his colleagues (Song, Kim and Ahn, 2015), recommend to those working with patients in the postnatal period to work from a perspective directed toward helping the woman to "become a mother", rather than generally urging her toward taking on her maternal role and responsibilities. One becomes a mother day by day. Advancement along that pathway of growth is a slow and gradual evolutionary process, and not merely the woman's acquisition of the new skills and abilities needed to manage the baby and his or her everyday needs.

Telephone Interventions of Support

The telephone interventions of support that have arisen over the last 20 years have reached a large number of new mothers, thanks to the widespread availability of the mobile telephone. Moreover, in the context of protecting the health of the population, the telephone also enables healthcare providers to reach patients who live a considerable distance from service centers, as well as those who are most disadvantaged (Wootton, 2001).

In the perinatal context, using the telephone to provide psychosocial support to women during pregnancy has had good results (Bullock et al., 1995). During the postpartum period, the telephone is, for example, particularly appreciated by users especially when it is possible to receive advice about breastfeeding and neonatal care (Osman et al., 2010; Wang, Chen, & Chen, 2008), as well as in situations where there is a risk of physical complications (David, 2010).

Telephone support can be proposed as a type of mutual assistance between peers, or offered by healthcare workers in the form of SMS (Jareethum et al., 2008) or telephone calls. The opportunities for intervention can be programmed or random. They can also be addressed to a specific population.

In their review of randomized clinical studies on the efficacy of telephone support aimed at some postnatal factors, including postpartum depression, Dennis and Kingston (2008) observed that, despite the fact that the studies have some limitations, this type of intervention has been shown to be able to significantly reduce depressive symptomatology. In particular in a more recent review, it was shown that women at high risk of depression who receive telephone support have lower mean depression scores in the period following the birth of the child, although there is no clear evidence that the recipients of such support will be less likely to have a diagnosis of depression (Lavender et al., 2013). The same authors conclude that, despite the benefits of reducing the scores linked to depressive symptomatology, extending the duration of breastfeeding, and increasing satisfaction with the postnatal care services received, the data currently available in the literature do not provide enough evidence to recommend an investment of resources in this type of intervention (Lavender et al., 2013).

At the same time, a more recent controlled randomized study (Osman et al., 2014) showed the effectiveness of two interventions to reduce postpartum stress in a group of first-time mothers: a video on postpartum stress, and the availability of a telephone line with round-the-clock personnel. In another randomized controlled study (Ngai et al., 2016), positive benefits from telephone interventions based on cognitive behavioral therapy were also shown to reduce distress scores at six weeks and six months after the birth of the child, thus facilitating the postpartum adaptation with positive consequences.

Altogether, these data demonstrate how this type of intervention can be promising especially in reducing stress and depressive symptoms in the first weeks after birth. In spite of this, in our opinion, further investigation is necessary to define with greater precision the specific aspects of potential telephone support to be given to new mothers. In other words, the optimal configuration of this type of intervention needs to be refined by further experimental studies. Specifications should set out whether the telephone support is provided by peers, or by healthcare workers; is delivered by SMS, or by telephone. Clarification about the frequency, the duration and the timing of the interventions is also necessary.

In-Home Interventions

In the Western context, the progressive reduction of the length of the hospital stay following the birth of the child, and the need to monitor maternal and child health during the postpartum period (42 days after the birth, according to the World Health Organization; OMS, 2005), including psychological health, have posed problems of how to provide assistance to the new mother in order to reduce postnatal mother-child complications. In reference to these operational guidelines, in numerous national contexts some of the assistance is currently being offered by territorial and community medical clinics. Home visits, carried out by healthcare personnel or by specially trained professionals (health visitors/home visitors), are widespread in all of the industrialized countries of the world. Despite all of this, to this day a clear, shared methodological definition of these interventions does not exist with respect to the duration, the number and frequency of visits, the procedures carried out or the profile of the personnel involved.

Even the term "home visiting" comes to be used differently depending on local context.

Dennis and Dowswell (2013), in their review of randomized and controlled studies that compared psychosocial and psychological interventions to the usual postnatal intervention approaches, found that among the psychosocial interventions, home visits carried out by trained expert professionals, similar to the nurses' repeated visits after childbirth, were among the most promising interventions for the prevention of postpartum depression. In particular, the results appeared to be better when the visits were repeated again and again during the postpartum period. This evidence of efficacy was especially observed in the women at risk of postpartum depression. Despite this, however, no sufficient elements emerged that would recommend the use of home visits in clinical practice in order to prevent the disorder.

More recently, in a meta-analytic review of randomized controlled studies which evaluated the effectiveness of diverse types of home-based interventions on the health of the mother and the child during the postpartum period (Yonemoto et al., 2017), it was shown that home visits following discharge from hospital have a limited effect on postpartum stress and its consequences, among which is postpartum depression. The home visits, however, do seem to have a greater influence on reducing the woman's use of infant health services. Beyond that, it was shown that an increase in the number of home visits encourages the woman to breastfeed exclusively. Lastly, home visits were found to increase women's satisfaction with postnatal care (Yonemoto et al., 2017).

In relation to home visits, therefore, a description of their effectiveness in reducing postnatal stress and preventing postpartum depression is difficult to identify definitively, precisely because of the heterogeneity of the methodologies adopted in the visits themselves.

Therefore, further studies are needed to identify standardized and effective operating procedures. It is also necessary to better understand if and how these interventions really influence the reduction of stress, or if they have the effect of mediating the effect of postpartum stress, and therefore consequently reducing the probability of developing postpartum depression.

The Postpartum Period and a Woman's Health Needs: Some Practical Recommendations

Assistance in the First Days after Childbirth

There are diverse aspects that can influence the manner in which a woman will handle the period following childbirth. Healthcare professionals must take this into account when meeting with the mothers so as to provide adequate assistance and support to meet the needs of each one. In fact, it is important that adequate training is at the center of standard assistance protocols adopted by healthcare units, preparing workers to recognize the peculiarities and specifics of each mother-baby pair and of the internal relations of the family in order to have a more flexible and the most individualized approach (Massey, Rising and Ickovics, 2006; Schmied et al., 2008; Yelland et al., 2007).

In his work to define the optimal model for assisting women in their first year after childbirth, Fahey emphasizes that there are three aspects which must be taken into consideration (Fahey and Shenassa, 2013).

The first aspect is the possibility/ability to recover from the pregnancy and the delivery. In fact, it takes about two months for the woman's body to regain its pre-pregnancy physiological condition, even though some studies show that women report concerns about the functioning of their bodies even six to twelve months after childbirth (Kanotra, D'Angelo and Phares, 2007). The length of time and the manner in which a woman regains the ability to carry out the duties that motherhood imposes upon her in a sufficiently adequate way are, in any case, distinctive and unique.

The second aspect is the woman's ability to find a compromise between her own individual needs, and those of the baby and the family. The perinatal period is in fact a transitional phase in which diverse relational, social and individual facets of the mother's world seek a new equilibrium and take on a revised significance.

During the first days and weeks that follow the birth, the central characteristic leading to a satisfactory adjustment is, for example, the ability of the woman to find a compromise that allows her to attend to the fundamental needs of the baby, but above all, to provide for her own basic needs to eat, to sleep and to bathe (Negron et al., 2013).

Generally, hospital workers and those engaged in providing home care concentrate their educational, assessment and support interventions primarily on the needs of the baby, rather than on those of the mother (Walker and Wilging, 2000). Moreover, those same mothers are often totally focused on the needs of the child and the family, and they fail to concern themselves with their own needs and their own physical and emotional health. Research carried out several years ago showed how, in the period following childbirth, the risk of the puerpera neglecting her own care escalated, with an increase in the possibility of beginning or reprising dangerous behaviors such as smoking, physical inactivity or erratic and irregular eating habits (Walker and Wilging, 2000). In particular, about one-third of the mothers reported that in the first two months after childbirth, their physical and emotional state interfered at least in part with their ability to take care of the newborn, with 42% of the new mothers disclosing a deterioration of their physical and/or emotional health. Fatigue, sleep that is frequently interrupted and the absence of any possibility of sleeping late during the postnatal period are associated with diverse disorders, including postpartum depression (Dennis and Ross, 2005). Postpartum depression, however, turns out to be associated with the difficulty in dealing with the transition to motherhood and looking after the newborn and the other members of the family (Wachs, Black and Engle, 2009).

It would be important in this regard for health workers to reassure women that during the postpartum period it is normal and recommended to take care of themselves too, and that they are not bad mothers if they seek to carve out some time to be able to take a shower, if they leave the newborn in the nursery for an hour (during their postpartum recovery in hospital) or with the husband in order to "unplug" (each in her own way) or if they get to the point of being unable to endure "waking up ten times in one night" and ask to have two hours to be able to sleep. What needs to be recognized and endorsed is that the women must be helped to take care of their own physical and emotional health in order to better look after their baby and their family.

A third element that must be kept in mind regarding the care of the mothers is that they are dealing with the so-called change in role, understood to be the process of redefining one's own identity, one's sense of self, one's goals and responsibilities. It is an itinerary that begins during pregnancy, but with the presence of the baby becomes a committed journey.

Rubin (1977) has defined three diverse phases which characterize this journey in the period immediately after childbirth.

The first phase is that in which the woman is focused on herself. She needs to repeatedly describe the experience of labor and delivery. She may have difficulty seeing the baby as hers, and she can appear passive and just barely inclined to take care of the baby. With reference to these aspects, it is important that staff be willing to listen to the woman so that her behaviors and needs—even to get away at certain times—are not misinterpreted as rejection directed toward the child.

In the second phase, which corresponds with the second to third day after the birth of the child, the mother is more involved in taking care of her own child, but may at the same time appear excessively anxious or worried, needing to be reassured that she is doing everything right, and needing to be guided and helped in taking care of the newborn. In these situations, it is good for the healthcare workers to approach these new mothers in a tactful, non-judgmental way because, in this phase, the woman can easily feel judged, leading to an experience of self-deprecation. Certainly, there are many phrases that the mother will remember as "written in stone" among those uttered by the healthcare workers during her hospital stay or in the first weeks postpartum. It is essential to remember that in this phase, the women are particularly vulnerable in emotional terms, and as a result, the words that are used by those who look after them (and, consequentially, the feelings that they convey) are of great importance and remain fixed in memory for a long time.

The third phase is characterized by accentuated emotional lability with moments of euphoria followed by moments of discouragement which usually last a few weeks, until the woman slowly and gradually adapts herself to a new normality that includes her own needs, those of the baby and those of family life.

Sense of Security

One aspect which appears to be significant when assisting the mother in the initial period following the birth of the child is the sense of security interpreted as a multidimensional concept (Persson et al., 2011).

The new mother's sense of security is associated with the nature of the assistance received after childbirth, social support, a sense of control, the attitude of the mother herself and her general well-being, and the support offered by the partner (Persson et al., 2007; Persson and Dykes, 2009). Some studies have shown, for example, that in the field of maternity assistance, the support offered during the postpartum period in general turns out to be the issue with which women express the greatest dissatisfaction (Brown et al., 2002; Walldenstrom and Rudman, 2008). In that regard, in their research Persson and his colleagues (Persson et al., 2011) identify three dimensions which are significant to the women's sense of security in the initial period after childbirth.

A first dimension is the support of staff, who must treat the woman as an individual bearer of needs, fears and problems, but also of resources. The women should therefore be supported and encouraged (Lundgren and Berg, 2007; Wilkins, 2006) in their capability of being "good enough" mothers. The women's need to receive increasingly individualized assistance collides, in fact, with the economic perspective of the healthcare system assigned to the task of providing routine care procedures and standardized, effective and functional guidelines. This is one of the factors that has led to a weakening of the relationship between the operating procedures of healthcare teams and the ever-increasing difficulty of individualizing and personalizing perinatal health and social-health care.

A more individualized approach, however, presupposes the availability of time and the ability to listen to the real needs of the patient, but that kind of availability is unfortunately often missing in the type of care offered by the public healthcare system (McKellar, Pincombe and Henderson, 2009; Persson et al., 2011).

A second dimension which reassures the woman is support provided by the family. This is one of the principal aspects that protect against the onset of emotional disorders during the postpartum period, including, in a particular way, postpartum depression.

During the hospital stay, the person who supports the woman can be her partner, as seen in some northern European countries. In that context, this presence, if requested by the woman, has been shown to be effective in augmenting the perception of security and increasing the patients' sense of satisfaction (Ellberg et al., 2006; Ellberg, Högberg and Lindh, 2010). It should be remembered, however, that the woman must always agree with the presence of the partner, just like the presence of other family members, and their presence must reflect her own genuine wishes (Forster, McLachlan and Rayner, 2008; Rudman and Waldenström, 2007). In other situations/cultures, those who provide support to the woman in the delivery room can also be another family member, an intimate friend, a private midwife or other birth partner.

A third dimension which influences the sense of security in the new mother is the possibility of being helped with taking care of herself and the baby.

Increasingly, women feel the need for better preparation with respect to the period after the birth. Before giving birth, the primiparas have no way of knowing what kinds of problems and critical issues they will encounter afterward. It is important, therefore, even during pregnancy, to provide the women with information on matters related to typical difficulties of the postnatal period (Deave, Johnson and Ingram, 2008; Fabian, Rådestad and Waldenström, 2005), setting up, for example, small discussion groups and facilitating the pregnant women's discussions of postnatal situations and guiding them to hypothesize possible solutions to the difficulties that might be encountered on their postnatal journey (Pearson et al., 2010).

It is also important for women to have a healthcare professional as a reference point, and to know whom to contact if they have difficulties. Persson et al. (2011), in reference to the new mother's sense of security, reaffirm the importance of planning a follow-up visit after discharge from hospital. For the women, it is indeed important to know they have this appointment at which they will be able to ask questions and express their uncertainties, and have someone that monitors their health and the health of their baby.

Finally, another aspect that is highlighted in some scientific works is that the central focus of new mothers proves to be the baby; in face of this, however, it is important that healthcare professionals also concentrate their attention on the difficulties of the mothers and their physical and emotional health (Persson et al., 2011).

Why Don't Women Seek Help during the Postpartum Period?

Seeking help for one's emotional difficulties and psychological symptoms involves a decision-making process that calls for the ability not only to recognize that one has a problem, but also to consciously decide to want to do something to solve the problem (Cornally and McCarthy, 2011). The decisional process is influenced by one's own beliefs and expectations with respect to the symptoms (Baines and Wittkowsky, 2013), by the stigma—understood as the subjective beliefs and perceptions of others about the symptoms/disorders (Clement et al., 2015)—and by cultural factors that influence the means by which one seeks help (Rüdell, Bhui and Priebe, 2008).

During the perinatal period, there are various barriers that intervene to obstruct the request for help. Dennis and Chung-Lee (2006), for example, in their systematic review of qualitative studies, have identified the following factors: the inability of the woman to reveal her own feelings; cultural obstacles; ignorance about the symptoms that characterize postpartum depression and/or the manner of getting help; the attitudes of family, friends and healthcare professionals. From an interesting work of meta-synthesis of qualitative studies on the search for support by UK women during the postpartum period, three relevant issues emerge specifically: the ability to identify the problem, the influence of healthcare professionals and the stigma (Button et al., 2017).

It does happen that many women are not aware of having a problem and are unable to interpret their symptoms. Some are indeed unable to communicate how they feel, while still others manage to talk only about somatic symptoms, but not those that concern their own emotional state (Edge, 2006; Parvin, Jones and Hull, 2004). When they undergo screening for the early detection of those at risk of perinatal psychopathology, many women hide how they really feel. Although the screening is, for some women, a way of revealing how they actually feel, for others the fact that there is no real connection with the health professional can make it difficult to open up and to disclose their true emotional state until they reach the breaking point and they feel they can no longer cope (Hanley and Long, 2006; Shakespeare, Blake and Garcia, 2003).

The role played by health professionals is fundamental in all of this. An open and non-judgmental attitude toward the lived experience and the feelings and emotions of the patient is a highly important factor that helps the woman to establish a relationship of trust and hope with the caregivers (Chew-Graham et al., 2009; Cooke et al., 2012). On the contrary, an approach that includes an aloof bedside manner and that is quick to advocate a certain direction of care can lead the new mother to avoid the suggested help altogether (Edge, 2011). Additionally, an excessive focus on the child and his or her needs, rather than on the mother's struggle to manage the situation, can lead the woman to feel she is neither understood nor supported (Cooke et al., 2012). In other words, the mother needs to feel she is included and accepted; she needs her problems to be acknowledged.

Studies show that continuity of care is such a significant element that women are more likely to seek help when they depend on the same health professional throughout the course of the full perinatal period (Raymond, 2009). In that regard, it has been shown that the model of maternity care most appreciated by women provides for assistance to be consistently delivered by the same health worker (Sandall et al., 2016).

The problem of the stigmatization of perinatal emotional disorders needs particular attention. The stigma manifests as a tendency to feel judged and to judge oneself in return, to normalize and minimize the symptoms, to attribute one's own distress to external factors and to experience anxiety regarding the consequences of the stigmatization (Button et al., 2017).

Globally, new mothers feel obliged to conform to an ideal of motherhood that is far from the woman's self-perception. The myth of the perfect mother often comes to be internalized (Raymond, 2009) as an ideal of self toward which a woman is drawn, with expectations so high that frustration and dissatisfaction inevitably follow. Discomfort and malaise are seen as a sign of one's inability to be a good mother (Ayers et al., 2015) and the sense of failure and fear of being judged by others sometimes triggers the women to hide their own internal uneasiness even from themselves. This creates a downward spiral in which the collapse of self-esteem and self-efficacy contributes to a lowering of mood with the consequence that stigmatization originating in the social context together with self-stigmatization can contribute to both the development and maintenance of postpartum depression (McLoughlin, 2013).

The guidelines issued by the National Institute for Health and Care Excellence (NICE) in this regard recommend that healthcare professionals give particular attention to potential stigma and to the shame that often is associated with perinatal mental health disorders. The guidelines further recommend that in antenatal classes, the issues of the transition to motherhood and of mental well-being should be extensively addressed (NICE, 2008).

Conclusions

The first weeks following the birth of one's child represent a crucial period in the life experience of every woman. Countless physical, psychological and relational demands characterize the lived postpartum experience. These demands can, in turn, take on the form of intense suffering, and extreme discomfort and distress. In the majority of cases, though, the difficulties of the postpartum period are distinguished by stress, and physical and emotional fatigue, and should not be overlooked and simplistically labeled as "maternity blues". In this delicate phase of transition, support should be as individualized as possible, and should ensure a continuity of the assistance provided during pregnancy. Programs should be attuned to the legitimate needs of each woman, of each mother-baby dyad and of each family, and focused not only on tangible and practical requirements, but also on the need for emotional help and support.

Some psychological and psychosocial support interventions have proved to be very useful, aimed above all at providing new mothers with information together with practical and emotional support so that they can better manage the many stressful elements of the postpartum period.

Finally, in the coming years, much work awaits those who concern themselves with maternity assistance: to dispel the social myth of the perfect mother so that women can ask for help to a greater extent while neither bearing the weight of stigma nor underestimating their own abilities as mothers.

References

Adewuya, A.O. (2005). The maternity blues in Western Nigerian Women: Prevalence and risk factors. *American Journal of Obstetrics and Gynecology, 193*, 1522–1525.

Albers, L.L. (2000). Health problems after childbirth. *Journal of Midwifery Women's Health, 45*(1), 55–57.

Alderdice, F., McNeill, J., & Lynn, F. (2013). A systematic review of systematic review of intervention to improve maternal mental health and well-being. *Midwifery, 29*(4), 389–399.

Attrill, B. (2002). The assumption of the maternal role: A developmental process. *The Australian Journal of Midwifery, 15*, 21–25.

Ayers, S., Fitzgerald, G., & Thompson, S. (2015). Brief online self-help exercises for postnatal women to improve mood: A pilot study. *Maternal Child Health Journal, 19*, 2375–2383.

Baines, T., & Wittkowski, A. (2013). A systematic review of the literature exploring illness perceptions in mental health utilising the self-regulation model. *Journal of Clinical Psychology in Medical Settings, 20*, 263–274.

Bandura, A. (1997). *Self-Efficacy: The Exercise of Control*. New York: Freeman.

Barclay, L.M., & Lloyd, B. (1996). The misery of motherhood: Alternative approaches to maternal distress. *Midwifery, 12*, 136–139.

Barrera, M. (1986). Distinctions between social support concepts, measures, and models. *American Journal of Community Psychology, 14*, 413–445.

Beck, C.T. (1991). Maternity blues research: A critical review. *Issues in Mental Health Nursing, 12*, 291–300.

Beck, C.T., Gable, R.K., Sakala, C., & Declerq, E.R. (2011). Posttraumatic stress disorders in new mothers: Results from a two-stage U.S. national survey. *Birth, 38*, 216–227.

Beeber, L.S., Schwartz, T., Holditch-Davis, D., Canuso, R., & Lewis, V. (2013). Parenting enhancement, interpersonal psychotherapy to reduce depression in low-income mothers of infants and toddlers: A randomized trial. *Nursing Research, 62*(2), 82–90.

Bener, A., Gerber, L.M., & Sheikh, J. (2012). Prevalence of psychiatric disorders and associated risk factors in women during their postpartum period. A major public health problem and global comparison. *International Journal of Women's Health, 4*, 191–200.

Bernard, R.S., Williams, S.E., Storfer Isser, A., Horowitz, S.M., Kooman, C., & Shaw, R.J. (2011). Brief cognitive behavioural intervention for maternal depression and trauma in the neonatal intensive care unit. A pilot study. *Journal of Traumatic Stress, 24*, 230–234.

Brown, S., Small, R., Faber, B., Krastev, A., & Davis, P. (2002). Early postnatal discharge from hospital for healthy mothers and term infants. *Cochrane Database of Systematic Reviews, 3*, CD002958.

Brown, S., Small, R., Faber, B., Krastev, A., & Davis P. (2010). Early postnatal discharge from hospital for healthy mothers and term infant. *Cochrane Database of Sisyematic Reviews, 3*. DOI: 10.1002/14651858.

Bryanton, J., & Beck, C.T. (2010). Postnatal parental education for optimizing infant general health and parent-infant relationships. *Cochrane Database Systematic Review, 20*(1), CD004068. Doi: 10.1002/14651858.

Bullock, L.F., Wells, J.E., Duff, G.B., & Hornblow, A.R. (1995). Telephone support for pregnant women: outcome in late pregnancy. *New Zealand Medical Journal, 108*, 476–478.

Buttner, M.M., Brock, R.L., & O'Hara, M.W. (2015). Patterns of women's mood after delivery: A growth curve analysis. *Journal of Affective Disorders, 174*, 201–208.

Buttner, M.M., O'Hara, M.W., & Watson, D. (2012). The structure of women's mood in the early postpartum. *Assessment, 19*, 247–256.

Button, S., Thornton, A., Lee, S., Shakespeare, J., & Ayers, S. (2017). Seeking help for perinatal psychological distress: a meta-synthesis of women's experiences. *British Journal of General Practice, 67*(663), e692–e699.

Byrom, A. (2013). Feeding guilt. *Practising Midwife,* Mar; *16*(3), 18, 20, 22–23.

Cheng, C.Y., & Li, Q. (2008). Integrative review of research on general health status and prevalence of common physical health conditions of women after childbirth. *Women's Health Issues, 18*, 267–280.

Cheng, C.Y., & Pickler, R.H. (2009). Effects of stress and social support on postpartum health of Chinese mothers in the United States. *Research in Nursing & Health, 32*, 582–591.

Chew-Graham, C.A., Sharp, D., Chamberlain, E., Folkes, L., & Turner, K.M. (2009). Disclosure of symptoms of postnatal depression, the perspectives of health professionals and women: A qualitative study. *BMC Family Practice, 10*(1), 7.

Clement, S., Schauman, O., Graham, T., Maggioni, F., Evans-Lacko, S., Bezborodovs, N., Morgan, C., Rüsch, N., Brown, J.S., & Thornicroft, G. (2015). What is the impact of mental health-related stigma on help-seeking? A systematic review of quantitative and qualitative studies. *Psychological Medicine, 45*, 11–27.

Cohen, S. (1988). Psychosocial models of the role of social support in the etiology of physical disease. *Health Psychology, 7*, 269–297.

Coleman, P., Nelson, E., & Sundre, D. (1999). The relationship between prenatal expectations and postnatal attitudes among first-time mothers. *Journal of Reproductive and Infant Psychology, 17*, 27–39.

Collins, N.L., Dunkel-Schetter, C., Lobel, M., & Scrimshaw, S.C. (1993). Social support in pregnancy: Psychosocial correlates of birth outcomes and postpartum depression. *Journal of Personality and Social Psychology, 65*, 1243–1258.

Cornally, N., & McCarthy, G. (2011). Help-seeking behaviour: A concept analysis. *International Journal of Nursing Practice, 17*, 280–288.

Cooke, S., Smith, I., Turl, E., Arnold, E., & Msetfi, R.M. (2012). Parent perspectives of clinical psychology access when experiencing distress. *Community Practice, 85*, 34–37.

Corwin, E.J., Brownstead, J., Barton, N., Heckard, S., & Morin, K., (2005). The impact of fatigue on the development of postpartum depression. *Journal of Obstetrics and Neonatal Nursing, 34*, 577–586.

Coyle, S.B. (2009). Health-related quality of life of mothers: A review of the research. *Health Care for Women International, 30*, 484–506.

Darvill, R.L., Skirton, H., & Farrand, P. (2010). Psychological factors that impact on women's experiences of first-time motherhood: A qualitative study of the transition. *Midwifery, 26*, 357–366.

David, S., Fenwick, J., Bayes, S., & Martin, T. (2010). A qualitative analysis of the content of telephone calls made by women to a dedicated 'Next Birth After Caesarean' antenatal clinic. *Women Birth, 23*, 166–171.

Deave, T., Johnson, D., & Ingram, J. (2008). Transition to parenthood: The needs of parents in pregnancy and early parenthood. *BMC Pregnancy Childbirth,* Jul 29; *8*, 30.

Declercq, E.R., Sakala, C., Corry, M.P., & Applebaum, S. (2006). *Listening to Mothers II: Report of the Second National U.S. Survey of Women's Childbearing Experiences.* New York: Childbirth Connection.

Declercq, E.R., Sakala, C., Corry, M.P., & Applebaum, S. (2013). *Listening to Mothers III: New Mothers Speak Out.* New York: Childbirth Connection.

Dennis, C.L., & Chung-Lee, L. (2006). Postpartum depression help-seeking barriers and maternal treatment preferences: A qualitative systematic review. *Birth, 33*, 323–331.

Dennis, C.L., & Dowswell, T. (2013). Interventions (other than pharmacological, psychosocial or psychological) for treating antenatal depression. *Cochrane Database Systematic Reviews,* Jul 31;(7):CD006795.

Dennis, C.L., & Hodnett, E. (2007). Psychosocial and psychological interventions for treating postpartum depression. *Cochrane Database Systematic Review,* Oct 17;(4):CD006116.

Dennis, C.L., Hodnett, E., Kenton, L., Weston, J., Zupancic, J., Stewart, D.E., & Kiss, A. (2009). Effect of peer support on prevention of postnatal depression among high risk women: Multisite randomised controlled trial. *BMJ, 338*, a3064.

Dennis, C.L., & Kingston, D. (2008). A systematic review of telephone support for women during pregnancy and the early postpartum period. *Journal of Obstetric, Gynecologic, & Neonatal Nursing, 37*, 301–314.

Dennis, C.L., & Ross, L. (2005). Relationships among infant sleep patterns, maternal fatigue, and development of depressive symptomatology. *Birth, 32*(3), 187–193.

Edge, D. (2006). Perinatal depression: Its absence among Black Caribbean women. *British Journal of Midwifery, 14*, 646–652.

Edge, D. (2011). It's leaflet, leaflet, leaflet then, "see you later": Black Caribbean women's perceptions of perinatal mental health care. *British Journal of General Practice, 61*, 256–262.

Ellberg, L., Högberg, U., & Lindh, V. (2010). We feel like one, they see us as two': New parents' discontent with postnatal care. *Midwifery, 25*, 463–468.

Ellberg, L., Högberg, U., Lundman, B., & Lindholm, L. (2006). Satisfying parents' preferences with regard to various models of postnatal care is cost-minimizing. *Acta Obstetricia et Gynecologica Scandinavica, 85*, 175–181.

Emmanuel, E.N., Creedy, D.K., St., John, W., & Brown, C. (2011). Maternal role development: The impact of maternal distress and social support following childbirth. *Midwifery, 27*, 265–272.

Emmanuel, E., & St John, W. (2010). Maternal distress: A concept analysis. *Journal of Advanced Nursing, 66*, 2104–2115.

Fabian, H.M., Rådestad, I.J., & Waldenström, U. (2005). Childbirth and parenthood education classes in Sweden. Women's opinion and possible outcomes. *Acta Obstetricia et Gynecologica Scandinavica, 84*, 436–443.

Fahey, J.O., & Shenassa, E. (2013). Understanding and meeting the needs of women in the postpartum period: The perinatal maternal health promotion model. *Journal of Midwifery Womens Health, 58*, 613–621.

Ferber, S.G. (2004). The nature of touch in mothers experiencing maternity blues: The contribution of parity. *Early Human Development, 79*, 65–75.

Forster, D.A., McLachlan, H.L., & Rayner, J. (2008). The early postnatal period: Exploring women's views, expectations and experiences of care using focus groups in Victoria, Australia. *BMC Pregnancy Childbirth*, Jul 22; *8*, 27.

Fossey, L., Papiernik, E., & Bydlowski, M. (1997). Postpartum blues: A clinical syndrome and predictor of postnatal depression? *Journal of Psychosomatic Obstetrics & Gynaecology, 18*, 17–21.

Fowles, E., & Walker, L. (2009). Maternal predictors of toddler health status. *Journal of Specialists in Pediatric Nursing, 14*, 33–40.

Gausia, K., Fisher, C., Ali, M., & Oosthuizen, J. (2009). Magnitude and contributory factors of postnatal depression: A community-based cohort study from a rural subdistrict of Bangladesh. *Psychological Medicine, 39*, 999–1007.

George, I. (2005). Lack of preparedness: Experiences of first-time mothers. *MCN American Journal of Maternal-Child Nursing, 30*, 251–255.

Glasheen, C., Richardson, G.A., & Fabio, A. (2010). A systematic review of the effects of postnatal maternal anxiety on children. *Archives of Women's Mental Health, 13*, 61–74.

Glavin, K., & Leahy-Warren, P. (2013). Postnatal depression is a public health nursing issue: Perspectives from Norway and Ireland. *Nursing Research & Practice, 2013*, 813409.

Grussu, P. (2016). *Il Maternity Blues*. In P. Grussu & A. Bramante, Manuale di Psicopatologia Perinatale. Erickson, Trento 47–61.

Grussu, P., & Quatraro, R.M. (2013). Maternity blues in Italian Primipara Women: Symptoms and mood states in the first fifteen days after childbirth. *Health Care for Women International, 324*, 556–576.

Hanley, J., & Long, B. (2006). A study of Welsh mothers' experiences of postnatal depression. *Midwifery, 22*, 147–157.

Harris, B. (1981). Maternity blues in East African clinic attenders. *Archives of General Psychiatry, 38*, 1293–1295.

Henshaw, C. (2003). Mood disturbance in the early puerperium: A review. *Archives of Women's Mental Health, 6*(Suppl.2), s33–s42.

Hill, P.D., & Aldag, J.C. (2007). Maternal perceived quality of life following childbirth. *Journal of Obstetric, Gynecologic, & Neonatal Nursing, 36*, 328–334.

Howell, E.A., Mora, P., & Leventhal, H. (2006). Correlates of early postpartum depressive symptoms. *Maternal and Child Health Journal, 10*(2), 149–157.

Hung, C.H. (2001). The construct of postpartum stress: A concept analysis. *Journal of Nursing (Nurses' Association of the Republic of China), 48*, 69–76.

Hung, C.H. (2006). Correlates of first-time mothers' postpartum stress. *Kaohsiung Journal of Medical Sciences, 22*, 500–507.

Hung, C.H., Lin, C.J., Stocker, J., & Yu, C.Y. (2011). Predictors of postpartum stress. *Journal of Clinical Nursing, 20*, 666–674.

Jareethum, R.[1], Titapant, V., Chantra, T., Sommai, V., Chuenwattana, P., & Jirawan, C. (2008). Satisfaction of healthy pregnant women receiving short message service via mobile phone for prenatal support: A randomized controlled trial. *Journal of the Medical Association of Thailand, 91*, 458–463.

Jones, T.L., & Prinz, R.J. (2005). Potential roles of parental self-efficacy in parent and child adjustment: A review. *Clinical Psychology Review, 25*, 341–363.

Kanotra, S., D'Angelo, D., Phares, T.M. et al. (2007). Challenges faced by new mothers in the early postpartum period: An analysis of comment data from the 2000 Pregnancy Risk Assessment Monitoring System (PRAMS) survey. *Maternal and Child Health Journal, 11*, 549–558.

Kendell, R.E., McGuire, R.J., Condor, Y., & Cox, J.L. (1981). Mood changes in the first three weeks after childbirth. *Journal of Affective Disorders, 3*, 317–326.

Kennerley, H., & Gath, D. (1989). Maternity blues I: Detection and measurement by questionnaire. *British Journal of Psychiatry, 155*, 356–362.

Lane, A., Keville, R., Morris, M., Kinsella, A., Turner, M., & Barry, S. (1997). Postnatal depression and elation among mothers and their partners: prevalence and predictors. *British Journal of Psychiatry, 171*, 550–555.

Lavender, T., Richens, Y., Milan, S.J., Smyth, R.M., & Dowswell, T. (2013). Telephone support for women during pregnancy and the first six weeks postpartum. *Cochrane Database Systematic Review*, Jul 18;(7):CD009338.

Lawrence, E., Nylen, K., & Cobb, R.J. (2007). Prenatal expectations and marital satisfaction over the transition to parenthood. *Journal of Family Psychology, 21*(2), 155–164.

Leahy-Warren, P., & McCarthy, G. (2011). Maternal parental self-efficacy in the postpartum period. *Midwifery, 27*, 802–810.

Leahy-Warren, P., McCarthy, G., & Corcoran, P. (2012). First-time mothers: Social support, maternal parental self-efficacy and postnatal depression. *Journal of Clinical Nursing, 21*, 388–397.

Leerkes, E.M., & Crockenberg, S.C. (2002). The development of maternal self-efficacy and its impact on maternal behavior. *Infancy, 3*, 227–247.

Lefkowitz, D.S., Baxt, C., & Evans, J.R. (2010). Prevalence and correlates of posttraumatic stress and postpartum depression in parents of infants in the Neonatal Intensive Care Unit. *Journal of Clinical Psychology in Medical Settings, 17*, 230–237.

Leigh, B., & Milgrom, J. (2007). Acceptability of antenatal screening for depression in routine antenatal care. *Australian Journal of Advanced Nursing, 24*, 14–18.

Lundgren, J., & Berg, M. (2007). Central concept in the midwife woman relationship. *Scandinavian Journal of Caring Science, 21*, 220–228.

Lundgren, I., & Wahlberg, V. (1999). The experience of pregnancy: A hermeneutical/phenomenological study. *Journal of Perinatal Education, 8*, 12–20.

Massey, Z., Rising, S.S., & Ickovics, J.R. (2006). Centering pregnancy group prenatal care: Promoting relationship-centered care. *Journal of Obstetric, Gynecologic, & Neonatal Nursing, 35*, 286–294.

McKellar, L., Pincombe, J., & Henderson, A. (2009). Encountering the culture of midwifery practice on the postnatal ward during action research: An impediment to change. *Women Birth, 22*, 112–118.

Mc Loughlin, J. (2013). Stigma associated with postnatal depression: A literature review. *British Journal of Midwifery, 21*, 784–791.

Meçe, D. (2013). Postpartum depression and marital relationship. *Academic Journal of Interdisciplinary Studies, 2*, 319–323.

Meleis, A.I., Sawyer, L.M., Im, E.O., Hilfinger Messias, D.K., & Schumacher, K. (2000). Experiencing transitions: An emerging middle-range theory. *ANS Advances in Nursing Science, 23*, 12–28.

Mercer, R.T. (2004). Becoming a mother versus maternal role attainment. *Journal of Nursing Scholarship, 36*, 226–232.

Mercer, R., & Walker, L.O. (2006). A review of nursing interventions to foster becoming a mother. *Journal of Obstetric, Gynecologic, & Neonatal Nursing, 35*, 568–582.

Miller, M.L., Kroska, E.B., & Grekin, R. (2017). Immediate postpartum mood assessment and postpartum depressive symptoms. *Journal of Affective Disorders, 207*, 69–75.

Nicolson, P., (1999). Loss, happiness and postpartum depression: The ultimate paradox. *Canadian Psychology, 40*, 162–178.

Negron, R., Martin, A., Almog, M., Balbierz, A., & Howell, E.A. (2013). Social support during the postpartum period: Mothers' views on needs, expectations, and mobilization of support. *Maternal and Child Health Journal, 17*, 616–623.

Newport, D.J., Hostetter, A., Arnold, A., & Stowe, Z.N. (2002). The treatment of postpartum depression: minimizing infant exposures. *Journal of Clinical Psychiatry, 63*, 31–44.

Ngai, F.W., Wong, P.W., Chung, K.F., & Leung, K.Y. (2016). The effect of telephone-based cognitive-behavioural therapy on parenting stress: A randomised controlled trial. *Journal of Psychosomatic Research, 86*, 34–38.

NICE (2007). Antenatal and postnatal mental health. Clinical guideline. *CG 45*. Available at: www.nice.org.uk/ nicemedia/live/11004/30431/30431.

NICE (2008). Antenatal care: Routine care for the healthy pregnant woman. *CG 62*. Available at: www.nice.org.uk/nicemedia/pdf/CG002.

Oakley, A., & Chamberlain, G. (1981). Medical and social factors in post-partum depression. *Journal of Obstetrics and Gynaecology, 1*, 182–187.

O'Hara, M.W., Schlechte, J.A., Lewis, D.A., & Wright, M.A. (1991). Prospective study of postpartum blues: Biologic and psychosocial factors. *Archives of General Psychiatry, 48*, 801–806.

O'Hara, M.W., Zekoski, E.M., Philipps, L.H., & Wright, E.J. (1990). Controlled prospective study of post-partum mood disorders: Comparison of childbearing and nonchildbearing women. *Journal of Abnormal Psychology, 99*, 3–15.

Osman, H., Chaaya, M., El Zein, L., Naassan, G., & Wick, L. (2010). What do first-time mothers worry about? A study of usage patterns and content of calls made to a postpartum support telephone hotline. *BMC Public Health,* Oct 15, *10*, 611.

Osman, H., Saliba, M., Chaaya, M., & Naasan, G. (2014). Interventions to reduce postpartum stress in first-time mothers: a randomized-controlled trial. *BMC Womens Health,* Oct 15, *14*, 125.

Parvin, A., Jones, C.E., & Hull, S.A. (2004). Experiences and understandings of social and emotional distress in the postnatal period among Bangladeshi women living in Tower Hamlets. *Family Practice, 21*, 254–260.

Paschetta, E., Berrisford, G., Coccia, F., Whitmore, J., Wood, A., Pretlove, S., & Ismail, K.M.K. (2014). Perinatal psychiatry disorders, *American Journal of Obstetrics and Gynecology, 3794*, 52–86.

Persson, E.K., & Dykes, A.K. (2009). Important variables for parents' postnatal sense of security: Evaluating a new Swedish instrument (the PPSS instrument). *Midwifery, 25*, 449–460.

Persson, E.K., Fridlund, B., & Dykes, A.K. (2007). Parents' postnatal sense of security (PPSS): Development of the PPSS instrument. *Scandinavian Journal of Caring Science, 21*, 118–125.

Persson, E.K., Fridlund, B., Kvist, L.J., & Dykes, A.K. (2011). Mothers' sense of security in the first postnatal week: Interview study. *Journal of Advanced Nursing, 67*, 105–116.

Pitt, B. (1973). Maternity blues. *British Journal of Psychiatry, 122*, 431–433.

Porter, C.L., & Hsu, H.-C. (2003). First-time mothers' perceptions of efficacy during the transition to motherhood: Links to infant temperament. *Journal of Family Psychology, 17*, 54–64.

Prost, A., Lakshminarayana, R., Nair, N., Tripathy, P., Copas, A., Mahapatra, R., & Costello, A. (2012). Predictors of maternal psychological distress in rural India: A cross-sectional community-based study. *Journal of Affective Disorders, 138*, 277–286.

Rallis, S., Skouteris, H., McCabe, M., & Milgrom, J. (2014). The transition to motherhood: towards a broader understanding of perinatal distress. *Women Birth, 27*, 68–71.

Rallis, S., Skouteris, H., Wertheim, E.J., & Paxton, S.J. (2007). Predictors of body image during the first year postpartum: A prospective study. *Women Health, 45*, 87–104.

Raphael-Leff, J. (2015). *The Dark Side of the Womb: Pregnancy, Parenting and Persecutory Anxieties.* London: Anna Freud Centre.

Raymond, J.E. (2009). Creating a safety net': Women's experiences of antenatal depression and their identification of helpful community support and services during pregnancy. *Midwifery, 25*, 39–49.

Razurel, C., Bruchon-Schweitzer, M., Dupanloup, A., Irion, O., & Epiney, M. (2011). Stressful events, social support and coping strategies of primiparous women during the postpartum period: A qualitative study. *Midwifery, 27*, 237–242.

Reck, C., Stehle, E., Reinig, K., & Mundt, C. (2009). Maternity blues as a predictor of DSM-IV depression and anxiety disorders in the first three months postpartum. *Journal of Affective Disorders, 113*, 77–87.

Reece, S.M. (1992). The parent expectations survey: A measure of perceived self-efficacy. *Clinical Nursing Research, 1*, 336–346.

Reece, S.M., & Harkless, G. (1998). Self-efficacy, stress, and parental adaptation: Applications to the care of childbearing families. *Journal of Family Nursing, 4*, 198–215.

Roberts, F. (1997). *Perinatal Nursing.* New York: McGraw Hill.

Robinson, G.E., & Stewart, D.E. (1993). Postpartum disorders. In N. Stotland & D. Stewart (Eds.). *Psychological aspects of women's health care: the interface between psychiatry and obstetrics and gynecology.* Washington, DC: American Psychiatric Press.

Rogan, F., Shmied, V., Barclay, L., Everitt, L., & Wyllie, A. (1997). Becoming a mother' – developing a new theory of early motherhood. *Journal of Advanced Nursing, 25*, 877–885.

Rondón, M.B. (2003). Maternity blues: Cross-cultural variations and emotional changes. *Psychiatry Update, 10*, 167–171.

Rubin, R., 1977. *Cognitive Style, in Roberts F., Perinatal Nursing 1977*. New York: McGraw Hill.

Ruchala, P.L., & Halstead, L. (1994). The postpartum experience of low-risk women: A time of adjustment and change. *Maternal-Child Nursing Journal, 22*, 83–88.

Rüdell, K., Bhui, K., & Priebe, S. (2008). Do 'alternative' help-seeking strategies affect primary care service use? A survey of help-seeking for mental distress. *BMC Public Health*, Jun 11; *8*, 207.

Rudman, A., & Waldenström, U. (2007). Critical views on postpartum care expressed by new mothers. *BMC Health Service Research*, Nov 5; *7*, 178.

Sandall, J., Soltani, H., Gates, S., Shennan, A., & Devane, D. (2016). Midwife-led continuity models versus other models of care for childbearing women. *Cochrane Database Systematic Reviews*, Apr 28;4:CD004667.

Schmied, V., Cooke, M., Gutwein, R., Steinlein, E., & Homer, C. (2008). Time to listen: Strategies to improve hospital-based postnatal care. *Women Birth, 21*, 99–105.

Shakespeare, J., Blake, F., & Garcia, J. (2003). A qualitative study of the acceptability of routine screening of postnatal women using the Edinburgh Postnatal Depression Scale. *British Journal of General Practice, 53*, 614–619.

Soifer, R. (1987). *Psicologia del Embarazo, Parto y Puerperio (Spanish Edition)*, Paperback.

Song, J.E., Kim, T., & Ahn, J.A. (2015). A systematic review of psychosocial interventions for women with postpartum stress. *Journal of Obstetric, Gynecologic, & Neonatal Nursing, 44*, 183–192.

Stein, G., Marsh, A., & Morton, J. (1981). Mental symptoms, weight changes, and electrolyte excretion in the first postpartum week. *Journal of Psychosomatic Research, 25*, 395–408.

Stern, D.N. (1985). *Il mondo interpersonale del bambino*. Torino: Bollati Boringhieri Editore.

Tarkka, M.J., & Paunonen, M. (1996). Social support and its impact on mother's experiences of childbirth. *Journal of Advanced Nursing, 23*, 70–75.

Thomson, G., Ebisch-Burton, K., & Flacking, R., (2015). Shame if you do—shame if you don't: Women's experiences of infant feeding. *Maternal and Child Nutrition, 11*, 33–46.

Tronick, E.Z., Bruschweiler-Stern, N., Harrison, A.M., Lyons-Ruth, K., Morgan, A.C., Nahum, J.P. et al. (1998). Dyadically expanded states of consciousness and the process of therapeutic change. *Infant Mental Health Journal, 19*, 290–299.

Tsukasaki, M., Ohta, Y., Oishi, K., Miyaichi, K., & Kato, N. (1991). Types and characteristics of short-term course of depression after delivery using Zung's Self-rating Depression Scale. *Japanese Journal of Psychiatry and Neurology, 45*, 565–576.

Vallino, D., & Macciò, M. (2004). *Essere neonati. Osservazioni psicoanalitiche*. Borla Edizioni.

Wachs, T.D., Black, M.M., & Engle, P.L. (2009). Maternal depression: A global threat to children's health, development, and behavior and to human rights. *Child Development Perspectives, 3*, 51–59.

Waldenström, U., & Rudman, A. (2008). Satisfaction with maternity care: How to measure and what to do. *Womens Health (Lond), 4*, 211–214.

Waldenstrom, U., Rudman, A., & Hildingsson, I. (2006). Intrapartum and postpartum care in Sweden: Wome's opinions and risk factors for not being satisfied. *Acta Obstetricia et Ginecologica Scandinavica, 85*, 551–560.

Walker, L.O., & Wilging, S. (2000). Rediscovering the "M" in "MCH": Maternal health promotion after childbirth. *Journal of Obstetric, Gynecologic, & Neonatal Nursing, 29*, 229–236.

Wang, S.F., Chen, C.H., & Chen, C.H. (2008). Related factors in using a free breastfeeding hotline service in Taiwan. *Journal of Clinical Nursing, 17*, 949–956.

Watanabe, M., Wada, K., Sakata, Y., Aratake, Y., Kato, N., Ohta, H., & Tanaka, K. (2008). Maternity blues as predictor of postpartum depression: A prospective cohort study among Japanese women. *Journal of Psychosomatic Obstetrics & Gynaecology, 29*, 206–212.

Werner, E.L., Miller, M., Osborne, L.M., Kuzava, S., & Monk, C. (2015). Preventing postpartum depression: Review and recommendations. *Archives of Women's Mental Health, 18*, 41–60.

Wilkins, C. (2006). A qualitative study exploring the support needs of first-time mothers on their journey towards intuitive parenting. *Midwifery, 22*, 196–180.

Winnicott, D.W. (1953). Transitional objects and transitional phenomena—A study of the first not-me possession. *The International Journal of Psycho-Analysis, 34*, 89–97.

Winnicott, D.W. (1958). *Collected Papers. Through Paediatrics to Psycho-Analysis*. London: Tavistock Publications; New York: Basic Books.

Wootton, R. (2001). Recent advances: Telemedicine. *BMJ, 323*, 557–560.

World Health Organization (2005). Promoting the health of mothers and newborns during birth and the postnatal period. Report of the collaborative Safe Motherhood pre-congress workshop, International Confederation of Midwives, Brisbane, Australia, 21–23 July.

Wrede, S., Benoit, C., Bourgeault, I.L., van Teijlingen, E.R., Sandall, J., & de Vries, R.G. (2006). Decentred comparative research: Context sensitive analysis of maternal health care. *Social Science and Medicine, 63*, 2986–2997.

Yelland, J., McLachlan, H., Forster, D., Rayner, J., & Lumley, J. (2007). How is psychosocial health assessed and promoted in the early postnatal period? Findings from a review of hospital postnatal care in Victoria, Australia. *Midwifery, 23*, 287–297.

Yonemoto, N., Dowswell, T., Nagai, S., & Mori, R. (2017). Schedules for home visits in the early postpartum period. *Cochrane Database Systematic Review*, Aug 2;8:CD009326.

Zauderer, C. (2009). Postpartum depression: How childbirth educators can help break the silence. *The Journal of Perinatal Education, 18*, 23–31.

9

Parental Emotional Experiences after Newborn Hospitalization

Lisa S. Segre and Sue L. Hall

When my husband and I walked out of the maternity ward after our daughter was born, we didn't look like the new parents. Other couples carefully carried swaddled bundles to their cars and nervously strapped them into their safety seats, while we held only our overnight bags—and a breast pump. My perfect pregnancy had ended five weeks early, and our 2-day-old daughter was in a neonatal intensive care unit (NICU). She was breathing through a tube, surrounded by other premature or sick newborns and the beeps of highly calibrated machines that keep them all alive. It would be three weeks before we'd be able to bring little Abigail home from the hospital.

(Epel, 2015)

Each year in the United States approximately 7.7% of newborns are hospitalized in a neonatal intensive care unit (NICU; Harrison & Goodman, 2015). Although estimates from around the world are not readily available, for most parents hospitalization is unexpected. Early on, parental reactions include fear, shock at the newborn's premature appearance, concern about whether the newborn will live, worry about painful procedures inflicted on the newborn, and ongoing distress in response to unfamiliar and highly technological equipment with distressing sights and sounds (American Academy of Pediatrics, 2015; Tahirkheli, Cherry, Tackett, McCaffree, & Gillaspy, 2014). As time on the NICU increases, additional common reactions include a perceived loss of their parental role to nurses and physicians, general anxiety, stress regarding mounting hospital bills, anger, guilt, loss, powerlessness, and sadness (American Academy of Pediatrics, 2015; Tahirkheli et al., 2014). Other situational stresses facing NICU parents include problems making arrangements to care for siblings, difficulties with transportation, and concerns about the need to return to work (Singer et al., 2012).

This chapter examines parental emotional experiences in response to newborn hospitalization. "Prevalence and Meaning of Emotional Distress in NICU Parents" section summarizes studies from around the world on the prevalence of emotional distress among NICU parents, compares these rates to those reported in parents of non-hospitalized, healthy newborns, and explores the significance of elevated symptoms for NICU parents. "Support for Emotionally Distressed Parents" section has a practical focus. First general support programs for NICU parents are described, including an overview of the newly issued guidelines for the psychosocial care of NICU parents, a description of procedures that can be incorporated into the infant's care in the NICU, and a description of a hospital-based general support program. A second focus of "Support for Emotionally

Distressed Parents" section is to summarize the status of research on interventions focused on emotional distress in NICU mothers, and to review issues surrounding post discharge support.

Prevalence and Meaning of Emotional Distress in NICU Parents

A recent systematic review of postpartum depression prevalence among women with preterm and low birth weight newborns noted that the sample characteristics of these studies, assessment points, measures, and cutoff scores for depression measures were too heterogeneous to quantitatively synthesize (Vigod, Villegas, Dennis, & Ross, 2010). The current chapter differs from that meta-analytic review in two important ways. First, this chapter reviews studies of both depression and anxiety symptoms in NICU parents, an approach that aligns with a multidimensional model of emotional distress, in which depression and anxiety are viewed as an overlapping disorder reflecting a tendency to experience negative emotions (Mineka, Watson, & Clark, 1998). Second, whereas the prior review focused broadly on preterm and low birth weight newborns, this chapter focuses specifically on parents of newborns who are hospitalized in an NICU and thus cannot go home with the new parents. As suggested by the experience of the parents in the opening quote, such hospitalization of a newborn is a uniquely stressful event. Indeed, hospitalization of a child is now recognized as a traumatic stress, not only to the infant but also to the infant's parents (Shah, Jerardi, Auger, & Beck, 2016).

To find the relevant epidemiological studies, PubMed was searched using a combination of keywords: NICU, maternal, paternal, parental, depression, anxiety, distress, emotional distress, depression symptoms, and anxiety symptoms. A large number of relevant U.S. studies were identified, so our analysis was limited to U.S. studies with samples of 100 or more participants. To address an international audience, a targeted search for epidemiological reports outside of the United States identified at least one study each from Canada, South America, Australia/New Zealand, Europe, and Asia.

Prevalence of Depression, Anxiety, and Posttraumatic Stress Symptoms

A meta-analysis of community samples of postpartum women estimated that 10% of newborn mothers reported depression symptoms at their first-month postpartum assessment (Gavin et al., 2005). One way to assess the relative prevalence of depression in NICU mothers is to compare this 10% estimate with the prevalence rates obtained in studies limited to NICU mothers. For NICU mothers, the prevalence of elevated depression symptoms is higher, ranging from 25% (Segre, McCabe, Chuffo-Siewert, & O'Hara, 2014) to 63% (Miles, Holditch-Davis, Schwartz, & Scher, 2007) in two studies from the United States. Such a comparison, while informative, is at best speculative. Although the estimates from community samples were for the first post partum month specifically, study assessments of NICU mothers varied from immediately after birth to one month postpartum. Additionally, the community sample prevalence estimate may include some NICU mothers.

No meta-analytic review was found that examined community samples for the rate of maternal anxiety symptoms during the first postpartum month specifically. However, a small, population-based study in Norway assessed anxiety symptoms in mothers ($N = 127$) and fathers ($N = 122$) of healthy, term infants zero to four days after birth (Skari et al., 2002). The results of this study indicate that when assessed via the State-Trait Anxiety Inventory (Spielberger, 1970), 12% of mothers and 11% of fathers scored within the elevated range. The rates of elevated symptoms of anxiety in the studies of NICU mothers were comparatively higher, ranging from 18% in New Zealand (Carter, Mulder, Bartram, & Darlow, 2005) to 47.4% in the United States (Shaw et al., 2014). Among the two studies that also assessed general symptoms of anxiety in NICU fathers, the prevalence of elevated anxiety symptoms was 11% in New Zealand (Carter et al., 2005) and 20% in China (Kong et al., 2013).

Both acute stress disorder and post-traumatic stress disorder (PTSD) are also seen in NICU parents. In a study by Lefkowitz, 35% of NICU mothers and 24% of fathers met criteria for acute stress disorder (Lefkowitz, Baxt, & Evans, 2010), while Shaw found that 28% of NICU parents had symptoms of acute stress disorder (Shaw et al., 2006). PTSD, although less frequent, is still not uncommon, ranging from 15% (Lefkowitz et al., 2010) to 23% (Feeley et al., 2011) to 30% (Shaw, Bernard, Storfer-Isser, Rhine, & Horwitz, 2013) in NICU mothers and 8% in NICU fathers (Lefkowitz et al., 2010).

Studies of emotional distress in NICU parents (which included a control group of parents of non-hospitalized, term newborns) provide a more accurate comparison of the relative rates of symptoms. Across these studies a similar pattern of results emerged. Specifically, the prevalence of elevated symptoms in the first postpartum month was higher for NICU mothers compared to non-NICU mothers, for NICU mothers compared to NICU fathers, and for NICU fathers compared to non-NICU fathers.

Fathers, who have been called the "forgotten parent," must work to manage their emotions after the birth of a preterm infant (Hugill, Letherby, & Lavender, 2013). In a smaller study of 35 NICU fathers, Mackley found that they remained significantly stressed throughout their baby's hospital stay, with their symptoms being independent of their infant's degree of illness (Mackley, Locke, Spear, & Joseph, 2010). Fully one-third of them were found to have persistently elevated scores on a depression scale at five weeks after their baby's birth.

Considered together, the available evidence from studies around the world supports the assertion that having a newborn hospitalized in the NICU is a stressful experience, resulting in clinically significant levels of emotional distress in some, but not all, NICU parents.

It is helpful, therefore, to know which parents are at highest risk for emotional distress. Although some NICU mothers with depression had no identifiable risk factors other than having an extremely premature infant (Rogers, Kidokoro, Wallendorf, & Inder, 2013), a number of other factors have been found to be associated with maternal depression. Parents of very preterm infants (less than 30–32 weeks) are most consistently identified as being at increased risk (Davis, Edwards, Mohay, & Wollin, 2003; Rogers et al., 2013; Singer et al., 2012). Other risk factors include higher levels of maternal stress in general (Davis et al., 2003), history of a traumatic birth (Cho, Holditch-Davis, & Miles, 2008), unmarried status (Miles et al., 2007), perception of maternal role loss (Miles et al., 2007; Rogers et al., 2013), worries about the child's health and survival (Cho et al., 2008), prolonged ventilation (Rogers et al., 2013), and infant rehospitalization (Miles et al., 2007). Carter found that NICU parents with anxiety were more likely to have had an NICU admission with a previous child and to be in a lower family income bracket. Once again, the degree of the infant's prematurity was associated with increased symptoms in both NICU mothers and NICU fathers (Carter, Mulder, Frampton, & Darlow, 2007).

While parents of extremely preterm infants experience depression and anxiety at higher rates than mothers of term infants, even parents of late preterm infants (34–36 weeks of gestational age) are at significant risk for emotional distress including both depression and anxiety (Brandon et al., 2011; Voegtline, Stifter, & The Family Life Project Investigators, 2010; Zanardo et al., 2011), rendering their infants to be a previously unrecognized vulnerable population (Zanardo et al., 2011). Rates of postpartum depression in parents of late preterm infants were the same in one study as rates for parents of preterm infants of other gestational ages (Hawes, McGowan, O'Donnell, Tucker, & Vohr, 2016). Among the causes of the increased parental distress in this group of parents are negative experiences during labor and delivery, worry about their infant's survival, and poorer infant health outcomes (Brandon et al., 2011). The increased occurrence of depression and anxiety in this group has been associated with disruptions in lactation performance (Zanardo et al., 2011), and with parents giving their infants higher ratings of negativity (Voegtline et al., 2010).

Shaw found that parents who developed acute stress disorder had associated factors that included female gender, alteration in parental role, family cohesiveness, and emotional restraint (Shaw et al., 2006). Factors that increase an NICU parent's risk for developing PTSD include being a primipara (Greene et al., 2015), giving birth by Cesarean section, having experienced previous pregnancy problems, and giving birth to a lower birth weight or lower gestational age baby (Callahan & Hynan, 2002). Additional factors include having one or more severe medical complications (Callahan & Hynan, 2002; DeMier, Hynan, Harris, & Manniello, 1996), a longer hospitalization (DeMier et al., 1996), concurrent life stressors, a dysfunctional coping style and higher maternal education (Shaw et al., 2013), and a family history of anxiety and depression (Lefkowitz et al., 2010). Mothers with PTSD are more likely to also have higher depressive symptoms (Cho et al., 2008). Another vulnerable population, although not specific to NICU parents but sure to be represented among NICU parents, is that of women with hypertensive disorder of pregnancy which may progress to pre-eclampsia and even eclampsia. These women were found by Porcel to have a four times elevated risk of PTSD when compared with women who had normotensive pregnancies, with the risk of screening positive increasing with the severity of the hypertensive condition (Porcel et al., 2013).

Significance of Distress in NICU Parents

Increased depression and anxiety symptoms in NICU parents, although not particularly surprising, raise important clinical issues. In 2016, the United States Preventive Services Task Force (USPSTF) revised the recommendation to screen all adults for depression by adding a specification for pregnant and postpartum women (Siu & US Preventive Services Task Force, 2016). Because this recommendation is limited to screening for depression only, many NICU parents with clinically significant levels of anxiety may be missed. Additionally, because the fear of losing a newborn is understandably distressing, an elevated depression or anxiety screening score might be considered normal for this population. However, some NICU parents score in the normal range on depression or anxiety screening scales, so an elevated score may indeed signal a need for help. Additionally, the studies considered in this review were those in which emotional distress was assessed early in the newborn's hospitalization. Two longitudinal studies found that the prevalence of distress among NICU mothers significantly decreases over a year (Miles et al., 2007; Singer et al., 1999), likely resolving as the newborn's health status improves. However, for parents of very preterm infants, elevated levels of depression and anxiety symptoms remain above expected levels throughout the newborn period and at six months (Pace et al., 2016).

Thus, an additional question emerges: does temporary emotional distress reflecting concern over a hospitalized newborn's health really need to be identified, labeled, and referred to formal treatment? The meaning of an elevated depression or anxiety scale score in NICU parents, early in the newborn's hospitalization, is thus unclear.

The results of two qualitative studies of the experiences of NICU mothers and NICU fathers provide one means to understand the emotional needs of these parents. In the first study, narrative interviews were conducted with six Swedish mothers whose infants were hospitalized in the NICU three years prior (Lindberg & Ohrling, 2008). Five common themes emerged from their reports. First, the unexpected birth was a shocking experience for which the mothers were not prepared, women felt robbed of the initial happiness they expected with the birth of their newborn, and these new mothers avoided mothers of full-term infants. Second, feelings of anxiety were pervasive, caused by constant worry about whether their newborn would survive or become ill. Third, they were often separated from the newborn and limited in their ability to take care of him/her, and this experience was stressful. Fourth, mothers—especially those with older children at home—felt torn between family life and staying with the newborn. Fifth, the mothers identified the importance of having support in the form of someone who knew about the newborn to listen to their thoughts and desires. The first four themes all pertain to emotional distress and the fifth indicates their need for support to cope with this distress.

The setting of the second qualitative study was an NICU in Dublin in the Republic of Ireland (Hollywood & Hollywood, 2011). Here, five NICU fathers were interviewed when their infants were between 34 and 42 weeks of age. Five common themes emerged from the fathers' descriptions of their experiences, including the emotional effects of the hospitalization, the realization of becoming a father to a premature baby, the importance of having accurate information, the difference between maternal and paternal roles, and the constraints imposed by work. Relevant to this chapter are the fathers' emotional reactions to the hospitalization, which included feeling anxious/fearful and helpless, aptly captured in one quote from the father of hospitalized twins: "It was initially the most scariest thing I had ever seen. When we walked in and saw them my legs were weak. I felt so helpless as I could do nothing for them" (Hollywood & Hollywood, 2011, p. 35).

These results from qualitative assessments poignantly underscore NICU parents' significant emotional stress, and the comments suggest supportive care could be helpful. With regard to the desire for help, in the qualitative study of mothers, women suggested that extra support is needed, particularly from someone who was knowledgeable about the well-being of their newborn. Bergstrom determined that mothers who experienced depression at one month after the birth of their NICU infant had an almost eight-fold risk of experiencing postpartum depression at four months. The risk was further increased to 60% for women who were not offered counseling during their infant's NICU stay (Bergstrom, Wallin, Thomson, & Flacking, 2012).

A particularly important reason to offer psychosocial support to NICU parents, whether it be from a social worker, psychologist, or psychiatrist—or even a bedside nurse—is that parent-infant bonding can be disrupted when parents are depressed or stressed, and their interactions with their infants may be less sensitive and less structured (Feeley et al., 2011). Parents may also have more negative evaluations of their baby's behavior (Voegtline et al., 2010). Both the severity of maternal depression (Singer et al., 1999) and the intensity of post-traumatic reactions among parents (Pierrehumbert, Nicole, Muller-Nix, Forcada-Guex, & Ansermet, 2003) predict worse developmental outcome among preterm infants, possibly mediated through the impairment of a strong, positive, interactive parent-infant relationship.

The next section thus provides an overview of newly issued guidelines for psychosocial care of NICU parents, as well as a descriptive overview of effective interventions specific to emotionally distressed NICU parents.

Support for Emotionally Distressed Parents

In the 1990s, the use of surfactants was a major advance in neonatology.[1] As predicted in a recent state-of-the-art report, fully incorporating parents into the newborn care is likely to be the next major advance (Hall et al., 2017). To capture this change in perspective about the increased importance of parents' roles, the authors of that report propose changing the unit's name from "Neonatal Intensive Care" to "Newborn Intensive Parenting" unit. In addition to this expansion from newborn to family focus, there is increased recognition that the intensive care nursery is a trauma center for parents, staff, and newborns that is associated with significant stress among all participants (Hynan & Hall, 2015).

In formal recognition of this stress, in 2014, the *National Perinatal Association* (NPA) convened a workgroup comprising NICU parents and multi-disciplinary clinicians. In a series of meetings, and based on a review of relevant literature as well as consensus-building discussions, this workgroup developed six guidelines for psychosocial care of NICU families (Box 9.1), published in a special issue of the *Journal of Perinatology* (Hynan & Hall, 2015). Although these recommendations

---

Box 9.1 National Perinatal Association's Six Guidelines for the Psychosocial Support of NICU Parents

Recommendations for involving the family in developmental care of the NICU baby

(Craig et al., 2015)

Recommendations for peer-to-peer support for NICU parents

(Hall, Ryan, Beatty, & Grubbs, 2015)

Recommendations for mental health professionals in the NICU

(Hynan et al., 2015)

Recommendations for palliative and bereavement care in the NICU: a family-centered integrative approach

(Kenner, Press, & Ryan, 2015)

NICU discharge planning and beyond: recommendations for parent psychosocial support

(Purdy, Craig, & Zeanah, 2015)

Recommendations for enhancing psychosocial support of NICU parents through staff education and support

(Hall, Cross et al., 2015).

---

are based on a U.S. perspective, the NPA views these recommendations as "a road map for how NICUs should be transformed" (Hynan & Hall, 2015, p. 51). Readers from around the world can thus examine their own NICU practices, evaluate needs within their own healthcare systems, and flexibly implement these recommendations.

Some of the NPA's recommendations for psychosocial support of NICU parents can be easily implemented in the NICU setting to further influence the development of positive parent-infant interactions, while simultaneously mitigating at least some of the stresses that contribute to parental depression and anxiety. Mehler found that mothers who saw their very low birth weight infants within three hours of the infant's birth had higher rates of secure attachment than mothers who did not have this early contact with their infants (Mehler et al., 2011). Flacking described how physical and emotional closeness between NICU infants and their parents is crucial to the well-being of both, and specifically to the brain development of the infant (Flacking et al., 2012). Flacking further suggested that NICU staff could increase and support parent-infant contact by providing family-centered care with generous visitation policies for parents, attending to details of the physical environment which can enhance parent-infant closeness (which could include single-family rooms to promote privacy and comfort), and encouraging early and prolonged skin-to-skin contact (Flacking et al., 2012).

Skin-to-skin care is probably the best way to support and strengthen parent-infant bonding. Mothers of NICU infants reported feelings of "being needed" and "feeling comfortable" with their infants regardless of the infant's health status during skin-to-skin holding (Johnson, 2007). Bigelow found that mothers of healthy, full-term infants who engaged in this practice for five hours a day for the first week, and two hours a day for the rest of the first month, had lower symptoms of maternal depression and less physiologic stress (Bigelow, Power, MacLellan-Peters, Alex, & McDonald, 2012). Feldman and colleagues completed a longitudinal study, following premature infants and their mothers over a decade, and determined that mothers who engaged in the skin-to-skin intervention for a period of 14 consecutive days compared with those whose infants received standard incubator care had increased maternal attachment behavior in the postpartum period and reduced maternal anxiety (Feldman, Rosenthal, & Eidelman, 2014). Further, their children had improved cognitive development from six months to ten years, and improved mother-child reciprocity at ten years. Stress scores for mothers were lowered in mothers who participated in the family-integrated model of care in a study by O'Brien and colleagues (O'Brien et al., 2013). In this model of care, parents spent a minimum of eight hours a day in the NICU, performing basic cares for their infants, attending rounds, and participating in educational sessions.

Encouraging parent-infant contact and parental involvement in their infant's care has long-lasting benefits not only for the parents, with lower occurrence of depression and anxiety, but also for their infants in terms of improved neurodevelopmental outcomes. There is great variability in whether NICUs offer parents formal psychological support (Alam, Ahlund, Thalange, & Clarke, 2010), and even fewer offer psychiatric support. In one program in which perinatal psychiatric services were made available in an NICU setting, mothers of very low birth weight infants were disproportionately likely to be referred with either depression or anxiety, related primarily to their infant's medical problems. Psychiatrists focused their interventions on promoting healthy parent-infant interactions to support bonding; most parents did not require long-term treatment (Friedman, Kessler, Yang, Parsons, & Friedman, 2013). In Penny's study of the use of a psychiatric consultation service in an NICU, one-sixth of NICU mothers were referred for service, with more than 25% requiring follow-up after NICU discharge (Penny, Friedman, & Halstead, 2017).

Clinical psychologists are becoming more involved in NICUs, as was suggested in the National Perinatal Association's recommendations for mental health professionals in the NICU (Hynan et al., 2015). Their role is usually dual: to provide emotional support to distressed parents as well as to the staff (Kraemer, 2006; Steinberg & Kraemer, 2010; Steinberg & Patterson, 2017). Steinberg and Kraemer described psychologists' work with staff as being an important way to help them "remain emotionally available even in the disorienting face of ambiguity and uncertainty" (Steinberg & Kraemer, 2010).

If formal psychological or psychiatric services are not available in individual NICUs, there are a number of other programs that can provide psychosocial support to parents. One excellent program consistent with many of the *NPA's* guidelines is the *March of Dimes' NICU Family Support Program*. Perhaps one of the most comprehensive hospital-based services for NICU families, the *NICU Family Support Program* is provided in more than 120 hospitals in the United States and Canada. Recognizing that many NICUs have already established some supportive services for families, and that the demographics served by each NICU can dramatically vary, the *NICU Family Support Program* is tailored to complement existing services and to serve the demographics of each hospital. A core component of the program includes sensitive and engaging educational materials. The most compelling of these educational materials is the "Parent Care Kit." A gift to each family, this kit contains brochures and videos to enhance a family's understanding of NICU life, including explanations of commonly used NICU equipment, procedures, and infant medical conditions. In line with the philosophy of a Neonatal Intensive Parenting Unit, these materials stress that parents are the primary caregivers and encourage their participation in their child's care. Perhaps, the loveliest gift in the kit is the special baby book that has been tailored to the NICU experience, and has places for NICU families to record both difficult and celebratory experiences. Some of these materials are available to the public through the *March of Dimes* website.[2] Finally, to support staff in their clinical care, the *March of Dimes* offers continuing education for NICU nursing staff through its perinatal nursing education program. In each participating hospital, the *NICU Family Support Program* is coordinated by the support specialist, a *March of Dimes* staff person who selects and provides program services at each site.

A descriptive evaluation of the *NICU Family Support Program* in eight hospitals used a telephone interview and survey methodology to assess views of NICU administrators ($N = 11$), clinical staff ($N = 502$), and families ($N = 216$) (L. G. Cooper et al., 2007). Based on participant responses, it is clear that the program was well received. NICU administrators valued the NICU family support specialist, as she was able to focus on education and support of families. NICU staff reported that the program enhanced the overall quality of NICU care and that, as a result of the program, parents were more informed, were less stressed, had increased confidence at discharge and had enhanced bonding with their infant. Almost two-thirds of families received help from the NICU family support specialist; and 83% of them indicated that this help reduced stress and made them feel more confident as parents. Although the program evaluation relied on descriptive outcomes, these results indicate that families value this supportive resource.

Although hospital-based programs offer support to emotionally distressed families, none specifically target parental emotional distress. A recent meta-analysis evaluated NICU-based interventions which used a randomized controlled trial methodology and also assessed maternal depression and anxiety outcomes (Mendelson, Cluxton-Keller, Vullo, Tandon, & Noazin, 2017). Interestingly, all of the interventions reviewed were presented as a depression/anxiety treatment option, even if emotional well-being was not the direct focus of sessions. For example, one educational intervention was shown to coincidentally reduce depression symptoms in NICU mothers, even though emotional distress was not the focus of the intervention sessions (Melnyk et al., 2006). Of the 12 interventions that were included in that meta-analytic review (Mendelson et al., 2017), only four directly targeted mother's emotional experiences. None of these four interventions resulted in statistically significant change in symptoms in NICU mothers relative to the comparison group. Thus, a critical need among emotionally distressed NICU parents, who may spend essentially all of their free time with their hospitalized newborn, is effective emotional support that directly addresses parental emotional distress, and that is delivered conveniently to the newborn's point of care. Although not yet validated specifically for NICU parents, two empirically supported interventions are promising because they can be provided conveniently at the newborn's point of care: Listening Visits and Acceptance and Commitment Therapy (ACT).

Listening Visits were developed for British home-visiting nurses (called health visitors) to provide a first-line, supportive approach for postpartum mothers with mild to moderately severe depression symptoms (Holden, Sagovsky, & Cox, 1989). As implied by the name, the central assumption of the Listening Visits intervention is that talking about feelings to an empathic and nonjudgmental professional is therapeutic. Key intervention components include empathic listening with collaborative problem solving. Considerable empirical support from European-based randomized controlled trials (P. J. Cooper, Murray, Wilson, & Romaniuk, 2003; Holden et al., 1989; Wickberg & Hwang, 1996) supported Britain's *National Institute of Clinical Excellence* in recommending Listening Visits as an evidence-based intervention for postpartum women with mildly to moderately severe depression symptoms (British Psychological Society, 2007). Yet, success in one healthcare setting does not guarantee success in a different country with a different healthcare system. So, from 2007 to 2012, a U.S.-based research team conducted an open as well as randomized controlled trial of Listening Visits. Its results validated this approach for impoverished mothers of term infants in U.S. community-based settings (Brock, O'Hara, & Segre, 2017; Segre, Brock, & O'Hara, 2015; Segre, Stasik, O'Hara, & Arndt, 2010).

To address the critical need for emotional support in mothers of hospitalized newborns, this U.S.-based research team also evaluated Listening Visits for the first time in the NICU. Here, Listening Visits was delivered in six, 30–50-minute sessions that were provided in a private hospital location, every two to three days by a doctorally prepared nurse. The intervention was non-directive, so the NICU mother chose the focus of each session. Two case studies of NICU mothers who received Listening Visits in the NICU-based open trial are available in a published report (Chuffo Siewert, Cline, & Segre, 2015). Results of the small ($N = 23$) open-trial evaluation in the NICU setting were promising (Segre, Chuffo-Siewert, Brock, & O'Hara, 2013). Emotional distress improved significantly from pre- to post-LV, as revealed by a reduction in symptom scores from 14.26 to 9.00 on the Edinburgh Postnatal Depression Scale (EPDS: Cox, Holden, & Sagovsky, 1987) as well a reduction of scores from 16.57 to 11.14 on the Beck Anxiety Scale (BAI: Beck, Epstein, Brown, & Steer, 1988). In addition, NICU mothers were willing to use this form of care: 78% of eligible depressed mothers opted to try the Listening Visits intervention. Finally, NICU mothers who received Listening Visits were very satisfied: 91.3% of mothers rated the quality of help received as excellent. Considered together, the numerous RCTs of Listening Visits, plus the positive outcomes from the first open-trial with NICU mothers, are promising results. Moreover, the fact that Listening Visits can be conveniently delivered in the NICU, by trusted nurses who are also knowledgeable about the newborn's medical conditions, suggests that this approach is particularly well suited to the NICU setting. These sentiments are captured by the views of one NICU mother who received Listening Visits during the open trial:

> I thought that they were very helpful. Whenever I had any concerns or questions it was nice to have a nurse listen. She was able to clarify any medically related questions and she was able to listen to my feelings. I can remember having those "hard" days where you think everything is going wrong and why? Having a nurse there to listen to me was nice for me to let out all my feelings and not be judged … She was there with me during my journey and experience at the NICU.

ACT is an evidenced-based treatment for depression, anxiety, and stress in general community populations (Hayes, Luoma, Bond, Masuda, & Lillis, 2006; Hofman, Sawyer, Witt, & Oh, 2010). ACT also seems particularly well suited to emotionally distressed NICU parents. The goal of ACT is to help individuals accept/be present with difficult feelings and thoughts resulting from uncontrollable life circumstances, such as the hospitalization of a newborn. At the same time, ACT teaches individuals to identify important life goals and engage fully in life, guided by their own goals and values rather than by reacting reflexively to difficult circumstances (Harris, 2009; Hayes et al., 2006).

Particularly noteworthy for the NICU setting are the wide range of ACT delivery formats shown to be effective in non-NICU settings, including brief forms ranging from 75 minutes to one-day workshops (Dindo, Recober, Marchman, Turvey, & O'Hara, 2012), web-based forms of delivery (Levin, Pistorello, Seeley, & Hayes, 2013), a self-help guide (Johnston, Foster, Shennan, Starkey, & Johnson, 2010), and even delivery via PowerPoint slides (Natstally & Dixon, 2012). ACT was also successfully adapted for prevention (Bach & Hayes, 2002; Levin et al., 2013). One ACT-informed particularly promising treatment for NICU parents is called *Take a Breath*. Developed by a Melbourne-based team (Rayner et al., 2016), *Take a Breath* targets emotionally distressed parents of infants and children hospitalized with life threatening illness or injury. The intervention is delivered in five, nine-minute weekly, online sessions that are led by a therapist. Three weeks after the fifth session, there is a sixth booster session. The sessions focus on introducing mindfulness principles, including breathing deeply, slowing down, observing feelings and thoughts, identifying and listing to values, and deciding what matters the most and doing it in line with values. The randomized controlled trial evaluation is currently underway. ACT for NICU parents is thus a promising direction for clinical research.

In summary, a wide range of hospital-based supportive services are typically available for emotionally distressed NICU families. Recently issued guidelines of the *National Perinatal Association* provide a roadmap for improving this care. As noted in this review, despite that emotional distress is prevalent in NICU parents, empirically supported treatments specifically targeting emotional distress are lacking. Two interventions, Listening Visits and ACT, offer promising approaches.

Post-Discharge Support

The period after discharge from the NICU is a time fraught with stress for parents who are bringing a vulnerable infant home, even if they have not previously experienced anxiety or depression. Child abuse occurs more frequently among preterm than full-term infants, and NICU mothers' psychiatric illnesses are often thought to place them at higher risk to engage in child abuse (Ishizaki, Nagahama, & Kaneko, 2013). Giving birth to a very low birth weight infant can impact parents' perceptions of their child and the nature of the parent-child relationship well into childhood. In a follow-up study of children who were eight years of age, Singer noted that those who were high-risk very low birth weight infants (those defined as weighing less than 1,500 grams and having bronchopulmonary dysplasia) were more likely to be perceived by their mothers as being more demanding, distractable, hyperactive, and less adaptable than low-risk infants in the same birth weight category and infants born at term. Parent-child conflict was actually lower in these families; the children were more compliant and dependent, and less likely to be involved in outdoor activities (Singer et al., 2007). Controlling and overprotective patterns of parent-child interactions in mothers of former preterm infants have been described, especially in mothers who experienced PTSD (Forcada-Guex, Borghini, Pierrehumbert, Ansermet, & Mueller-Nix, 2011; Wightman et al., 2007). This reaction may be in response to parents' views that their formerly medically fragile child remains "vulnerable" (Allen et al., 2004). Perception of ongoing child vulnerability was more common among mothers who displayed anxiety at their infant's hospital discharge (Allen et al., 2004). Therefore, preparing parents for discharge—beginning from the time of admission to the NICU—is critically important for the family's future functioning.

Mothers of higher-risk NICU infants who were queried six weeks after their infant's discharge reported higher levels of emotional distress and depressive symptomatology than mothers of lower-risk infants, indicating a need to pay attention to factors related to the infant's condition when planning discharge, as well as to parental factors. Mothers' dissatisfaction with social support from their partners, other family, and friends also predicted their depressive symptoms at follow-up (Bennett & Slade, 1991). Parents who experienced emotional distress or mental health disorders during their NICU stay perceived themselves to be less ready for discharge (McGowan et al., 2017), and could therefore be targeted for focused attention prior to discharge. Immigrant mothers and single mothers of preterm infants are also at risk for depressive symptoms after their infant's discharge, and interventions that reduce stress and increase family functioning as well as social support may be helpful in reducing their risk (Ballantyne, Benzies, & Trute, 2013). Preparing parents for discharge through educational/behavioral programs that increase their involvement with their infant during the hospital stay, such as the Creating Opportunities for Parent Empowerment (COPE) program, can decrease the depression and anxiety they experience two months after their infant's discharge (Melnyk, Crean, Feinstein, & Fairbanks, 2008). Primary care providers can further support parents after discharge by engaging them in screening for postpartum depression at well-child visits (Gjerdingen, Crow, McGovern, Miner, & Center, 2009), and making necessary referrals for further services as indicated.

Conclusions

In examining the postnatal emotional experiences of parents of hospitalized newborns, several key points emerge. First, emotional distress is prevalent in NICU parents. Second, although general support is often provided through hospital-based programs like the *NICU Family Support Program* of the *March of Dimes*, validated treatments that specifically target emotional distress in NICU parents are lacking. Third, although anxiety or depression can be considered a normal reaction to the hospitalization of a newborn that will dissipate as the newborn's health improves, reports from

NICU mothers and NICU fathers indicate that they would value the opportunity to talk. Additionally, there are many ways to involve parents in the care of their infants in the NICU which can help minimize their feelings of depression and anxiety; similarly, targeted supportive services provided to particularly high-risk families prior to discharge can be helpful. Finally, and perhaps most importantly, because emotional distress is normative, parents may not perceive the need for formal treatment from a mental-health specialist, which is likely a stigmatized and inconvenient form of care. Instead, treatments delivered in the NICU setting, by trusted professionals such as nurses, who are also knowledgeable about the medical condition of the newborn, may be an optimal first-line supportive approach to emotional distress in this population. Another reason to embrace this model of care is the paucity of professional mental health services currently available in NICUs. To conclude, the emotional experiences of parents of hospitalized newborns and the kind of support that they would value are best captured by a quote from one NICU mother who reads a news release about the Listening Visits open trial:

> I spent almost every day of my twins' 47-day NICU stay by myself with no one to talk to. No friends would go with me. I still sit with anxiety over a year later. I didn't make friends in the NICU as my twins were their own roommates. Anytime I see NICU things on TV, I burst into tears and it hurts. If only I had someone to talk to then, I wouldn't cringe so much [now].

Notes

1 Surfactant, a naturally produced substance, provides a coating for alveoli—air sacs within the lungs. Without it, the air sacs open but have difficulty remaining open because they stick together.
2 March of Dimes NICU Family Support Program: www.marchofdimes.org/complications/the-nicu-family-support-program.aspx.

References

Alam, J., Ahlund, S., Thalange, N., & Clarke, P. (2010). Psychological support for parents in UK tertiary-level neonatal units—a postcode lottery. *Archives of Disease in Childhood, 95*, A104. doi:10.1136/adc.2010.186338.224

Allen, E. C., Manuel, J. C., Legault, C. L., Naughton, M. J., Pivor, C., & O'Shea, M. (2004). Perception of child vulnerability among mothers of former premature infants. *Pediatrics, 113*, 267–273. doi:10.1542/peds.113.2.267

American Academy of Pediatrics. (2015). Common parent reactions to the NICU. Retrieved from www.healthychildren.org/English/ages-stages/baby/preemie/pages/Common-Parent-Reactions-to-the-NICU.aspx

Bach, P., & Hayes, S. C. (2002). The use of Acceptance and Commitment Therapy to prevent the rehospitalization of psychotic patients: A randomized controlled trial. *Journal of Consulting and Clinical Psychology, 70*, 1129–1139. doi:10.1037//0022-006X.70.5.1129

Ballantyne, M., Benzies, K. M., & Trute, B. (2013). Depressive symptoms among immigrant and Canadian born mothers of preterm infants at neonatal intensive care. *BMC Pregnancy and Childbirth, 13*, S11. doi:10.1186/1471-2393-13-S1-S11

Beck, A. T., Epstein, N., Brown, G., & Steer, R. A. (1988). An inventory for measuring clinical anxiety: Psychometric properties. *Journal of Consulting and Clinical Psychology, 56*(6), 893–897. doi:10.1037/0022-006X.56.6.893

Bennett, D. E., & Slade, P. (1991). Infants born at risk: Consequences for maternal post-partum adjustment. *British Journal of Medical Psychology, 64*, 159–172. doi:10.1111/j.2044-8341.1991.tb01653.x

Bergstrom, E.-B., Wallin, L., Thomson, G., & Flacking, R. (2012). Postpartum depression in mothers of infants cared for in a Neonatal Intensive Care Unit-Incidence and associated factors. *Journal of Neonatal Nursing, 18*(4), 143–151. doi:10.1016/j.jnn.2011.11.001

Bigelow, A., Power, M., MacLellan-Peters, J., Alex, M., & McDonald, C. (2012). Effect of mother/infant skin-to-skin contact on postpartum depressive symptoms and maternal physiological stress. *41*, 369–382. doi:10.1111/j.1552-6909.2012.01350.x

Brandon, D. H., Tully, K. P., Silva, S. G., Malcolm, W. F., Murtha, A. P., Turner, B. S., & Holditch-Davis, D. (2011). Emotional respones of mothers of late-preterm and term infants. *Journal of Obstetric, Gynecologic, & Neonatal Nursing, 40*(6), 719–731. doi:10.1111/j.1552-6909.2011.01290.x

British Psychological Society. (2007). *Antenatal and postnatal mental health: The NICE guideline on clinical management and service guidance.* Leicester (UK): National Collaborating Centre for Mental Health (UK) Retrieved from www.ncbi.nlm.nih.gov/books/NBK54487/.

Brock, R. L., O'Hara, M. W., & Segre, L. S. (2017). Depression treatment by non-mental-health providers: Incremental evidence for the effectiveness of Listening Visits *American Journal of Community Psychology, 59*, 172–183.

Callahan, J. L., & Hynan, M. T. (2002). Identifying mothers at risk for postnatal emotional distress: Further evidence for the validity of the perinatal posttraumatic stress disorder questionnaire. *Journal of Perinatology, 22*, 448–454. doi:10.1038/sj.jp.7210783

Carter, J. D., Mulder, R. T., Bartram, A. F., & Darlow, B. A. (2005). Infants in a neonatal intensive care unit: Parental response. *Archives of Disease in Childhood: Fetal and Neonatal Edition, 90*(2), F109–F113. doi:10.1136/adc.2003.031641

Carter, J. D., Mulder, R. T., Frampton, C. M. A., & Darlow, B. A. (2007). Infants admitted to a neonatal intensive care unit: Parental psychological status at 9 months. *Acta Paediatrica, 96*, 1286–1289. doi:10.1111/j.1651-2227.2007.00425.x

Cho, J., Holditch-Davis, D., & Miles, M. S. (2008). Effects of maternal depressive symptoms and infant gender on the interactions between mothers and their medically at-risk infants. *Journal of Obstetric and Gynecological Neonatal Nursing, 37*, 58–70. doi:10.1111/j.1552-6909.2007.00206.x

Chuffo Siewert, R., Cline, M., & Segre, L. (2015). Implementation of an innovative nurse-delivered depression intervention for mothers of NICU infants. *Advances in Neonatal Care, 15*(2), 104–111. doi:10.1097/ANC.0000000000000146

Cooper, L. G., Gooding, J. S., Gallagher, J., Sternesky, L., Ledsky, L., & Berns, S. D. (2007). Impact of family-centered care initiative on NICU care, staff and families. *Journal of Perinatology, 27*, S32–s37. Retrieved from www.nature.com/jp/journal/v27/n2s/pdf/7211840a.pdf doi:10.1038/sj.jp.7211840

Cooper, P. J., Murray, L., Wilson, A., & Romaniuk, H. (2003). Controlled trial of the short-and long-term effect of psychological treatment of post-partum depression. I. Impact on maternal mood. *British Journal of Psychiatry, 182*(5), 412–419. doi:10.1192/bjp.182.5.412

Cox, J. L., Holden, J. M., & Sagovsky, R. (1987). Detection of postnatal depression: Development of the 10-item Edinburgh Postnatal Depression Scale. *British Journal of Psychiatry, 150*(6), 782–786. doi:10.1192/bjp.150.6.782

Craig, J. W., Glick, C., Phillips, R., Hall, S. L., Smith, J., & Browne, J. (2015). Recommendations for involving the family in developmental care of the NICU baby. *Journal of Perinatology, 2015*, S5–S8. doi:10.1038/jp.2015.142

Davis, L., Edwards, H., Mohay, H., & Wollin, J. (2003). The impact of very premature birth on the psychological health of mothers. *Early Human Development, 73*(1–2), 61–70. doi:10.1016/S0378-3782(03)00073-2

DeMier, R. L., Hynan, M. T., Harris, H. B., & Manniello, R. L. (1996). Perinatal stressors as predictors of symptoms of posttraumatic stress in mothers of infants at high risk. *Journal of Perinatology, 16*, 276–280.

Dindo, L., Recober, A., Marchman, J. N., Turvey, C., & O'Hara, M. W. (2012). One-day behavioral treatment for patients with comorbid depression and migraine: A pilot study. *Behavior Research and Therapy, 50*, 537–543. doi:10.1016/j.brat.2012.05.007

Epel, S. (2015). Leaving baby at the NICU: A parent's survival guide for when a preemie needs intensive care. *Parenting.* Retrieved from www.parenting.com/article/leaving-baby-behind.

Feeley, N., Zelkowitz, P., Cormier, C., Charbonneau, L., Lacroix, A., & Papageogiou, A. (2011). Posttraumatic stress among mothers of very low birthweight infants at 6 months after discharge from the neonatal intensive care unit. *Applied Nursing Research, 24*, 114–117. doi:10.1016/j.apnr.2009.04.004

Feldman, R., Rosenthal, Z., & Eidelman, A. I. (2014). Maternal-preterm skin-to-skin contact enhances child physiologic organization and cognitive control across the first 10 years of life. *Biological Psychiatry, 75*, 56–64.

Flacking, R., Lehtonen, L., Thompsen, G., Axelin, A., Ahiqvist, S., Moran, V. H., … The SCENE group. (2012). Closeness and separation in neonatal intensive care. *Acta Paediatrica, 101*, 1032–1037. doi:10.1111/j.1651-2227.2012.02787.x

Forcada-Guex, M., Borghini, A., Pierrehumbert, B., Ansermet, F., & Mueller-Nix, C. (2011). Prematurity, maternal posttraumatic stress and consequences on the mother–infant relationship. *Early Human Development, 87*, 21–26. doi:10.1016/j.earlhumdev.2010.09.006

Friedman, S. H., Kessler, A., Yang, S. N., Parsons, S., & Friedman, H. (2013). Delivering perinatal psychiatric services in the neonatal intensive care unit. *Acta Paediatrica, e392–397.* doi:10.1111/apa.12323

Gavin, N. I., Gaynes, B. N., Lohr, K. N., Meltzer-Brody, S., Gartlehner, G., & Swinson, T. (2005). Perinatal depression: A systematic review of prevalence and incidence. *Obstetrics and Gynecology, 106,* 1071–1083.

Gjerdingen, D., Crow, S., McGovern, P., Miner, M., & Center, B. (2009). Postpartum depression screening at well-child visits: Validity of a 2-question screen and the PHQ-9. *Annals of Family Medicine, 7,* 63–70. doi:10.1370/afm.933

Greene, M. M., Rossman, B., Patra, K., Kratovil, A. L., Janes, J. E., & Meier, P. (2015). Depressive, anxious and perinatal post-traumatic distress in mothers of very low birth weight infants in the NICU. *Journal Developmental Behavioral Pediatrics, 36,* 362–370. doi:10.1097/DBP.0000000000000174

Hall, S. L., Cross, J., Selix, N. W., Patterson, C., Segre, L., Chuffo-Siewert, R., ... Martin, M. L. (2015). Recommendations for enhancing psychosocial support of NICU parents through staff education and support. *Journal of Perinatology, 35,* S29–S36. doi:10.1038/jp.2015.147

Hall, S. L., Hynan, M. T., Phillips, R., Lassen, S., Craig, J. W., Goyer, E., Hatfield, R., & Cohen, H. (2017). The Neonatal Intensive Parenting Unit (NIPU): An Introduction. *Journal of Perinatology* epub ahead of print. doi:10.1038/jp.2017.108

Hall, S. L., Ryan, D. J., Beatty, J., & Grubbs, L. (2015). Recommednations for peer-to-peer support for NICU parents. *Journal of Perinatology, 35,* S9–S13. doi:10.1038/jp.2015.143

Harris, R. (2009). *ACT made simple.* Oakland, CA: New Harbinger Press.

Harrison, W., & Goodman, D. (2015). Epidemiologic trends in neonatal intensive care, 2007–2012. *Journal of the American Medical Association, 169,* 855–862. doi:10.1001/jamapediatrics.2015.1305

Hawes, K., McGowan, E., O'Donnell, M., Tucker, R., & Vohr, B. (2016). Social emotional factors increase risk of postpartum depression in mothers of preterm infants. *The Journal of Pediatrics, 179,* 61–67. doi:10.1016/j.jpeds.2016.07.008

Hayes, S. C., Luoma, J. B., Bond, F. W., Masuda, A., & Lillis, J. (2006). Acceptance and Commitment Therapy: Model processes and outcomes. *Behavior Research and Therapy, 44,* 1–25. doi:10.1016/j.brat.2005.06.006

Hofman, S. G., Sawyer, A. T., Witt, A. A., & Oh, D. (2010). The effect of mindfulness-based therapy on anxiety and depression: A meta-analytic review. *Journal of Consulting and Clinical Psychology, 78,* 169–183. doi:10.1037/a0018555

Holden, J. M., Sagovsky, R., & Cox, J. L. (1989). Counselling in a general practice setting: controlled study of health visitor intervention in treatment of postnatal depression. *British Medical Journal, 298*(Jan.), 223–226. doi:10.1136/bmj.298.6668.223

Hollywood, M., & Hollywood, E. (2011). The lived experiences of fathrs of a premature baby on the neontal intensive care unit. *Journal of Neonatal Nursing, 17,* 32–40. doi:10.1016/j.jnn.2007.05.004

Hugill, K. G., Letherby, T. R., & Lavender, T. (2013). Experiences of fathers shortly after the birth of their preterm infants. *Journal of Obstetric and Gynecological Neonatal Nursing, 42,* 655–663. doi:10.1111/1552-6909.12256

Hynan, M. T., & Hall, S. L. (2015). Psychosocial program standards for NICU parents. *Journal of Perinatology, 35,* 51–54. doi:10.1038/jp.2015.141

Hynan, M. T., Steinberg, Z., Baker, L., Cicco, R., Geller, P. A., Lassen, S., ... Stuebe, A. (2015). Recommendations for mental health professionals in the NICU. *Journal of Perinatology, 35,* S14–S18.

Ishizaki, Y., Nagahama, T., & Kaneko, K. (2013). Mental health of mothers and their premature infants for the prevention of child abuse and maltreatment. *Health, 5,* 612–616. doi:10.4236/health.2013.53A081

Johnson, A. N. (2007). The maternal experience of Kangaroo Holding. *Journal of Obstetric and Gynecological Neonatal Nursing, 36,* 568–573. doi:10.1111/j.1552-6909.2007.00187.x

Johnston, M., Foster, M., Shennan, J., Starkey, N. J., & Johnson, A. (2010). The effectiveness of an acceptance and commitment therapy self-help intervention for chronic pain. *Clinical Journal of Pain, 26,* 393–402. doi:10.1097/AJP.0b013e3181cf59ce

Kenner, C., Press, J., & Ryan, D. J. (2015). Recommendations for palliative and bereavement care in the NICU: a family-centered integrative approach. *Journal of Perinatology, 35,* S19–S23. doi:10.1038/jp.2015.145

Kong, L.-P., Cui, Y., Qiu, Y.-F., Han, S.-P., Yu, Z.-B., & Guo, Z.-R. (2013). Anxiety and depression in parents of sick neonates: a hospital based study. *Journal of Clinical Nursing, 22,* 1163–1172. doi:10.1111/jocn.12090

Kraemer, S. B. (2006). So the cradle won't fall: Holding the staff who hold the parents in the NICU. *Psychoanalytic Dialogues, 16,* 149–164.

Lefkowitz, D. S., Baxt, C., & Evans, J. R. (2010). Prevalence and correlates of posttraumatic stress and postpartum depression in parents of infants in the neonatal intensive care unit (NICU). *Journal Clinical Psychology in Medical Settings, 17*(3), 230–237. doi:10.1007/S10880-010-9202-7

Levin, M., Pistorello, J., Seeley, J. R., & Hayes, S. C. (2013). Feasibility of a prototype web-based Acceptance and Commitment Therapy prevention program for college students. *Journal of American College Health, 62*, 20–30. doi:10.1080/07448481.2013.843533

Lindberg, B., & Ohrling, K. (2008). Experiences of having a prematurely born infant from the perspective of mothers in northern Sweden. *International Journal of Circumpolar Health, 67*, 461–471. doi:10.3402/ijch.v67i5.18353

Mackley, A. B., Locke, R. G., Spear, M. L., & Joseph, R. (2010). Forgotten parent: NICU paternal emotional response. *Advances in Neonatal Care, 10*, 200–203. doi:1097/ANC.0b013e3181e946f0

McGowan, E., Du, N., Hawes, K., Tucker, R., O'Donnell, M., & Vohr, B. (2017). Maternal mental health and neonatal intensive care unit discharge readiness in mothers of preterm infants. *The Journal of Pediatrics*. Retrieved from www.sciencedirect.com/science/article/pii/S0022347617301622 doi:10.1016/j.jpeds.2017.01.052

Mehler, K., Wendrich, D., Kissgen, R., Roth, B., Oberthuer, A., Pillekamp, F., & Kribis, A. (2011). Mothers seeing their VLBW infants within 3 h after birth are more likely to establish a secure attachment behavior: Evidence of a sensitive period with preterm infants? *Journal of Perinatology, 31*, 404–410. doi:10.1038/jp.2010.139

Melnyk, B. M., Crean, H. F., Feinstein, N. F., & Fairbanks, E. (2008). Maternal anxiety and depression after a premature infant's discharge from the neonatal intensive care unit: Explanatory effects of the creating opportunities for parent empowerment program. *Nursing Research, 57*, 383–394. doi:10.1097/NNR.0b013e3181906f59

Melnyk, B. M., Feinstein, N. F., Alpert-Gillis, L., Fairbanks, E., Crean, H. F., Sinkin, R. A., … Gross, S. J. (2006). Reducing premature infants' length of stay and improving parents' mental health outcomes with the Creating Opportunities for Parent Empowerment (COPE) Neonatal Intensive Care Unit Program: A randomized controlled trial. *Pediatrics, 118*, e1414–e1427. doi:10.1542/peds.2005-2580

Mendelson, T., Cluxton-Keller, F., Vullo, G. C., Tandon, D., & Noazin, S. (2017). NICU-based interventions to reduce maternal depression and anxiety symptoms: A meta-analysis. *Pediatrics, 139*, e20161870. doi:10.1542/peds.2016-1870

Miles, M. S., Holditch-Davis, D., Schwartz, T. A., & Scher, M. (2007). Depressive symptoms in mothers of prematurely born infants. *Journal of Developmental & Behavioral Pediatrics, 28*(1), 36–44. doi:10.1097/01.DBP.0000257517.52459.7a

Mineka, S., Watson, D., & Clark, L. A. (1998). Comorbidity of anxiety and unipolar mood disorders. *Annual Review of Psychology, 49*, 377–412.

Natstally, B. L., & Dixon, M. R. (2012). The effect of a brief Acceptance and Commitment Therapy intevention on near-miss effect in problem gamblers. *The Psychological Record, 62*, 677–690.

O'Brien, K., Bracht, M., Macdonell, K., McBride, T., Robson, K., O'Leary, L., … Lee, S. K. (2013). A pilot cohort analytic study of Family Integrated Care in a Canadian neonatal intensive care unit. *BMC Pregnancy and Childbirth, 13*, S12. doi:10.1186/1471-2393-13-S1-S12.

Pace, C. C., Spittle, A. J., Molesworth, C. M.-L., Lee, K. J., Northam, E. A., Cheong, J. L. Y., … Anderson, P. J. (2016). Evolution of depression and anxiety symptoms in Parents of Very Preterm Infants during the Newborn Period. *JAMA Pediatrics, 170*, 863–870. doi:10.1001/jamapediatrics.2016.0810

Penny, K. A., Friedman, S. H., & Halstead, G. M. (2017). Psychiatric support for mothers in the Neonatal Intensive Care Unit. *Journal of Perinatology*, 451–457.

Pierrehumbert, B., Nicole, A., Muller-Nix, C., Forcada-Guex, M., & Ansermet, F. (2003). Parental post-traumatic reactions after premature birth: Implications for sleeping and eating problems in the infant. *Archives of Disease in Childhood: Fetal and Neonatal Edition, 88*, 400–404.

Porcel, J., Feigal, C., Poye, L., Postma, I. R., Zeeman, G. G., Olowoyeye, A., … Wilson, M. (2013). Hypertensive disorders of pregnancy and risk of screening positive for Posttraumatic Stress Disorder: A cross-sectional study. *Pregnancy Hypertension: An International Journal of Women's Cardiovascular Health, 3*, 254–260. doi:10.1016/j.preghy.2013.07.004

Purdy, I. B., Craig, J. W., & Zeanah, P. (2015). NICU discharge planning and beyond: Recommendations for parent psychosocial support. *Journal of Perinatology, 35*, S24–S28. doi:10.1038/jp.2015.146

Rayner, M., Muscara, F., Dimovski, A., McCarthy, M. C., Yamada, J., Andersson, V. A., … Nicholson, J. M. (2016). Take a breath: Study protocol for a randomized controlled trial of an online group intervention to reduce traumatic stress in parents of children with a life threatening illness or injury. *BMC Psychiatry, 16*. doi:10.1186/s12888-016-0861-2

Rogers, C. E., Kidokoro, H., Wallendorf, M., & Inder, T. E. (2013). Identifying mothers of very preterm infants at-risk for postpartum depression and anxiety before discharge. *Journal of Perinatology, 33*(3), 171–176. doi:10.1038/jp.2012.75

Segre, L. S., Brock, R. L., & O'Hara, M. W. (2015). Depression treatment for impoverished mothers by point-of-care providers: A randomized controlled trial. *Journal of Consulting and Clinical Psychology, 83*(2), 314–324. doi:10.1037/a0038495

Segre, L. S., Chuffo-Siewert, R., Brock, R. L., & O'Hara, M. W. (2013). Emotional distress in mothers of preterm hospitalized infants: A feasibility trial of nurse-delivered treatment. *Journal of Perinatology, 33*(12), 924–928. doi:10.1038/jp.2013.93

Segre, L. S., McCabe, J. E., Chuffo-Siewert, R., & O'Hara, M. W. (2014). Depression and anxiety symptoms in mothers of newborns hospitalized on the neonatal intensive care unit. *Nursing Research, 63*(5), 320–332. doi:10.1097/NNR.0000000000000039

Segre, L. S., Stasik, S. M., O'Hara, M. W., & Arndt, S. (2010). Listening visits: An evaluation of the effectiveness and acceptability of a home-based depression treatment. *Psychotherapy Research, 20*(6), 712–721. doi:10.1080/10503307.2010.518636

Shah, A. N., Jerardi, K. E., Auger, K. A., & Beck, A. F. (2016). Can hospitalization precipitate toxic stress? *Pediatrics, 137*, e20160204. Retrieved from http://pediatrics.aappublications.org/content/pediatrics/137/5/e20160204.full.p

Shaw, R. J., Bernard, R. S., Storfer-Isser, A., Rhine, W., & Horwitz, S. M. (2013). Parental coping in the Neonatal Intensive Care Unit. *Journal of Clinical Psychology in Medical Settings, 20*, 135–142. doi:10.1007/s10880-012-9328-x

Shaw, R. J., Deblois, T., Ikuta, L., Ginzburg, K., Fleisher, B., & Koopman, C. (2006). Acute stress disorder among parents of infants in the neonatal intensive care nursery. *Psychosomatics, 47*, 206–212. doi:10.1176/appi.psy.47.3.206

Shaw, R. J., Lilo, E. A., Storfer-Isser, A., Ball, M. B., Proud, M. S., Vierhaus, N. S., … Horwitz, S. M. (2014). Screening for symptoms of postpartum traumatic stress in a large sample of mothers with preterm infants. *Issues in Mental Health Nursing, 35*, 198–206. doi:10.3109/01612840.2013.853332

Singer, L. T., Fulton, S., Kirchner, H. I., Eisengart, S., Lewis, B., Short, E., … Baley, J. (2012). Longitudinal predictors of maternal stress and coping after very low-birth-weight birth. *Archives of Pediatrics and Adolescent Medicine, 164*, 518–524. doi:10.1001/archpediatrics.2010.81

Singer, L. T., Fulton, S., Kirchner, L., Eisengart, S., Lewis, B., Short, E., … Baley, J. (2007). Parenting very low birth weight children at school age: Maternal stress and coping. *The Journal of Pediatrics, 151*, 463–469. doi:10.1016/j.jpeds.2007.04.012

Singer, L. T., Salvator, A., Guo, S., Collin, M., Lilien, L., & Baley, J. (1999). Maternal psychological distress and parenting stress after the birth of a very-low-birth-weight infant. *Journal of the American Medical Association, 281*(0), 799–805. doi:10.1001/jama.281.9.799

Siu, A. L., & US Preventive Services Task Force. (2016). Screening for depression in adults: US Preventive Services Task Force recommendation statement. *Journal of the American Medical Association, 315*, 380–387. doi:10.1001/jama.2015.18392

Skari, H., Skreden, M., Malt, U. F., Dalholt, M., Ostensen, A. B., Egeland, T., & Emblem, R. (2002). Comparative levels of psychological distress, stress symptoms, depression and anxiety after childbirth-a prospective population-based study of mothers and fathers. *BJOG: An International Journal of Obstetrics and Gynecology, 109*, 1154–1163. doi:10.1111/j.1471-0528.2002.00468.x

Spielberger, C. D. (1970). *STAI manual for the state-trait anxiety inventory*. Palo Alto: Consulting Psychologists Press.

Steinberg, Z., & Kraemer, S. (2010). Cultivating a culture of awareness: Nurturing reflective practices in the NICU. *Zero to Three, November*, 15–21.

Steinberg, Z., & Patterson, C. (2017). Giving voice to the psychological in the NICU: A Relational Model. *Journal of Infant, Child and Adolescent Psychotherapy, 16*, 25–44. doi:10.1080/15289168.2016.1267539

Tahirkheli, N. N., Cherry, A. S., Tackett, A. P., McCaffree, M. A., & Gillaspy, S. R. (2014). Postpartum depression on the neonatal intensive care unit: Current perspectives. *International Journal of Women's Health, 6*, 975–987. doi:10.2147/IJWH.S54666

Vigod, S. N., Villegas, L., Dennis, C.-L., & Ross, L. E. (2010). Prevalence and risk factors for postpartum depression among women with preterm and low-birth-weight infants: A systematic review. *BJOG: An International Journal of Obstetrics and Gynecology, 117*, 540–550.

Voegtline, K. M., Stifter, C. A., & The Family Life Project Investigators. (2010). Late-preterm birth, maternal symptomatology, and infant negativity. *Infant Behavior and Development, 33*, 545–554. doi:10.1016/j.infbeh.2010.07.006

Wickberg, B., & Hwang, C. P. (1996). Counselling of postnatal depression: A controlled study on a population based Swedish sample. *Journal of Affective Disorders, 39*(3), 209–216. doi:10.1016/0165-0327(96)00034-1

Wightman, A., Schluchter, M., Dennis, D., Andreias, L., Taylor, H. G., Klein, N., … Hack, M. (2007). Parental protection of extremely low birth weight children at age 8 years. *Journal of Developmental & Behavioral Pediatrics, 28*, 371–326. doi:10.1097/DBP.0b013e3180330915

Zanardo, V., Gambina, I., Begley, C., Litta, P., Cosmi, E., Giustardi, A., & Trevisanuto, D. (2011). Psychological distress and early lactation performance in mothers of late preterm infants. *Early Human Development, 87*, 321–323. doi:10.1016/j.earlhumdev.2011.01.035

10

Emotional and Practical Needs in Postpartum Women

The Role of Family and Friend Support and Social Networks

Wendy Davis, Kimberly McCue, Brenda Papierniak,
Christena Raines, and Lita Simanis

The role of social support is critical to the healing process for a mother suffering from postpartum mental illness. This chapter will explore in great detail the types of support that mothers benefit from on the road to recovery from postpartum mood and anxiety disorders. A large body of psychological and maternal mental health literature documents the link between social support and mothers who experience postpartum mood and anxiety disorders. In order to provide a comprehensive look at the types of support that have been shown to meet the emotional and practical needs of postpartum women, this chapter will provide an overview of social support and categorize the support specific to partners, family, and social networks. Furthermore, it will provide a review of the institutional support and operational guidelines for effectively responding to the affective and emotional needs of new mothers and their families in the postnatal period. Lastly, a review of the literature examining the roles of social support as it relates to specific diagnoses in the postnatal period highlights the symptomatology differences in postpartum mood disorders, anxiety and obsessive–compulsive disorder (OCD), and postpartum psychosis.

Within the broader mental health research, social support is defined as the social resources that one would perceive to be available, or the support that is actually provided (Reid and Taylor, 2015). Throughout mental health literature, there are two types of social support that emerge and garner the most attention: emotional support and instrumental support (Hopkins and Campbell, 2008; Reid and Taylor, 2015; Thoits, 2011). Emotional support is defined as providing one with gestures of love, esteem, encouragement, and empathy causing the individual to feel valued (Thoits, 2011), while instrumental support is the offer or actions of assisting someone with tasks and responsibilities (Thoits, Reid, and Taylor, 2015). An abundance of evidence has emerged in the literature demonstrating that social support has been shown to be a protective factor in the risk for major depression (Kawachi and Berkman 2001; Thoits, 2011) and shown to play a helpful role in reducing the risk of postpartum depression (PPD) (Xie et al., 2009; Webster et al., 2011). Reid and Taylor (2015) concluded that the direct protective effects of social support are, in and of themselves, as powerful as some of the most salient stressors in increasing risk of PPD. This study also found that support from an intimate partner (compared to support from friends and family) appears to be uniquely beneficial and highly significant for married women (Reid and

Taylor, 2015). With regard to family and friend support, all women gained significant protection from such care. Of interest, intimate partner support had a greater impact on PPD for both married and cohabiting women compared to friend and family support and was equal in magnitude to friend and family support for single women (Reid and Taylor, 2015).

Social support is a complex and multifaceted concept that incorporates companionship, appraisal, informational and instrumental support, as well as perceived information leading one to believe that they are cared for, loved, esteemed, and a member of a network of mutual obligations (Cobb, 1976). Social support involves both social relationships that are embedded, such as relationships with family members or friends, and those that are created (Dennis, 2003). A large-scale systematic review and meta-analysis of qualitative and quantitative studies of interventions for postpartum mental health (Morrel et al., 2016) found that social support was one of the four major strategies (educational intervention, pharmacological interventions, complementary and alternative medicine, and social support) for enhancing both the prevention and treatment of postpartum mental health disorders. This same review found evidence ranked high to moderate for improving postpartum recovery when partners provided instrumental or practical support. Instrumental support was described as task-focused such as taking over most duties of the household, for example, cooking, cleaning and caring for the children. Conversely, this meta-analysis found that lack of support and understanding from a partner as well as feelings of abandonment from partner were high to moderate predictors of maternal mental health issues (Morrel et al., 2016).

Role of Partner Support

Support of a partner during recovery from postpartum mood and anxiety disorders can be accomplished in a multitude of ways to make mom feel that her physical and emotional well-being is a priority. A partner's willingness to understand the signs and symptoms of postpartum mental illness and openness to psychoeducation regarding the symptoms and treatment options can lead to the likelihood that mom will be open to treatment herself.

Social Networks

Social networks and relationships have been shown to be an integral part of health and mediating stress (Heaney and Israel, 2008). Being part of a social network may produce positive psychological states such as having a sense of purpose, belonging, and a recognition of self-worth, which in turn may increase motivation for self-care as well as modulate the brain's response to stress (Cohen et al., 2000, in Morrell et al., 2016). Social network members can have a positive influence on mental health by role-modeling healthy behaviors (Berkman in Morrell et al., 2016). Being part of a social network enhances the likelihood of accessing various forms of social support, which in turn protects against distress (Lin et al., 1999 in Dennis Dowswell, 2013).

> The term social network refers to the web of social relationships that surround individuals. The provision of social support is one of the important functions of social relationships. Thus, the term social network refers to linkages between people that may or may not provide social support...
>
> *(Heaney and Israel, 2008, p. 190)*

There are many dimensions to social networks including informal, formal, structural, interactional, functional, as well as components within these dimensions that can be used to further delineate structure and function (Rice et al., 2001). For the purposes of this chapter, formal social networks will be defined as a social network that provides social support and is embedded in a formal organizational or institutional structure (Heaney and Israel, 2008), while informal social networks will be defined as a non-family–based social relationship outside of a formal organizational or institutional structure. The Cochrane review by Dennis and Dowswell (2013) states psychosocial interventions for PPD:

> …both professionally-based (average RR 0.78, 95% CI 0.60 to 1.00) and lay-based (average RR 0.70, 95% CI 0.54 to 0.90) interventions appeared beneficial in reducing the risk to develop depressive symptomatology at last assessment.

It is important to note that the results seen in these studies include measuring received social support in contrast with perceived social support and these elements are part of a social network as well. Perceived social support is considered available if needed, while received social support is support that has been recently provided. The majority of studies that show improved results were from perceived support both for mental health in general and for PPD in particular. Glazier et al. (2004), Haslam et al. (2006), Horenstein and Cohen (2008), and Thoits in Reid and Taylor (2015), with a notable exception from Gebuza et al. (2014), show an increase in life satisfaction in the third trimester of pregnancy and in postpartum correlated with increased received support.

Social networks provide emotional, informational, or practical supports within their structures. While research is able to delineate these varying elements of social support and social networks, clinically the lines are often not so clear. For example, a formal support group running at a hospital that provides emotional, informational, received, and interactional support may find that members form sub-networks of informal practical support: offering one another baby goods or child care.

Informal social networks have been shown to have a positive effect in postpartum on reduction of depressive symptoms and parental self-efficacy in first-time mothers (Leahy-Warren, McCarthy, and Corcoran, 2012). These informal social networks can come in the form of friends, neighbors, online relationships, and informal groups that develop alongside more structured activities such as story times for children at libraries. A multitude of informal social networks for the support of new parents exist that are currently unstudied, such as Mommy and Me Groups, Stroller Strides®, church groups, and Mom and baby yoga classes. These groups are worth noting because of their prevalence and potential benefits to mother's social networks.

Among the most studied of the informal social networks are peer supports. The definition of peer support has been thoroughly reviewed by Dennis (2003), who writes:

> Through an in-depth examination of the literature, three critical attributes emerged repeatedly in the descriptors of peer interventions: emotional, informational, and appraisal support. These attributes are the supportive functions of peer relationships and may be differentially useful for various stressors and health outcomes. It is noteworthy to mention that instrumental support does occur rarely as a supportive function in peer relationships but due to its infrequency it is not a defining attribute.
>
> *(p. 325)*

Assessing a mother's social support and social network during pregnancy and providing resources for her may help improve outcomes. Morikawa et al. (2015) found that having limited available support persons during pregnancy is predictive of PPD and that psychosocial interventions focusing on the social support network are effective in preventing PPD, especially for mothers with depression during pregnancy. One intervention with promising results is telephone-based peer support, as described in Dale et al. (2008) for health improvement and in Dennis and Kingston (2008) for PPD in particular with women at high risk for PPD (Dennis et al., 2009). Another study of teenage mothers by Boath et al. (2013) concluded: "Peer support gave these young women an opportunity to compare their experiences of motherhood, with others in a similar situation, gain knowledge and advice and discuss some of the primary difficulties they had experienced as parents," which led the teenage mothers to report that peer support was one of their most valued resources.

Peer support can be categorized as both informal and formal depending on how it is delivered. One version of formal peer support would be peer support that is provided by a peer specialist. A study specific to peer specialists in PPD that included home visits for 12 weeks showed no better results for those receiving the home-based peer support than controls (Letourneau et al., 2011). Similar results for lay person home visits were seen by Morrell et al. (2000), where the addition of home visits by a community support worker had no protective effect on PPD. However, more research is needed in this area for the perinatal period, as peer specialists have been shown to have positive impacts for other mental health diagnoses (Solomon, 2004).

Other formal support networks include support groups. Support group structures are varied as well, including peer-led, professionally led, in-person, online, and other types of support groups. While therapy groups, which are more structured than support groups, have a strong evidence base showing positive outcomes, support groups would benefit from further research. Studies that have looked at professionally led peer support groups have had methodological weaknesses, and self-help groups have lacked robust investigation (Dennis, 2003).

Online support groups have been shown to provide a way to receive reassurance, validation, and hope from peers as a source of instrumental, informational, and emotional form of social support in a safe way (Evans et al., 2012). A study specifically exploring an online forum for lesbian mothers with PPD also revealed that instrumental, informational, and emotional forms of support were exchanged in a safe setting, allowing mothers to receive reassurance and validation without fear of stigma and social rejection that can come from heterosexism (Alang and Fomotar, 2015). Given the growing use of online platforms for social connections, and the growing body of research on the benefits of online social support, clinicians should be aware of reliable and reputable online resources for support to provide to their patients.

Support groups may be found as part of institutional or formal supports such as within an agency, hospital, clinic, or non-profit agency. Other institutional supports may include telephone warmlines or hotlines, lactation consultants, visiting nurses, perinatal educators, and more. However, research on the benefits of these supports in the reduction or prevention of postpartum mood disorders is lacking and warrants investigation. In the Cochrane review by Dennis (2013), antenatal classes teaching about PPD provided no preventative effect and are not a recommended intervention, but professionally based home visits show promising results.

Given that we know that women with a family history of depression are less at risk for PPD than their counterparts who perceive little or no support from their social networks during pregnancy and after birth (O'Hara and Swain, 1996), as well as the benefits of strong social networks (Heaney and Israel, 2008), it is imperative that we continue to find the best resources for women to be able to empower them with tools for improved postpartum outcomes.

Special Considerations

Clinicians working with women who struggle with perinatal mental health concerns must take into account the diversity and individual treatment needs of those women. Evidence-based approaches must be developed to best treat and understand multicultural and spiritual issues, as well as the special needs of adolescent mothers, LGBTQ mothers, and adoptive mothers. These unique needs can all have a potential impact on a mother's available support system and types of supports she receives.

Multicultural and Spiritual Understanding of Supports

Much of the research on perinatal mental health has been focused on Caucasian women. Women of color are as likely if not more so to suffer from perinatal mental health concerns but are less likely to seek support through formal services than Caucasian mothers. Many African American and Latina mothers with postpartum mood and anxiety disorders who do seek services are much less satisfied with the formal services they receive (Keefe, Brownstein-Evans, and Rouland Polmanteer, 2016). Women of color report experiencing prejudice from many of their healthcare providers and will often rely on informal sources of support such as churches and spiritual centers.

African American families are more involved in their religious and spiritual communities. This connection and involvement offers a unique resource for social supports and coping with stressors they may experience. "Religious and spiritual experiences are especially salient during and after pregnancy because many religious traditions attach spiritual significance to childbirth, parenthood, and family" (Cheadle et al., 2015, p. 283). The rituals that are often attached to important life events such as baptisms, weddings, and burials can serve as a time where people come together to celebrate with their family and community which further solidifies their identity and links to their community. Churches can also serve as a community center where they help to educate and address social and health concerns of their community. Bringing in health professionals who offer a variety of health screenings and educational programming on a number of health topics directly to the church community has shown to have positive health outcomes.

In Middle East and Arable countries, men remain close with their mothers. A woman who experiences a poor relationship with her mother-in-law can be at higher risk for perinatal mental health disorders. According to Haque, Azimeh, and Breene (2015), daughters-in-law and grandchildren's lives are greatly influenced by the mother-in-law.

> Women's dependence on patriarchal kin relations, undesired gender of the baby, death of one's father before age of 13, polygamy, poor relationship with the in-law family, and having a relative with an alcohol problem are also factors unique to these studies.
>
> *(Haque et al., 2015)*

According to Kim-Godwin (2003), some Middle Eastern women still practice a variety of postpartum rituals including a 40-day period of resting where others will come to their home to help with the new mother as she takes care of the baby. Her supports will help with any other children and the household. The mother's usual activities and diet may be restricted during this time as well.

Interventions for those struggling with perinatal mental health disorders must take into consideration the importance of pregnancy and postpartum cultural expectations and traditions as well as a new mother's cultural identity. It is also crucial for medical professionals and mental health clinicians to understand the barriers that women of different cultures face in seeking treatment for perinatal mental health disorders. Those barriers may include difficulties in the family, social economic factors, lack of knowledge or understanding about perinatal mental health, difficulty obtaining care, and language barriers. Providing basic psychoeducation about perinatal mental health – including describing typical symptoms, sharing statistics, and educating patients that they are not at fault and that perinatal mental health disorders are treatable. This can be ways for healthcare professionals to increase the trust and likelihood that these patients will seek outside supports if needed.

Adolescent Mothers and Supports

Adolescent mothers are at higher risk for experiencing symptoms of depression, and the rates of PPD in adolescent mothers are possibly double that of older mothers (Mollborn and

Morningstar, 2009). The pressures of pregnancy in adolescence can be experienced very differ-ent between mothers in early adolescence versus those in late adolescence. How pregnancy and motherhood is experienced by a 13-year-old versus an 18-year-old is likely to look quite different. Upadhya and Ellen (2011) hypothesize that factors related to social disadvantages in later adoles-cence have less influence because there is more opportunity and capacity for forming healthy peer and romantic relationships.

Young mothers can experience far more challenges due to lack of resources and less social support. "Loneliness, an exceedingly unpleasant and distressing experience resulting from per-ceived deficiencies in a person's relationships, is an important aspect of well-being for adolescents in general" (Hudson et al., 2016). A common concern for new adolescent mothers is the social isolation from family, peers, and the infant's father especially as they tend to the many mothering expectations placed on them which can exacerbate their feelings of loneliness. An adolescent's mother and her male partner when available can play a significant role in postpartum adjustment. However, these supports can also add to a mother's stress level if there is inconsistency with sup-port or if high levels of conflict are experienced. Adolescent mothers surveyed during pregnancy tended to overestimate the support that would be available to them during the postpartum period.

> Antenatal predictions of support were significantly higher than those realized 6 months postpartum. This impacted on a number of essential daily activities in mothercrafting. The findings suggest that pregnant teenagers over-estimate and idealize the supports networks available to help them care for their child.
>
> *(Quinlivan, Franzcog, Luehr, and Evans, 2004)*

Difficulty with coping, low levels of support, or low levels of perceived support tend to correlate with depressive symptomatology in adolescent mothers. Programs that include assistance with outlining and understanding the daily expectations of mothering and how to cope with those expectations would benefit adolescent mothers and may serve to lower the rates of perinatal men-tal health disorders. Adolescent mothers indicated that emotional and financial support was most needed but they often did not feel these supports were available to them. "Their main source of any support was their own mother, followed by the father of their unborn child" (Quinlivan, Franzcog, Luehr, and Evans, 2004). Some of the social service programs that have shown to be successful with adolescent mothers include visits by home nurses and volunteers that offer educa-tion and support as well as in-home counseling support to assess for and to provide needed mental health support. "Adolescent mothers may need extra education about the meaning of infant be-havior to decrease frustration if her infant is fussy or cries despite her care" (Secco et al., 2007). Support programs that offer groups with other adolescent mothers can normalize their experience as a new mother and serve to offer a buffering effect. They may also help a mother learn to cope in healthy ways with the difficulties of a new infant such as crying and fussy behaviors. Support groups specifically geared toward grandparents of adolescent parents have also been shown to have a positive impact on the adolescents feeling of support and overall outcomes.

Sexual Minorities (LGBTQ)

The research for women in the sexual minority and PPD is limited and does not generally include the difference between subgroups such as lesbian and bisexual women. The existing research does indicate that the rates of PPD may be higher among lesbian mothers compared to heterosexual mothers (Flanders, Gibson, Goldberg, and Ross, 2016, p. 300). There can be multiple factors socially that contribute to this including social isolation and the stressors often felt as a minority population that also has a stigmatized identity. Goldberg and Smith (2011) found that among newly parenting lesbian and gay adoptive couples there were higher rates of depression and anxiety due to internalized homophobia; however, when couples experienced their neighborhoods as "gay-friendly," they experienced lower rates of depression. Flanders, Gibson, Goldberg, and Ross (2016) found

> women who had sex with individuals of more than one gender in the past 5 years, but were currently partnered with a man, reported higher EPDS scores that women partnered with men who had only sex with men in the last 5 years.

Sexual minority women not currently partnered and those who were partnered with women did not experience this same effect as per Flanders, Gibson, Goldberg, and Ross (2016) research.

Operational Guidelines for Social Support in the Perinatal Period

Social support refers to the social resources that one perceives to be available to them, or that are actually provided to them. Social support might be provided by family, friends, religious communities, self-help groups, mother's groups, or formally by trained social support volunteers or group facilitators. When providers facilitate connection and utilization of social support systems, they offer a key preventive element in the stressful perinatal and postpartum period. Whether we facilitate emotional support or instrumental support, new parents learn skills to ask for help and also understand that social support is part of a healthy family system. Clinical providers have an essential role and can be effective by helping new parents assess their needs, practice communication skills to ask for help from spouse, friends, and family, or by connecting them with formal social support resources.

When a society has limited integrated social support structures, healthcare and medical systems can be key resources to develop and introduce more organized formal social support systems that are external to the family. A psychoeducational approach, which teaches families the traditional value of social support and gives suggestions for development of their support system, can increase protective factors to buffer the stressors of the transition to parenthood. In traditional societies, community members observe and experience social support as a regular part of family life, while modern societies tend to emphasize and value independence and self-reliance (Posmontier and Horowitz, 2004). Women and families who have developed strong skills related to modern independence and vocational achievement might find that they are isolated when a new baby enters their family, during a time in which traditionally the protective factors of social support are essential to healthy adjustment.

There are a number of assessment tools available to the care provider to assess a patient's quality of life (QoL) and level of social support, such as the Social Support Questionnaire (SSQ), the Maternal Postpartum Quality of Life (MAPP-QOL) tool, and others (Hill, Aldag, Hekel, Riner, and Bloomfield, 2006). Helping women identify their own needs and expectations surrounding support can improve their ability to mobilize support. A provider must determine what, if any, formalized tools they will use in their assessments to obtain the information that can guide their treatment and referral process. Assessing a mother's emotional and practical needs is separate from her mental health assessment. A provider may choose to ask interview-style questions about support such as "If you needed a ride to an appointment, could you find someone to drive you?" or, for a new mother, "If you needed to take a nap, who could you call to help watch the baby?" Alternately, a provider may choose to have such questions in written form for the patient to complete.

Completing a written or verbal assessment also has an educational value, as the questions themselves instruct the mom that such help and a social support system can be a normal experience for new parents. Questions to elicit and assess social support elements should include questions about practical, emotional, and instructional support: e.g., help with chores or errands, help with meals, relying on somebody to listen to you, being able to relax with somebody, being able to share fears and worries, asking advice about taking care of the baby, having help with childcare.

Effective formal social support systems have a referral network of mental health providers and groups in place. Organizations like Postpartum Support International provide resources to develop support networks and referral networks specific to the perinatal period. Supporters are trained to provide social support through email and telephone, and in more recent times through text and Facebook Messenger. Peer supporters are trained to offer support, not clinical advice, and to understand the limits of their roles in supporting families and preventing crisis. Peer supporters are trained to assess the needs of those who have reached out to them, and to refer them to treatment providers when needed. Providing emotional support and connecting with local resources are an effective first step to treatment for families. Successful social support networks will keep a resource list that includes prescribers, psychologists, groups, lactation counselors, and support services such as doulas and nurses.

Examples of perinatal social support services include:

- Telephone helplines
- In-person support groups
- Support coordinators through organized groups
- Peer support specialists
- Online video support groups
- Social media support (e.g., closed Facebook groups)
- Night nurse
- Doula
- Home visitors
- Faith-based support

In the field of perinatal mental health, organized social support systems specific to perinatal mental health have become a visible means of support for pregnant and postpartum women and, more recently, fathers. Peer support groups have developed internationally, both online and in communities. According to Postpartum Support International, social support providers from groups and organizations should be trained and accountable in key aspects of services to perinatal families and should have resources for continuing education and consultation. Most importantly, they should understand the roles and limits of social support and how it differs from medical care. Additionally, they should understand the range and symptoms of perinatal mental health disorders, know appropriate resources including treatment options, understand culturally related differences and burdens, use active listening skills, endeavor to provide support free of judgment and bias, and use an appropriate confidentiality policy. Social support groups can provide a unique connection with others who are experiencing or have recovered from similar distress. However, it is important that group facilitators and moderators are trained and have a consistent and coherent system of response to group conflict, distress, and crisis (Davis, Raines, Indman, Meyer, and Smith, 2018).

Facilitating effective social support for those suffering with a perinatal mental health disorder serves two purposes. The primary effect is the reduction of stress and fatigue when families have practical or instrumental social support. However, there is second effect when we connect a new parent with other empathetic supporters who have lived through the challenges of a perinatal mental health crisis. Social support structures provide an opportunity to experience a sense of belonging and relationship to others with similar experiences, bringing relief and reduction of isolation. Additionally, social support is available every day and typically at no cost, which prevents isolation and escalation of distress. When there is no connection to a community of social support, a patient in treatment is at risk of seeing herself only as an ill patient. Pregnant and postpartum women report feeling empowered and less ashamed after communication with other mothers who will share the challenges of motherhood and empathize with their experiences (Valtchanov, Parry, Glover, and Mulcahy, 2014). By providing an emerging family with social support, we reduce their isolation and increase essential elements of well-being during the vulnerable transition to new parenthood.

References

Alang, S. M., & Fomotar, M. (2015). Postpartum depression in an online community of lesbian mothers: Implications for clinical practice. *Journal of Gay & Lesbian Mental Health*, *19*(1), 21–39.

Berkman, L. F., & Kawachi, I. (2000). *Social Epidemiology*. New York: Oxford University Press.

Boath, E. H., Henshaw, C., & Bradley, E. (2013). Meeting the challenges of teenage mothers with postpartum depression: Overcoming stigma through support. *Journal of Reproductive and Infant Psychology*, *31*(4), 352–369.

Cheadle, A. C. D., Dunkel Schetter, C., Gaines Lanzi, R., Reed Vance, M., Sahadeo, L. S., & Shalowitz, M. U. (2015). Spiritual and religious resources in African American women: Protection from depressive symptoms after childbirth. *Clinical Psychological Science*, *3*(2), 283–291.

Cobb, S. (1976). Social support as a moderator of life stress. *Psychosomatic Medicine*, *38*(5), 300–314. doi:10.1097/00006842-197609000-00003

Cohen, S., Underwood, L., & Gottlieb, B. H. (2000). *Social Support Measurement and Intervention: A Guide for Health and Social Scientists*. Oxford: Oxford University Press.

Dale, J., Caramlau, I. O., Lindenmeyer, A., & Williams, S. M. (2008). Peer support telephone calls for improving health. *The Cochrane Library*, 4.

Davis, W. N., Raines, C., Indman, P., Meyer, B. G., & Smith, A. (2018). History and purpose of postpartum support international. *Journal of Obstetric, Gynecologic & Neonatal Nursing*, *47*(1), 75–83.

Dennis, C. L. (2003). Peer support within a health care context: A concept analysis. *International Journal of Nursing Studies*, *40*(3), 321–332.

Dennis, C. L., & Dowswell, T. (2013). Psychosocial and psychological interventions for preventing postpartum depression (Review). *The Cochrane Collaboration*, *2*, 1–211.

Dennis, C. L., Hodnett, E., Kenton, L., Weston, J., Zupancic, J., Stewart, D. E., & Kiss, A. (2009). Effect of peer support on prevention of postnatal depression among high risk women: Multisite randomised controlled trial. *BMJ*, *338*, a3064.

Dennis, C. L., & Kingston, D. (2008). A systematic review of telephone support for women during pregnancy and the early postpartum period. *Journal of Obstetric, Gynecologic, & Neonatal Nursing*, *37*(3), 301–314.

Evans, M., Donelle, L., & Hume-Loveland, L. (2012). Social support and online postpartum depression discussion groups: A content analysis. *Patient Education and Counseling*, *87*(3), 405–410.

Flanders, C., Gibson, M., Goldberg, A. E., & Ross, L. E. (2016). Postpartum depression among visible and invisible sexual minority women: A pilot study. *Archives of Women's Health*. *19*(2), 299–305.

Glazier, R. H., Elgar, F. J., Goel, V., & Holzapfel, S. (2004). Stress, social support, and emotional distress in a sample of pregnant women. *Journal of Psychosomatic Obstetrics and Gynecology*, *25*, 247–255.

Gebuza, G., Kazmierczak, M., Mieczkowska, E., Gierszewska, M., & Kotzbach, R. (2014). Life satisfaction and social support received by women in the perinatal period. *Advances in Clinical and Experimental Medicine*, *23*, 611–619.

Gjerdingen, D. K., McGovern, P., Attanasio, L., & Kozhimannil, Katy. (2014). Maternal depressive symptoms, employment, and social support. *The Journal of the American Board of Family Medicine*, (1) 87–96.

Goldberg, A. E., & Smith, J. Z. (2011). Stigma, social context, and mental health: Lesbian and gay couples across the transition to adoptive parenthood. *Journal of Counseling Psychology*, *58*(1), 139–150.

Haque, A., Azimeh, N., & Breene, K. (2015). Prevalence and risk factors of postpartum in Middle Eastern/ Arab women. *Journal of Muslim Mental Health*, *9*(1).

Haslam, D. M., Pakenham, K. I., & Smith, A. (2006). Social support and postpartum depressive symptomatology: The mediating role of maternal self-efficacy. *Infant Mental Health Journal*, *27*, 276–291.

Heaney, C. A., & Israel, B. A. (2008). Social networks and social support. *Health Behavior and Health Education: Theory, Research and Practice*, *4*, 189–210.

Hill, P. D., Aldag, J. C., Hekel, B., Riner, G., & Bloomfield, P. (2006). Maternal postpartum quality of life questionnaire. *Journal of Nursing Measurement, 14*(3), 205.

Hopkins, J., & Campbell, S. B. (2008). Development and validation of a scale to assess social support in the postpartum period. *Archives of Women's Mental Health, 11*(1), 57–65.

Horenstein, J., & Cohen, S. (2008). Social support. In R. E. Ingram (ed.), *The International Encyclopedia of Depression*. New York: Springer Publishing Company.

Hudson, D. B., Campbell-Grossman, C., Kupzyk, K. A., Brown, S. E., Yates, B.C., Hanna, K. M. (2016). Social support and psychosocial well-being among low-income, adolescent, African American, first-time mothers. *Clinical Nurse Specialist, 30*(3):150–158.

Kawachi, I., & Berkman, L. F. (2001). Social ties and mental health. *Journal of Urban Health, 78*(3), 458–467.

Keefe, R. H., Brownstein-Evans, C., & Rouland Polmanteer, R. S. (2016). Having our say: African American and Latina mothers provide recommendations to health and mental health service providers working with new mothers living with postpartum depression. *Social Work in Mental Health, 14*, 497–508.

Kim-Godwin, Y. S. (2003). Postpartum beliefs and practices among non-western cultures. *The American Journal of Maternal/Child Nursing, 28*(2), 74–78.

Leahy-Warren, P., McCarthy, G., & Corcoran, P. (2012). First-time mothers: Social support, maternal parental self-efficacy and postnatal depression. *Journal of Clinical Nursing, 21*, 388–397.

Letourneau, N., Stewart, M., Dennis, C. L., Hegadoren, K., Duffett-Leger, L., & Watson, B. (2011). Effect of home-based peer support on maternal–infant interactions among women with postpartum depression: A randomized, controlled trial. *International Journal of Mental Health Nursing, 20*(5), 345–357.

Lin, N., Ye, X., & Ensel, W. M. (1999). Social support and depressed mood: A structural analysis. *Journal of Health and Social Behavior, 40*(4), 344–359.

Morikawa, M., Okada, T., Ando, M., Aleksic, B., Kunimoto, S., Nakamura, Y., … Ozaki, N. (2015). Relationship between social support during pregnancy and postpartum depressive state: A prospective cohort study. *Scientific Reports*, 10520, Published online 2015 May 29.

Mollborn, S., & Morningstar, E. (2009). Investigating the relationship between teenage childbearing and psychological distress using longitudinal evidence. *Journal of Health and Social Behavior, 50*, 310–326.

Morrell, C. J., Spiby, H., Stewart, P., Walters, S., & Morgan, A. (2000). Costs and effectiveness of community postnatal support workers: Randomised controlled trial. *BMJ, 321*(7261), 593–598.

Morrell, C. J., Sutcliffe, P., Booth, A., Stevens, J., Scope, A., Stevenson, M., … Ren, S. (2016). A systematic review, evidence synthesis and meta-analysis of quantitative and qualitative studies evaluating the clinical effectiveness, the cost-effectiveness, safety and acceptability of interventions to prevent postnatal depression. *Health Technology Assessment, 20*(37).

O'Hara, M. W., & Swain, A. M. (1996). Rates and risk of postpartum depression-a meta-analysis. *International Review of Psychiatry, 8*(1), 37–54.

Posmontier, B., & Horowitz, J. A. (2004). Postpartum practices and depression prevalences: Technocentric and ethnokinship cultural perspectives. *Journal of Transcultural Nursing, 15*(1), 34–43.

Quinlivan, J. A., Franzcog, Luehr, B., & Evans, S. F. (2004). Teenage mother's predictions of their support levels before and actual support levels after having a child. *Journal of Adolescent Gynecology, 17*, 273–278.

Reid, K. M., & Taylor, M. G. (2015). Social support, stress and maternal postpartum depression: A comparison of supportive relationships. *Social Science Research, 54*, 246–262.

Rice, J. J., Sheehan, D., Brown, S., & Cuff, M. (2001). Capturing community capacity: The role of informal and formal networks in supporting families with young children. In K. L. Brock and K. G. Banting (eds.), *The Non-profit Sector and Government in a New Century*. Montreal & Kingston: McGill-Queen's University Press.

Secco, M. L., Profit, S., Kennedy, E., Walsh, A., Letourneau, N., & Stewart, M. (2007). Factors affecting postpartum depressive symptoms of adolescent mothers. *Journal of Gynecological, Neonatal Nurses, 36*, 47–54.

Solomon, P. (2004). Peer support/peer provided services underlying processes, benefits, and critical ingredients. *Psychiatric Rehabilitation Journal, 27*(4), 392.

Thoits, P. A. (2011). Mechanisms linking social ties and support to physical and mental health. *Journal of Health and Social Behavior, 52*, 145–161.

Upadhya, K. K., & Ellen, J. M. (2011). Social disadvantages as a risk for first pregnancy among adolescent females in the United States. *Journal of Adolescent Health, 49*(5), 538–541.

Valtchanov, B. L., Parry, D. C., Glover, T. D., & Mulcahy, C. M. (2014). Neighborhood at your fingertips: Transforming community online through a Canadian social networking site for mothers. *Gender, Technology and Development, 18*(2), 187–217.

Webster, J, Catherine, N., Catherine, V., Noelle, C., Lisa, F. 2011. Quality of life and depression following childbirth: Impact of social support. *Midwifery.* 27, 745–749.

Xie, R. H., He, G., Koszycki, D., Walker, M., & Wen, S. W. (2009). Prenatal social support, postnatal social support, and postpartum depression. *Annals of Epidemiology, 19*(9), 637–643.

11

Breastfeeding and Weaning

Parental Well-Being and Psychological Distress

Jenny Perkel

Optimal breastfeeding is one of most effective interventions in reducing infant and child mortality (Jones et al., 2003). Evidence suggests that breastfeeding could save over 800,000 children's lives annually (Victora et al., 2016). Breastfeeding has been associated with increased intelligence, education attainment at adulthood, productivity, earning capacity and social development (Victora et al., 2015). Optimal breastfeeding as recommended by the World Health Organization (WHO, 2003) includes immediate initiation of breastfeeding, exclusive breastfeeding for six months and continued breastfeeding for at least two years with optimal complementary feeding from six months of age.

In the developed world, most new parents are aware of these and other facts about the huge benefits of breastfeeding. For some, this knowledge can help inspire and motivate them to breastfeed and encourage them to persevere during the difficult initial stages. But for other new mothers, this knowledge serves only to make them feel a substantial amount of guilt, shame and persecutory anxiety if for some reason they are not able to offer their infants a satisfactory breastfeeding experience. There are various complicated maternal emotions around breastfeeding, depending on each mother-infant dyad's actual experience. For some mothers breastfeeding is a highly positive experience but for others it is difficult, traumatic and emotionally draining.

Understanding the Link between Breastfeeding and Maternal Depression

One of the arguments for encouraging – sometimes even pressurising – women to breastfeed is the well-documented link between breastfeeding and lower rates of postnatal depression. Amongst others, a Japanese study by Nishioka et al. (2011) found that postpartum depression was associated with changing to bottle and formula feeding before six months postpartum. Dias and Figueiredo (2015), in a systematic review of the literature of breastfeeding and maternal depression, concluded that both pregnancy and postpartum depression are associated with a shorter duration of breastfeeding. Importantly however, Dias and Figueiredo do highlight the need for further studies to clarify the association between this link. Do mothers stop breastfeeding because they are depressed or does breastfeeding protect mothers against depression? Or are mothers more likely to become depressed if they are not successful in their attempts to breastfeed? In the author's clinical experience, mothers who fail in their attempts to breastfeed despite a sincere wish to do so often feel intense distress and disappointment. This can contribute towards postpartum depression. Some studies such as that conducted by Pope et al. (2016) actually found no link between breastfeeding attempt/duration and postpartum depression. Wading through the data, it seems that the link between breastfeeding and depression is a complicated one, and a qualitative approach might be more helpful in understanding the association. Perinatal mental health consultants should approach this topic with an open mind and sensitivity, bearing in mind the subjective experience of each patient, including the experience of the father and baby.

Physiology and Breastfeeding

There is a physiological component to why breastfeeding is usually emotionally satisfying for mothers and promotes the bond between infants and mothers. Daws and de Rementaria (2015) remind us that the love hormone, oxytocin, is released not only during breastfeeding, but during sex as well. This hormone supports bonding between the mother and the infant (and between the couple during sex). It assists in promoting a feeling of tranquility and it is supposed to induce sleep. In addition to oxytocin, prolactin and vasopressin are released during breastfeeding. These add to the feelings of protectiveness and love. These hormones theoretically should improve the attachment between the breastfeeding mother and her baby, and they usually do. However, there are other factors – discussed later in this chapter – that can stand in the way of this attachment, despite the 'best efforts' of oxytocin and her associates.

Breastfeeding: Getting Started

The mother-infant relationship in the early days and weeks revolves around feeding. Much of the day and night is taken up with feeding at first and it can be one of the biggest challenges facing mother and baby in the beginning of a child's life. It is the *first dance* in a way. Mother and baby are given the task of accomplishing something together that is absolutely vital for the child's growth and survival. Breastfeeding exclusively from the mother for the first few months is ideal for most babies. Breastfeeding where there are no complications or difficulties can certainly be protective for maternal mental health. But where problems arise that lead to the infant losing weight or failing to thrive, it can escalate maternal anxiety dramatically because of the terror that the mother is not able to keep her baby alive. Anxiety related to feeding problems may also be linked to the maternal underlying aggression (often unconscious) towards the baby for not taking the feeds well, or for causing the mother discomfort, pain, stress and extreme inconvenience. This underlying aggression – particularly if it is not acknowledged – can play an important role in the development of both anxiety and depression, and in some severe cases even postpartum psychosis.

Breastfeeding is more easily and successfully established when the new mother is able and willing to spend a considerable amount of time in *practising* it during the first few days and weeks after the birth. Mother and baby are breastfeeding novices in the beginning and it takes time to develop the skill. It is a bit like learning a new sport. Breastfeeding can sometimes cause physical pain and stiffness in the new mother because of the tension and the unfamiliarity of the position. Pain can develop in the nipple area, especially if the baby is not latching correctly. Once it is established, however, breastfeeding usually becomes easy for both mother and baby. Unless there are mental or physical health concerns, it is often worth persevering if possible, despite the initial discomfort.

Box 11.1 Psychological Benefits of Breastfeeding

Physical closeness and skin-to-skin contact promote attachment

Immediate relief to satisfy a hungry baby as opposed to having to wait while bottles are being prepared

Breast milk is always available

Breastfeeding empowers mothers

Breastfeeding is a reminder that all mothers are indispensable to their babies

Financial benefits

Breastfed babies and their mothers are more mobile, as long as they are together

---

Box 11.2 The Perinatal Consultant's Tips for Breastfeeding Mothers

Offer the breastfeeding as soon after the birth as possible

Only let the nursing staff give your newborn baby complementary feeds in the nursery if it is medically indicated. Ask your paediatrician's advice

Room in with your newborn baby in the hospital and try to breastfeed exclusively in the beginning

Breastfeeding is about supply and demand. The more you breastfeed, the more breast milk will be produced

Put your baby on the breast or express breast milk if you want to stimulate a greater supply of milk

If the baby does not suck, after a few days the breast would not produce milk

A low-stress environment facilitates the flow of breast milk

Breast milk supply is known to dwindle during times of stress

---

Box 11.3 The Perinatal Consultant's Tips for Bottle-Feeding Mothers

Offer a dummy to a baby in distress

Offer the bottle if the dummy does not help

Sucking itself is psychologically beneficial at this stage of development

Refusing to offer a feed to a hungry baby can result in problems in the relationship between mother and baby

The feeding atmosphere should be quiet, intimate, affectionate and loving

There should be few distractions

A low-stress environment with no time constraint allows the baby to relax and digest her food

---

Clinical Case Study 11.1

Samantha was born via emergency Caesarean Section after a highly stressful and potentially life-threatening labour experience involving cord prolapse. Her mother was exhausted and rather tearful after her ordeal. The nursing staff, thinking they were being helpful, took the baby to the nursery so that the mother could rest. Samantha was brought to her mother every three hours so that she could try to latch. She seemed hungry, though, so she was given complementary formula feeds in the nursery. Very quickly, she began to understand that the bottle feeds were much easier to take than the breast and she became reluctant to take the breast. Samantha lost much more than the expected weight loss after the birth and she had not regained it after three days. Unfortunately, due to sterilisation problems in the nursery, Samantha picked up a slight infection from an infected teat and it was transmitted to the mother's breast and she developed mastitis. This meant that not only did she feel terribly ill but she struggled even more to breastfeed because the pain was unbearable. After five weeks of pain, misery and conflict between mother and baby, the breastfeeding was abandoned altogether and the switch was made to formula. Although this meant that the benefits of breastfeeding had been lost, it was a better option for this particular mother-infant pair because Samantha started to pick up weight, and the battle was over.

When Samantha was given the bottle, the feeding problems were over. However, the whole experience could have been different. Although it seemed like a sensitive response from the nursing staff to give the mother a rest – soon after the birth – they could have handled it more effectively. If mother and baby had been roomed in together in hospital and the nursing staff had helped them with latching every couple of hours, they would have had a much stronger chance of getting the breastfeeding going. The practice of giving complementary feeds is controversial and it should be reserved for cases where it is medically indicated.

'Rooming in' together in the hospital after having given birth can help to develop the bond between mother and baby, and it will also strengthen the chances of breastfeeding successfully. This is likely to facilitate attachment. A hungry baby is an unhappy, stressed-out baby. Allowing the baby to feed more often and for longer periods of time in the beginning usually results in a greater production and supply of milk. The danger of doing this though is that the nipples might become sore, enflamed and cut.

When Things Go Wrong

Feeding problems are exceptionally stressful for the mother, as are they for the infant. Hunger is acutely uncomfortable and distressing, especially for a younger baby. Infants who take their feeds well with little or no conflict with their mothers are very fortunate. A smooth and easy early breastfeeding relationship powerfully strengthens a baby's developing mind. It forms an essential part of the beginnings of psychological growth. It also forms the basis of relating to others later. But, unfortunately, things do not always go well with feeding for a number of reasons. Problems with breastfeeding often arise during the first few days and weeks of life. This can set up difficulties that may persist and could even disrupt breastfeeding to such an extent that it has to be abandoned, as was evident in the case study mentioned above. An important part of the perinatal mental health consultant's job is to offer some wisdom and guidance as to when to support continued efforts to breastfeed and when to support moving to bottle feeding, either with expressed breast milk or with formula milk.

There are a myriad of issues that can contribute to maternal feelings of discomfort around breastfeeding. Some mothers do not like to lose their freedom or their independence. This might be true for unplanned or unwanted pregnancies. It can also be true for very young mothers who do not feel ready for the overwhelming everyday demands of motherhood. Some mothers might be highly anxious about the effect that breastfeeding will have on the appearance of their breasts and their sexual desirability. They might not like feeling like a dairy cow as opposed to a sex goddess. Some mothers are concerned about losing their partner's love or his sexual interest. A sizzling sexual moment can be somewhat dampened when breast milk starts leaking … a stark reminder that a passionate sex life and breastfeeding often do not go hand in hand.

Some fathers discourage breastfeeding because it positions them outside of the mother-infant pair and can make them feel excluded and resentful. Jealousy and rivalry experienced by the father might give rise to marital conflict or estrangement between the couple. Often, there is such an intense bond between the breastfeeding mother and her baby and she is so immersed in Winnicot's 'Primary Maternal Preoccupation' that the object of the mother's cathexis is the baby, not the father. It can feel like the mother has fallen out of love with the father in favour of the baby. For a new father who is emotionally insecure or narcissistically vulnerable, this can cause high levels of distress that might result in various difficulties such as him seeking sexual or emotional gratification and intimacy outside of the marriage.

The primal intimacy of breastfeeding that can be so gratifying for mothers can also be experienced as psychologically threatening for various reasons. Grieving the loss of someone close to the new mother can make her feel too vulnerable and emotionally fragile to breastfeed. She can feel too raw, exposed and wounded to allow herself to be suckled from. In fact, an unresolved loss may stand in the way of either parent developing a close and loving connection with their baby. New mothers can also feel attacked, devoured and mutilated by their babies who can sometimes suck on the breast with a force that has to be experienced to be believed. This can make a psychologically vulnerable mother feel as though breastfeeding could harm or destroy her.

Breast versus Bottle

There is undoubtedly no argument amongst medical and mental health professionals that *breast is best*. The health benefits are enormous and the psychological benefits are just as substantial. Breastfeeding can be emotionally rewarding, empowering and confidence-boosting for mothers, partly because of the bonding process, the deep connection between mother and infant, hormonal release and the realisation that a baby can grow and develop purely on the nourishment that comes from her mother's body. It can be highly satisfying for mothers who can breastfeed successfully, and, by contrast, it can feel like an acutely painful loss for those who long to but cannot breastfeed.

Some mothers are deeply committed to breastfeeding, but for a multitude of reasons – often to do with the latch or the baby's muscle weakness – they struggle to get breastfeeding established. The sadness, disillusionment and distress that they can experience are exacerbated by the pressure that is put onto mothers to breastfeed at all costs. People generally know that breastfed babies are at an advantage and not being able to breastfeed successfully can lead to high levels of guilt and shame, as well as an acute feeling of being a failure as a mother. This, coupled by other factors, may contribute towards mood disturbances and perhaps even postpartum depression.

For those more robust mothers who are less conflicted and tortured by feelings of disappointment, guilt and shame when breastfeeding fails, they may discover that the use of formula and bottles is a good enough substitute. Most babies are relieved to be offered a bottle after a frustratingly unsuccessful attempt at breastfeeding. An easy, unconflicted bottle-feeding experience is better than a mutually distressing breastfeeding struggle. In fact, bottle feeding has some definite advantages. It is easier to regulate and bottle-fed babies stay full for longer and are generally easier to feed according to some kind of time-based schedule. In addition, new parents can share the load and the experience of feeding their baby with one another and with others. It is also easier to see exactly how much the baby is drinking. This can be highly desirable, particularly for anxious parents, when almost everything else about a young infant is unpredictable and uncontrollable.

When Bottle Feeding Is Preferable

Despite the well-documented and widely accepted fact that breastfeeding is superior to bottle feeding, there are times in the author's experience that it is advisable for a mother to stop breastfeeding, in favour of formula and the bottle. These occasions are usually when the mental health of the mother is at risk.

Clinical Case Study 11.2

Susan is a 30-year-old woman with severe, debilitating obsessive compulsive disorder. During the pregnancy, her obsessive compulsive symptoms escalated and her anxiety levels increased substantially. Her psychologist became aware of the significant threat to Susan's mental health. As a result, the psychologist advised Susan to introduce formula bottles in the first few weeks after birth. Although there is a danger of the infant preferring the bottle to the breast and hence refusing the breast if it has not been established before the bottle is introduced, the psychologist believed that this was the lesser threat than the mother becoming consumed by the stress of being tied to her baby, without the possibility of respite. As a result of this advice, Susan's husband was able to offer formula bottles from the first week of the baby's life and Susan was given time to rest and focus on her own state of mind. Susan's inclination would have been to have devoted herself totally to her baby, and breastfeeding exclusively is likely to have depleted her internal resources to such an extent that it may have severely compromised her mental health.

A formula-and-bottle–fed infant is not necessarily exclusively reliant on the mother only. The father and other caregivers can be much more involved when the infant is fed with formula and bottles. This can provide a stressed or psychologically unstable mother with much needed support and respite from the relentless demands of motherhood. It can mean that sedation and other psychotropic drugs can be taken at night, with the aim of providing her with much needed sleep, so that either the father or another caregiver can feed and care for the infant during the night.

Often mothers who are battling with their mental health wrestle with their own exceptionally high standards and expectations of themselves to provide the very best care of their infants. This might mean that they are determined to express breastmilk at the same time as attempting – often at huge emotional cost to the mother – to breastfeed. The time-consuming cycle of breastfeeding (often unsuccessfully), expressing milk, sterilising and preparing bottles, winding the infant after feeds and trying to get the baby to sleep can be a relentless and exhausting process that continues almost all day and most of the night, for weeks and even months on end. This gruelling process can be frustrating and draining to the extent that it contributes dramatically to a depressive postpartum illness. It is clearly not beneficial to the mental health of the mother and the infant, nor the relationship between them. It also does nothing to benefit the relationship between the parents, nor for the state of mind of siblings.

Clinical Case Study 11.3

Wendy is a new mother in her 40s. She is devoted to her four-month-old baby after having struggled with infertility for four years. The gratitude she feels about having finally been given the opportunity to be a mother has contributed towards her being totally dedicated to her infant, which includes her determination to breastfeed. Unfortunately, despite the lactation consultants, the postnatal nursing support, paediatrician involvement and sheer determination on her part, Wendy and her new baby have not been

---

(Continued)

able to breastfeed exclusively and her baby is not gaining weight as she should. Wendy's frustration, fatigue and disappointment has given way to despair and hopelessness. A depressed mood with anxiety and suicidal thoughts has led her to consultation with a psychologist. After six consultations, Wendy – with the help of her psychologist – has decided to stop breastfeeding and use formula bottles instead. Psychiatric consultation and psychotropic medication have been part of the treatment plan, and Wendy's state of mind has substantially improved as a result.

When the Choice to Bottle Feed Is Psychologically Motivated

Mothers who make the choice not to breastfeed – despite not having given it a fair chance – usually have powerful psychological motivations for making that choice. Perinatal mental health practitioners should take the time to consider these motivations, as it may in fact be in the best interests of both mother and child for that baby to be bottle-fed. Women in the past have fought long and hard feminist battles for the right to make choices in their own lives. There is a strong argument that the choice not to breastfeed should be respected, although it should, if possible, be explored with the aim of clarifying and understanding the new mother's decision. Practical circumstances such as maternal career or work demands can influence mother's choices not to breastfeed. But perinatal psychologists are often aware that there are some mothers who are reluctant to disclose and talk about their personal feelings about why they stop breastfeeding, or do not even make an attempt to breastfeed at all. Sometimes, it is about the aversion to intimacy.

Clinical Case Study 11.4

Zinzi's baby was three months old. Breastfeeding was highly evocative for Zinzi. She found it hard to sit down and feed her baby, apparently because she had such a busy life. She would rush through the breastfeeding while talking on the phone at the same time. She did not look at her baby while he was feeding and she did not allow herself and her baby to take the time to connect quietly and to bond during the breastfeeding. She felt awkward and uncomfortable having a baby drink from her own body. It made her feel like an animal. She just hoped and prayed each time that it would soon be over. The only thing that kept Zinzi breastfeeding was guilt. She knew it was important for her baby and she did not want to be a bad mother. A family friend referred Zinzi to a parent-infant psychologist. She began to understand that her reluctance to be close and connected to her baby was linked to her difficult relationship with her own mother who had been harsh and cruel to her when she was a child. Thankfully, after about six consultations Zinzi found it in herself to stop rushing and start tuning into her baby, especially during breastfeeding. She discovered the joy of breastfeeding as the priceless time when she and her baby could bond together.

Clinical Case Study 11.5

Nolundi was a 30-year-old first-time mother who baffled the nursing staff at the maternity ward in the hours and days after the birth of her first child. The nursing staff was available to support and assist new mothers with breastfeeding. They had been well educated about the substantial, irrefutable advantages of breastfeeding. But they noticed that Nolundi looked troubled and upset each time they encouraged her to try to latch the baby onto the breast. The hospital-scheduled three to four hourly feeds were not given to this baby unless the nursing staff intervened and actively helped the mother to put her baby on the breast. Nolundi repeatedly requested to use bottles and formula and she did not resist picking up her baby, holding her close and comforting her when she was crying. The social worker was called in and she came to understand that Nolundi had a reluctance to expose her body and to get so close and naked with her baby. It gave her an uncomfortable feeling that she felt bad even talking about. Once bottles and formula were provided, Nolundi kept to the feeding schedule. At three months of age during her follow-up visit to the well-baby clinic, mother was apparently doing well and her bottle-fed baby was thriving.

In the previous case example, the mother's fears of intimacy – and perhaps unwelcome sexual feelings – were not explored or resolved in a therapeutic context, but the immediate potential crisis of feeding was resolved by allowing the mother to use formula bottles instead of breastfeeding.

Bottle Feeding for Other Reasons

Certain medication and maternal illness such as cancer can sometimes contraindicate breastfeeding. HIV-positive mothers should seek medical advice about whether breastfeeding or bottle feeding is preferable under their particular circumstances. In some instances, HIV-positive mothers are advised by their medical team to breastfeed because of the benefits of increased immunity and sometimes, in certain socio-economic areas, because of the possibility of poor water quality and subsequent health risks to the infant. But a mother might formula-bottle feed for reasons such as previous breast surgery or breast cancer. Under these circumstances, the psychologist or perinatal consultant may advise that the mother give most of the bottle feeds herself if possible in the first three months to facilitate bonding with her infant. The same is true for adopted babies. It is easier to have more separateness from the infant when a mother does not breastfeed. The psychologist should use his or her clinical judgement about whether this mother-infant pair would benefit from either more or less separateness from one another during this crucial time. A baby whose father is available to give bottle feeds has the benefit of being able to establish a close bond with the father early on. This is likely to promote feelings of well-being in the father, and it may lessen the load on the mother.

Keeping the Infant Alive

According to Stern (1985), a mother – particularly a new mother – carries the psychological burden of believing she is responsible for keeping her baby alive. It is true that babies cannot survive without a mother (or substitute mother) to take care of them. Feeding is central to a baby's survival. It also occupies a huge part of a mother and a baby's day and night in the beginning. If there are problems with feeding, everyday life becomes fraught with anxiety and frustration for both the mom and the baby. At a deep psychological level, the mother's fear is that her baby will die because she is not able to feed him. This fear is amplified if the baby is not gaining weight normally or if he is sickly. With good reason, mothers are often quite focused on worrying about their children's eating well beyond babyhood. It is true that nutrition plays an essential role in the physical and emotional health of children. But perhaps the concern that mothers continue to have about their children's eating patterns is a remnant of the early days of knowing that babies need a mother's milk (or substitute) in order to survive.

Schedule versus Demand Feeding

Most psychoanalytic clinicians – following Fraiberg (1975) – believe that forcing a hungry baby to wait for a feed because it is too early for its scheduled time to feed causes extreme stress and rage in the infant. It also creates unnecessary and perhaps destructive conflict between mother and baby. This is especially true for young babies under three or four months of age and it is the psychological component of why demand feeding is encouraged in the early weeks and months of the infant's life. As the infant grows, from the second part of the first year onwards, she becomes more and more able to tolerate frustration and she develops some understanding of and control over her impulses. Time schedules for feeding are often more appropriately introduced then. Battles between mothers and their babies over feeding during the early weeks and months of life are very stressful for both of them. However, hospital and nursing staff are well aware of the importance of documenting three or four hourly scheduled feeds, partly because of the danger that the infant will not receive those feeds without a schedule and documentation. Failure to monitor scheduled neonate feeds on maternity wards has from time to time had fatal consequences. So perhaps the origins – and the wisdom – of scheduling and feeding routines might be linked to this. At least if a baby is receiving her feeds every four hours, she is certain to be fed and not forgotten about.

Raphael-Leff (2014), in her enlightening descriptions of the different parenting style camps (who are often at war with one another in the new parent circles), reminds us of the benefits and drawbacks and the deeper meaning behind the *Regulator* and *Facilitator* approaches to feeding and caring for infants. In addition to being fully aware of these dynamics and patterns that can so dramatically influence infant care and feeding, the perinatal consultant should be mindful of the fact that an infant is in the oral phase of psychological development, and consequently she needs to feed and suck. During the oral phase, the psychological task is the development of trust. The experience of being offered nourishment in response to hunger is crucial for that development of trust. For the infant, having her needs met in this crucial way promotes a belief that the mother – and the world in general – is, for the most part, reliable, comforting, restorative and supportive.

Hunger is highly distressing for young babies. It will take some time and life experience before she learns that she can trust that her hunger will eventually be satisfied. Some mothers are extremely distressed by the intensity of outrage and agony her baby seems to experience when she wants a feed. This can become more complicated and upsetting when the new mother is trying to make her baby wait until a prescribed time before she offers a feed. New mothers are often advised by others to wait a prescribed time (say, three or four hours) between feeds. The younger your baby is, the less she can manage this. Obviously, if a distressed baby has just had a feed, hunger is probably not the issue. But many babies seem to need their feeds much more often than they *should*. Two-hourly feeds are common amongst young breastfed infants, despite what the parenting books say. Clearly, these babies have not read the books!

Particularly for young, breastfed babies, feeding on demand (when she is hungry) makes psychological sense. As the baby grows she becomes more and more able to tolerate frustration, and develops some understanding of and control over her impulses. So more rigid schedules for feeding can be introduced more successfully after the first few months. Depending on her own schedule, her other commitments and her emotional and physical capacity, the mother may feel that she cannot really be 100% available to her baby. Feeding on demand is very time-consuming and some new mothers feel as though their life needs to be more organised and predictable.

The breastfeeding relationship is a highly dependent relationship. For mothers who have an aversion to being needed and relied on, this can feel unpleasant and even frightening. They might want to get away from what is felt to be a needy, greedy creature. These mothers may have a powerful need to be independent and a great fear of their own dependency. Perinatal psychologists are familiar with many of these issues and their role is to assist these mothers to navigate the postnatal time in a way that promotes physical and mental health as best as possible, not only for the mother, but for the father, the infant and the whole family.

Operational Guidelines for Situations Involving Mothers and Fathers in Distress

> Most of us have been dragged kicking and screaming to the realization that what really works in psychotherapy is the relationship between therapist and client. That's what does the work.
>
> *(Stern, 2008)*

A psychologically vulnerable mother who has had a previous history of mental illness – anxiety, depression, eating disorders, substance abuse or psychotic illness – should be monitored carefully during the first year or so of each of her infant's life. Feeding concerns can offer perinatal mental health consultants an opportunity to make sure that these vulnerable mothers are monitored. Since Selma Fraiberg's psychotherapy in the kitchen and later Dilys Daws's weighing scales at well-baby clinics, infant mental health clinicians have been looking for ways in which to help new parents to see that their physical and practical concerns about their babies are often reflective of deeper psychological issues. Often perinatal mental health practitioners and other health consultants are invited to assist the new parents with problems related to feeding their new baby. These feeding difficulties can be explored from a practical perspective, but they can offer the clinician an opportunity to address issues related to the mental state of the mother, the father, the infant and the relationships in the family.

Illness, Colic and Reflux

When there are feeding difficulties, consultation with a medical doctor is essential in order to rule out any possible physical problems the infant might have. Anatomical abnormalities could interfere with sucking. Infants with underlying illnesses or developmental problems often have weak sucking reflexes and they fail to gain weight. Psychological issues should be addressed alongside but not without medical investigation. Colic can be the source of great discomfort for the infant and it can account for an extremely stressful and traumatic feeding experience for the first few months after birth. Some premature babies have an immature sucking reflex. Gastro-oesophageal reflux is notorious for causing feeding problems. Babies who suffer from this can be underweight and undernourished. Alternatively, feeding can relieve the pain caused by the burning of stomach acid that is regurgitated into the oesophagus, in which case she will probably want to feed a great deal. Some reflux babies are overweight and feel unwell as a result of drinking too much milk.

Sometimes the inclination is to attribute the feeding difficulties to the mother's 'stress' or her otherwise unsatisfactory attitude towards her infant. This is usually not helpful for a mother who is already feeling exhausted, inadequate, incompetent and anxious about her baby. Infant feeding problems, as they are later in life, can be a sign of deeper issues. They can reflect important fears and concerns in the parents, deeper dynamics within the mind of the mother, and complexities in the relationship between mother and infant, the baby's father, the maternal grandmother and others. There are various avenues through which new parents can find their way to a mental health professional. One of those avenues is feeding difficulties, and – sometimes linked to that – inadequate weight gain of the infant.

Failure to Thrive: More than Food

Professor Astrid Berg from the Division of Child and Adolescent Psychiatry at Red Cross Hospital has done some groundbreaking work with mothers and infants in a clinic in Khayelitsha which services an impoverished part of Cape Town (Berg, 2007). Those babies who are found to be failing to thrive for no apparent reason are referred to Prof. Berg, and she, together with her translator, provides an opportunity for the mother to talk about her experience of being a mother to her baby. Berg has noted that when infants fail to make the expected weight gains at certain times, this can be usefully addressed from a parent-infant mental health perspective. Failure to thrive, says Berg, can be examined from the perspective of the family dynamic, conflict within the mind of the mother and the effect of problematic attachment with the infant. Is the reason for the failure to gain weight physical (and illness), practical (no money for food), or is it a symptom of disordered attachment or depression in mother and child? Berg has described how parent-infant psychotherapy can bring to light the real reason behind the infant failing to gain weight, which will be explored during the course of the consultations. She has drawn our attention as infant mental health practitioners to the fact that when babies fail to gain weight, this can be an important indicator of a disturbance in the parent-infant relationship. Two thirds of the mother-infant dyads referred to Berg's clinic in Khayelitsha presented with a failure to gain adequate weight. Two thirds of those dyads were found to have a mental health problem, often involving depression.

Berg (2007) has noted that both the motherhood constellation and the father in the mind of the mother need to be addressed. She has offered some useful guidelines for mental health practitioners around infantile weight gain issues:

- an accepting and open therapeutic attitude
- observation of parent-infant interaction and infant
- information about relationships with the baby's father and the maternal grandmother
- containment of feelings as well as concrete suggestions and advice where appropriate.

Depth of Intervention: What Is the Best Approach?

Deep psychoanalytic work is often not indicated when working with parents of young infants. The ideal approach is to address the psychological problems with the aim of holding the mind of the parents (particularly the mother) together as cohesively as possible. But this is not always easy, particularly because having a baby can be extremely evocative. Being a new mother – or father – can stir up previously repressed ideas and impulses and bring about a precarious mental state. One such example is that of sexual feelings evoked by breastfeeding.

New mothers sometimes report embarrassment, revulsion or sensuality – perhaps leading to sexual arousal – associated with breastfeeding. The intimacy of the breastfeeding experience can be too psychologically threatening for some women to manage and it can make them feel shameful, embarrassed or claustrophobic. It can make certain women feel as though they are committing a sexual crime against their baby, resulting in extreme guilt and horror. Pressure to breastfeed in the face of these sensitive and delicate feelings can threaten the new mother's mental health and put her at risk for postpartum depression, anxiety and even psychosis.

Clinical Case Study 11.6

Jane was a 17-year-old first-time mother who fell pregnant unexpectedly, much to the disappointment of her family. Jane was already feeling judged and unsupported and she was determined to prove that she could take care of her baby. But her mood declined steadily over the first four months postpartum.

She was suffering from insomnia, her concentration and memory were impaired and she was constantly tearful and anxious. She breastfed her baby because she knew the benefits, but she was haunted by her private feelings of being sexually aroused during breastfeeding. This was not something she was able to discuss with anyone until the nursing sister at the baby clinic found an opportunity to talk alone with Jane. A referral was made to a psychologist, and Jane was able to express — to her great relief — the concern she had about her intolerable feelings. With the support of the psychologist, Jane continued breastfeeding and her child continued to thrive.

Mother-Infant Food Battles

Breastfeeding and bottle feeding can be the setting for significant power struggles between a mother and an infant. The introduction of solids into an infant's diet can potentially bring all sorts of new challenges to the mother–infant dyad. Some mothers become very preoccupied with the nurturing, feeding aspect of motherhood, sometimes fuelled by extreme anxiety about keeping the baby alive and healthy. When the infant begins to take solids, mothers sometimes spend a substantial amount of time in cooking, liquidising and preparing food for the child. Books have been written with copious amounts of recipes for appetising meals for infants. But infants often eat very small amounts, particularly in the beginning, and the carefully prepared meals are often rejected. The time and money wasted is annoying for some mothers, and they can feel frustrated and angry and anxious. But — besides the fact that babies often just do not eat much — there are also important psychological reasons why infants often reject food and why their parents can feel so upset about this.

An infant, particularly during the second part of the first year, is in the process of discovering her own autonomy. She begins to realise that she does not have to be controlled by her caregivers. She is navigating the power of saying 'no' to her caregivers, especially her mother. For the mother, having her position of power challenged is hard. She feels rejected and unappreciated. She also feels deeply worried that her child is not being nourished in the way she should be, and there will be serious health consequences as a result of her refusing her feeds, either breast, bottle or solids. This difficult phase of assertiveness is necessary and even psychologically strengthening as the infant is developing her own mind and her own identity.

Feeding is a strong point of contact between a mother and an infant, particularly if she is the primary caregiver and their relationship is close. It is often the scene for much of the inevitable power struggle that must take place in order for her to grow. Sometimes it is appropriate to be in charge of her eating behaviour, but sometimes it is more helpful to allow her to find her own way. If she does not want her mashed butternut now, it might be more constructive and psychologically sensible to leave it and perhaps offer it again in an hour or two. If she wants to scoop the mashed banana up with her hands instead of using a spoon, that is probably more psychologically beneficial than fighting with her mother over the banana. For mothers and fathers with high standards of cleanliness and hygiene or if there is a strong need to be in control, this can be highly stressful.

If feeding or mealtimes become associated with intense conflict, it is time to reassess and make changes. Often the food dynamic is less intense between fathers and their children, perhaps because they were less involved with feeding in the early months. Substitute caregivers often have more success with feeding older babies than mothers for this very reason. Babies and young children who reject their food can be making a statement to their mothers and caregivers. The perinatal consultant's role is to help to decode that and to find the meaning behind what the child is communicating in the rejection of feeds.

It can be irritating and evocative when an infant refuses and rejects feeds of any kind. The mother can feel as though her nurturance is not wanted. But this early food refusal is often the beginning of a long process of normal and healthy separation from the mother: refusing to wear shoes, refusing a hug or a kiss, refusing to be seen in public with her parents and so on. There are many times, from early infancy and beyond, when a mother will feel rejected by her child. It begins with food and then it becomes about other things. When a baby starts saying no, it can sometimes indicate that the healthy, normal process of becoming an individual with independent thoughts and will is underway.

Box 11.4 The Perinatal Consultant's List of Practical Tips for Parents

Do not go to a great deal of trouble preparing gourmet meals for your baby. You will be lucky if she eats two spoons of it

Simple, nutritious food that is easy to prepare is a more sensible option

Mashed banana, steamed vegetables and natural yoghurt are all perfectly healthy

---

Letting Go: The Process of Weaning

According to Lubbe (1995) weaning is about letting go of the old and moving on to the new. It creates an emotional turbulence that is intense because of the huge mental burden placed on the mother-infant dyad as they navigate the path of letting go of the highly valuable breastfeeding dance they have created together.

Most of the literature and much of the advice given to mothers about weaning take the form of simplistic, formulaic instructional pieces, for example, 'How to wean your baby off the breast in five easy steps' or 'When is it time to start solids?' In contrast, the more psychologically informed academic articles talk about the weaning process (if not done under ideal circumstances) as being filled with loss, emotional pain and trauma for the baby, sometimes with lasting implications. These are important and relevant, but there is a lot more to weaning that has more to do with an important psychological process.

The psychological task of weaning a child from his mother is that they successfully navigate the adaptive and appropriate separation between them. Winnicott (1957) believed that, for the most part, no baby is completely ready for weaning. The early merger between mother and child is loosened gradually, little by little, over the weeks, months and years. The infant needs to navigate the path away from the mother towards age-appropriate independence. This process continues into adulthood, but the early weaning process is intense and evocative in the first three or four years of her life. Moving from breastfeeding to bottle feeding, then from bottle feeding to a 'sippy cup', starting solids, sleeping alone, mom going back to work, and starting play school or crèche are all part of the broader weaning process. The ways in which mother and infant (and other caregivers) manage and respond to this process of separation is what makes weaning interesting and sometimes difficult. For some mothers and infants, the weaning process is extremely fraught.

Klein (1936) understood weaning as a kind of mourning process. For some mother-infant dyads, it feels as though the mourning that is required in order to wean successfully is too traumatic and painful and cannot be endured. This creates a situation that feels to be impossible. The infant appears to resist weaning and the mother is paralysed by her terror and torment about the grief and suffering she would cause to her baby (or herself) by forcing the baby to the next level of weaning, whether it be breast to bottle, relinquishing the bottle, sleeping alone, etc.

Clinical Case Study 11.7

Sia is a single mother whose only child, Bongi, was conceived with donor sperm. Sia's own mother was psychiatrically ill and the relationship between mother and daughter had broken down years before the birth of Sia's child. There were significant problems with getting breastfeeding established, but after a few months, breastfeeding became a rewarding and satisfying experience for Sia and Bongi. However, it became clear as Bongi began to grow that there were some attachment and sep-aration difficulties. When Bongi was 19 months old, Sia knew that he had to be weaned from the breast but she seemed not to have the capacity to cause him any distress. Bongi would scream and cry relentlessly for the breast, particularly at night. He would continue his tormented, heartbroken crying for many hours at a time, causing considerable distress for Sia. It felt like an impossible situation for Sia because although she understood – from an intellectual perspective – the value of weaning Bongi from the breast at that stage of his development, she felt paralysed by his torment and she did not want him to suffer.

Sia was determined not to neglect her own child in the way she herself had been deprived. She felt she was in the position to offer him what she did not receive as a child and she did not want to hurt him or shatter his trust. She quoted much of the popular literature – written by mothers and perinatal specialists who have positioned themselves as extreme facilitators – arguing that breastfeeding can and should continue well past the first two years of life. This substantiated her belief that it was actually in her child's best interests not to be weaned and to continue with the merger with his mother well into the toddler years. Sia became increasingly frustrated, exhausted and depressed. She was exasperated with her child for 'demanding the breast throughout the night' and for crying relentlessly unless he was offered the breast.

Sia's own repressed, disavowed hostility towards her child and her consequent anxiety and depres-sion became a concern for her psychotherapist. The hatred and anger that had been kept unconscious since before the birth started to surface in moments of violent rage, sometimes leading to her having to leave Bongi alone in a room for fear of deliberately hurting him. It was only when this reached levels that shocked Sia that she finally was able to hear what her psychotherapist had been trying to say to her for many months: it's time to let go and give Bongi an opportunity to find his way without the breast. Sia stopped breastfeeding at that point, but she felt herself to be a failure and she was concerned that she had damaged her child mentally. She was not able to bear the pain and the loss of the merger and she believed that Bongi lost her breastfeeding experience. The psychotherapy process continues as new mothering challenges present themselves to Sia as she and Bongi navigate the developmental process together.

The Timing and Pace of Weaning

Weaning can be particularly complicated for those mothers who fall into the category of what Leff calls 'Facilitators' (Raphael Leff, 2014). Amongst the general parent public, this is often referred to as 'Attachment Parenting'. From the perspective of a Facilitator parent, weaning can be seen as traumatic and the tendency is to delay it for as long as possible. These Facilitator mothers often participate in organisations which offer highly valuable breastfeeding support to mothers. From this perspective, a substantial amount of significance is attached to bonding and breastfeeding, and the value of separation and weaning can sometimes be under-emphasised. Facilitator mothers can be inclined to use this ideological position as grounds to substantiate why they are not able or willing to wean their infants until they are much older than what is developmentally appropriate.

Those mothers in the opposite camp described by Leff (2014) as the 'Regulator' mothers subscribe to more strict, rigid, scheduled or routine-bound approaches to parenting and feeding. Weaning for the Regulator mother can often feel like a bit of a relief and it usually happens earlier and with more precision. Bion (1959) reminds us that it is only in the absence of the breast that the child begins to grow psychologically. Children of regulator parents can sometimes benefit in this way: their parents allow them to experience separation that might not be so fraught with ambivalence and complexity. They might, however, be weaned too early because of the mother's intolerance for the dependency that breastfeeding requires. But what does 'too early' actually mean?

Parents often ask us as psychologists or perinatal consultants when and how to wean their babies. But there is not one answer of course, as it depends on family and work circumstances, family relationships and dynamics, physical and mental health of the mother, both parents' perspectives and wishes, and the infant's needs. This is yet another example of the dilemma facing the mental health practitioner when the patient really wants advice and formulas. As with other aspects of working in the perinatal arena, a more effective approach is usually to steer the parents towards finding their own solutions, using the psychologists' knowledge and insight as a guide. Recognising and interpreting a parent's feelings of helplessness is often useful, as is helping parents to find a space in their own minds to think about what is useful for their child. But sometimes it makes sense to offer some practical advice (Dugmore, 2007).

The author and some 'Babies in Mind' colleagues have had discussions about the link between weaning and trauma. Although it can be highly challenging for some mothers and babies, we are not convinced that weaning is always associated with trauma. However, it can be challenging. Weaning and separation bring inevitable losses for both the infant and the mother. Relinquishing a blissful merger with another person is painful, but necessary. Separation often goes hand in hand with disappointment, frustration and loss. Sometimes mothers and their babies resist weaning and separation in attempt to hold onto the state of oneness. Some mothers struggle to say 'no' when their babies clearly need to separate.

Hopkins (1996) has warned about the dangers of what she calls 'too good mothering'. A mother who fails to recognise the importance of being able to disappoint and frustrate her infant or child creates significant difficulties for the child that may take the form of arrested psychological development or a tendency for the child (later on) to reject the mother in attempt to create much needed and long overdue separation. Sometimes, a protracted, extended breastfeeding experience can be an example of too good mothering. It can be an indication that the mother and child are having difficulty separating from one another. However, this is not always the case. It can also be a reflection of other factors, some of which are practical, and, in particular, socio-economic. Breastfeeding is cheaper than formula milk, cow's milk and solid food so where poverty is an issue, it makes sense that breastfeeding continues for longer. It is perhaps for this reason that the World Health Association recommends continued breastfeeding up to two years of age or beyond and the American Academy of Pediatrics (AAP) recommends that breastfeeding continue for at least 12 months, and thereafter for as long as mother and baby desire.

Conclusion

Sometimes those who try the hardest to be a good mother and those who sacrifice the most for their babies are the ones who are most psychologically and psychiatrically debilitated by the experience of early motherhood. Raphael Leff's Facilitator mothers (2014) can be at risk for depression and anxiety if they find themselves breastfeeding almost continuously throughout the day and much of the night, exhausting themselves beyond what they can bear. Their perinatal mental health consultants can help them to acknowledge and face up to their ambivalence, which in turn can free them up to put limits on the amount of energy and time they give to their babies. Those Regulator mothers (Raphael Leff, 2014) who set up rigid (bottle) feeding schedules might also be struggling with various mental health issues to do with anxiety and the attempt to control and bring order to the chaos that babies bring. They can also be highly distressed when their babies do not operate according to the provided schedule. The consultant can assist these mothers in addressing their anxiety and perhaps in exploring ways in which the bond between mother and baby can be strengthened.

Breastfeeding – when it goes well – often plays an integral role in facilitating the powerful bond between mother and baby. This blissful merger is highly protective for the baby in that it promotes a feeling of emotional security, connectedness and trust. This trust is understood as being the basis of mental health. But a conversation about breastfeeding should probably always be accompanied by a discussion about weaning. Sometime from the second half of the first year of life, the merger between mother and child should be followed by a gradual process of weaning. This process is all about separation and independence. It can be associated with varying amounts of sadness, fear and pain, but it is also extremely exciting and positive for a child. As long as it is not forced onto a child before she is ready, age-appropriate independence at every stage of development is filled with joy and delight. It is what makes the world come alive. By the age of about two years, children should no longer be cocooned safely for long periods of time with their breastfeeding mothers, except perhaps when they are ill, distressed or recovering from trauma. They should be exploring and discovering the exciting world that exists outside of the mother.

References

Berg, A. (2007). Ten years of parent-infant psychotherapy in a township in South Africa. What have we learnt? In M. P. Monzo (Ed.) *Innovations in Parent-Infant Psychotherapy*. Karnac: UK.

Bion, W. R. (1959). Attacks on linking. *International Journal of Psycho-Analysis*, 40: 308–315.

Daws, D., & de Rementaria, A. (2015). *Finding Your Way with Your Baby: The Emotional Life of Parents and Babies*. UK: Routledge.

Dias, C., & Figueiredo, B. (2015). Breastfeeding and depression: A systematic review of the literature. *Journal of Affective Disorders*, 171: 142–154.

Dugmore, N. (2007). The Tavistock short course for work with under-fives: The model and its applicability for private practitioners in South Africa. *Psychoanalytic Psychotherapy in South Africa*, 15: 71–84.

Fraiberg, S., Adelson, E., & Shapiro, V. (1975). Ghosts in the nursery. *Journal of the American Academy of Child Psychiatry*, 14: 387–421.

Hopkins, J. (1996). The dangers and deprivations of too good mothering. *Journal of Child Psychotherapy*, 22(3): 407–422.

Jones, G., et al. (2003). How many child deaths can we prevent this year? *Lancet*, 362(9377): 65–71. View ArticlePubMedGoogle Scholar.

Klein, M. (1936). Weaning. In R.E. Money-Kyrle (Ed.) *The Works of Melanie Klein*, Vol 1. London: Hogarth Press, 1975.

Lubbe, T. (1995). Who will let go first? Some observations on the struggles around weaning. Congress of infant mental Health Proceedings. Cape Town: South Africa.

Nishioka, E., Haruna, M., Ota, E., Matsuzaki, M., Murayama, R., Yoshimura, K., & Murashima, S. (2011). A prospective study of the relationship between breastfeeding and postpartum depressive symptoms appearing at 1–5 months after delivery. *Journal of Affective Disorders*, 133: 553–559.

Pope, C., Mazmanian, D., Bedard, M., & Sharma, V. (2016). Breastfeeding and postpartum depression: Assessing the influence of breastfeeding Intention and other Risk Factors. *Journal of Affective Disorders*, 200: 45–50.

Raphael-Leff, J. (2014). *The Dark Side of the Womb: Pregnancy, Parenting and Persecutory Anxieties*. UK: Anna Freud Centre.

Stern, D. (1985). *The Interpersonal World of the Infant*. UK: Karnac.

Stern, D. (2008). The clinical relevance of infancy. *Infant Mental Health Journal*, 29(3): 177–188.

Victora, C. G., et al. (2016). Breastfeeding in the 21st century: Epidemiology, mechanisms, and lifelong effect. *Lancet*, 387(10017): 475–490. View ArticlePubMedGoogle Scholar.

Victora, C. G., Horta, B. L., de Mola, C. L., Quevedo, L., Pinheiro, R. T., Gigante, D. P., & Barros, F. C. (2015). Association between breastfeeding and intelligence, educational attainment, and income at 30 years of age: A prospective birth cohort study from Brazil. *The Lancet Global Health*, 3(4): e199–e205. doi: 10.1016/S2214-109X(15)70002-1

WHO. (2003). *Global Strategy for Infant and Young Child Feeding*. Geneva: WHO. Google Scholar.

Winnicott, D. (1957). *The Child, the Family and the Outside World*. UK: Penguin.

Part IV
Risk of Psychopathology and Prevention

12

Depression, Anxiety, and Psychological Distress in the Perinatal Period

Jeannette Milgrom and Alan W. Gemmill

Introduction

Depressive and anxiety disorders are characterised by intense sadness, loss of enjoyment and constant, uncontrollable worry. Enduring symptoms of depression and anxiety in the postnatal period can have a particularly pervasive effect due to the simultaneous demand placed on new mothers of caring around the clock for a highly dependent newborn infant. Antenatally, depressed women are additionally coping with substantial physical changes and, in some cases, a difficult pregnancy with possible medical complications.

Symptoms of depression and anxiety in the perinatal period (the period from pregnancy until 12 months postpartum) are experienced by women from all social backgrounds (Dennis & Chung-Lee, 2006) and are frequently co-morbid in their occurrence (Falah-Hassani, Shiri, & Dennis, 2017; Wisner et al., 2013). While the majority of women (85%) will experience the transitory 'postnatal blues' during the very early postpartum period (Pearlstein, 2008), some perinatal women experience a more enduring mental disorder, or a range of sub-clinical symptoms that may not formally meet diagnostic criteria, but nevertheless cause considerable psychological distress, impairment of daily functioning and reduced quality of life (Coates, Ayers, & de Visser, 2014; Da Costa, Dritsa, Rippen, Lowensteyn, & Khalife, 2006; de Tychey et al., 2008; Rallis, Skouteris, McCabe, & Milgrom, 2014; Weinberg et al., 2001).

Perinatal Depression

The prevalence of depression with sufficient symptoms and severity to meet diagnostic criteria for a depressive disorder has been estimated at around 10% at each trimester of pregnancy (Gavin et al., 2005). The best meta-analytic estimates suggest that 13% of women meet criteria for minor depression and 7% for major depression at three months postpartum and the period prevalence of a major or minor depressive episode from delivery to 12 months postpartum could be as high as 53.7% (Gavin et al., 2005).

As depression during pregnancy (antenatal depression) is a strong predictor of postnatal depression, many postnatal women identified with depression will have been depressed during pregnancy (Leigh & Milgrom, 2008). In addition, symptoms of antenatal and postnatal depression have a wider impact, not only profoundly affecting a woman's emotional well-being but also being associated with poorer antenatal self-care and a variety of obstetric complications and pregnancy outcomes (Andersson, Sundström-Poromaa, Wulff, Åström, & Bixo, 2004; Couto et al., 2009; Dayan et al., 2006; Zhao et al., 2016; Zuckerman, Amero, Bauchner, & Cabral, 1989).

There are also potential negative consequences for a woman's infant and her partner (Don & Mickelson, 2012; Murray, Fearon, & Cooper, 2015). It has long been recognised that maternal depression interferes with interactions between mother and infant, which can have long-term implications for child development at least into late adolescence (Milgrom, Westley, & Gemmill, 2004; Murray et al., 2010, 2015). Perinatal mental health difficulties can also impact on the woman's partner and their relationship (Barnes, 2006; Don & Mickelson, 2012; Milgrom & McCloud, 1996).

Diagnosis of Perinatal Depressive Disorders

In terms of clinical classification, the Diagnostic and Statistical Manual of Mental Disorders (DSM-IV) listed a 'specifier' for postpartum depression as a depressive episode having an onset within four weeks of childbirth (American Psychiatric Association, 2000). The DSM-5 updated and renamed this to specify depression with 'peripartum onset', which now includes pregnancy (American Psychiatric Association, 2013). However, the DSM specifier does not reflect the terminology most commonly applied in practice by both clinicians and researchers. A pragmatic, commonly applied, definition of perinatal depression is an episode of a major or minor depressive disorder with an onset either during pregnancy or during the first year postpartum (Milgrom & Gemmill, 2014). Here, we summarise the possible range of depressive disorders that women may be diagnosed with in the perinatal period, according to the current DSM classification (American Psychiatric Association, 2013), whether or not the peripartum onset specifier is applied.

MAJOR DEPRESSIVE DISORDER

In the current DSM classification, for a diagnosis of major depressive disorder, a woman must have five or more of the following symptoms in the preceding two-week period: depressed mood/irritability; diminished interest in activities; significant weight or appetite change; sleeping problems, e.g. insomnia or hypersomnia; psychomotor agitation and/or retardation; fatigue; feelings of worthlessness/guilt; inability to think clearly or concentrate; recurrent thoughts of death and/or suicide. At least one of the first two symptoms (depressed mood/irritability; diminished interest in activities) must be present.

OTHER SPECIFIED DEPRESSIVE DISORDER AND UNSPECIFIED DEPRESSIVE DISORDER

For a diagnosis of Other Specified Depressive Disorder symptoms characteristic of a depressive disorder must be present which cause clinically significant distress or impairment in important areas of functioning (e.g. social, occupational) but do not fully meet criteria for any other depressive disorder (American Psychiatric Association, 2013).

In the previous DSM-IV (American Psychiatric Association, 2000), there was a possible diagnosis of Minor Depression, in a subsection called 'Depression Not Otherwise Specified', of which one example is Minor Depression. Diagnosis of Minor Depression, in essence, required at least two symptoms one of which had to be either depressed mood/irritability or diminished interest in activities.

In the current DSM-5, under Other Specified Depressive Disorders, a diagnosis of 'Depressive Episode with Insufficient Symptoms' is the closest to the previous DSM-IV classification of 'Minor Depression' and requires, in essence, at least two symptoms – one of which needs to be depressed mood.

In the current classification, diagnosis of Unspecified Depressive Disorder uses the same criteria as Other Specified Depressive Disorder, but would be used where a clinician chooses not to specify the reason that diagnostic criteria for another depressive disorder are not fully met, typically where there is insufficient time or information available (e.g. presentation in a hospital emergency department).

Perinatal Anxiety

The prevalence of anxiety symptoms and disorders in perinatal women is receiving increasing interest (Ayers, Coates, & Matthey, 2015; Dennis, Falah-Hassani, & Shiri, 2017; Mauri et al., 2010; Meades & Ayers, 2011; Rallis et al., 2014). Anxiety appears to be at least as common as depression. The best available meta-analyses report an overall prevalence of diagnosed anxiety disorders in pregnancy of 15.2% (Dennis et al., 2017) with 4.1% being a generalised anxiety disorder (GAD). The prevalence of anxiety disorders over the first six months postpartum is 9.9% with GAD representing 5.7%. These symptoms are frequently co-morbid with depression (Milgrom, Ericksen, Negri, & Gemmill, 2005; Ross & McLean, 2006; Dennis, Falah-Hassani, Brown, & Vigod, 2016; Wisner et al., 2013). For example, a recent meta-analysis found that over first 24 weeks postpartum, the prevalence of co-morbid anxiety symptoms and mild to severe depressive symptoms was 8.2% and the prevalence of a clinical diagnosis of co-morbid anxiety and depression was 4.2% (Falah-Hassani et al., 2017).

Furthermore, for some perinatal women, anxiety problems can emerge which are very specifically focused on the perinatal context, such as fear and worry about the birth itself (Ayers et al., 2015). A 2015 review of this developing area of interest (Brunton, Dryer, Saliba, & Kohlhoff, 2015) reported numerous pregnancy-specific anxiety scales (Alderdice, McNeill, Gargan, & Perra, 2017; Staneva, Morawska, Bogossian, & Wittkowski, 2016; Weis, Lederman, Walker, & Chan, 2017).

Diagnosis of Perinatal Anxiety Disorders

The diagnostic characteristics of some of the more common anxiety disorders occurring in the perinatal period are summarised below. In all cases, symptoms must cause clinically significant distress or impairment in important areas of functioning, occur for at least six months and not be attributable to the effects of a substance, a medical condition or another mental disorder (American Psychiatric Association, 2013).

GENERALISED ANXIETY DISORDER

This is the most commonly reported anxiety diagnosis in the perinatal period. A woman must have excessive anxiety or worry that she finds difficult to control about a number of events or activities resulting in significant distress or impairment in functioning. This must be accompanied by at least three of the following symptoms occurring on most days for six months: restless or feeling keyed up or on edge, being easily fatigued, difficulty concentrating/mind going blank, irritability, muscle tension, sleep disturbance (American Psychiatric Association, 2013).

SOCIAL ANXIETY DISORDER

Symptoms of 'marked fear' or anxiety of at least one social situation characterise this diagnosis. Anticipation of potential scrutiny, negative evaluation by others or causing offence to others in these situations almost always provoke anxiety and fears that are out of proportion leading to the situation either being avoided or endured with intense discomfort.

SPECIFIC PHOBIA

For a diagnosis of a Specific Phobia, when a woman is presented with a specific object or situation she almost always responds with marked fear or anxiety. The object or situation almost always provokes disproportionate anxiety and is either avoided or endured with intense difficulty and this occurs for at least six months.

PANIC DISORDER

For a diagnosis of Panic Disorder (American Psychiatric Association, 2013), a woman must present with recurrent and unexpected panic attacks. Panic attacks are marked by a fear or intense discomfort, reaching its peak within minutes where four or more of the following symptoms are present: palpitations, pounding heart, accelerated heart rate; sweating; trembling or shaking; shortness of breath; feelings of choking; chest pain/discomfort; nausea/abdominal distress; feeling dizzy, unsteady, light-headed or faint; chills or heat sensations; paraesthesias (numbness/tingling); derealisation or depersonalisation; fear of losing control/'going crazy'; fear of dying. The attacks must be followed by a least a month of persistent worry about additional attacks and their consequences or there must be a significant and maladaptive change in behaviour related to the attacks (American Psychiatric Association, 2013).

Other Related Disorders

Obsessive-Compulsive Disorder

Women meeting criteria for a diagnosis of Obsessive-Compulsive Disorder must present with symptoms of both obsessions (defined as unwanted and persistent thoughts, urges or images that cause marked anxiety or distress which the woman attempts to ignore, suppress or neutralise using another thought or action) and compulsions (repetitive behaviours or cognitions that the individual feels driven to complete in response to an obsession aimed at reducing or preventing anxiety and distress). The symptoms must be either time-consuming (more than an hour) or result in clinically significant distress and/or impairment in social, occupational or other important areas of functioning (American Psychiatric Association, 2013).

Post-Traumatic Stress Disorder (PTSD)

A diagnosis of PTSD is not uncommon in perinatal women and there continues to be considerable research on this topic (James, 2015; Kim et al., 2015; Shlomi Polachek, Dulitzky, Margolis-Dorfman, & Simchen, 2016; Simpson & Catling, 2016). Alcorn, Ayers and others (Alcorn, O'Donovan, Patrick, Creedy, & Devilly, 2010; Ayers, Jessop, Pike, Parfitt, & Ford, 2014; Ayers & Pickering, 2001) reported that between 1% and 7% of perinatal women may attract a diagnosis and many more report symptoms not meeting criteria. Ayers (Ayers, 2007) in a small qualitative study found that

> women with posttraumatic stress symptoms reported more panic, anger, thoughts of death, mental defeat, and dissociation during birth; after birth, they reported fewer strategies that focused on the present, more painful memories, intrusive memories, and rumination, than women without symptoms.

For some, longer term effects can include emotional detachment from their babies and partners and fear of future pregnancies (Vossbeck-Elsebusch, Freisfeld, & Ehring, 2014). The key feature of PTSD is an exposure to actual or threatened death, serious injury or sexual violence (American Psychiatric Association, 2013). Childbirth can clearly be trigger factor for some women, with potentially life-threatening events, unexpected caesarean and pain experiences. However, traumatic birth experience may be mitigated by increasing a sense of control and providing social support after the birth (Furuta, Sandall, Cooper, & Bick, 2016).

To attract a diagnosis of PTSD, one or more of the following intrusive symptoms must be present for at least a month, beginning after the traumatic event: recurrent, involuntary and intrusive distressing memories of the event; recurrent distressing dreams about the event; dissociative reactions; intense or prolonged psychological distress at exposure to internal or external cues that symbolise or represent the event; marked physiological reactions to internal or external cues that symbolise or represent the event.

A further diagnostic criterion is avoidance of stimuli associated with the traumatic event as evidenced by: avoidance of distressing memories, thoughts and feelings related to the event; or avoidance of external reminders that arouse memories, thoughts or feelings related to the event.

At least two of the following negative alterations in cognition and mood associated with the event must be present: inability to remember an important aspect of the event; persistent and exaggerated negative beliefs or expectations about oneself; persistent, distorted cognitions about the cause of consequences of the event; persistent negative emotional state; markedly diminished interest in participation in significant activities; feelings of detachment or estrangement from others; persistent inability to experience positive emotions

Lastly, a woman must present with marked alterations in arousal and reactivity associated with the event as evidenced by two or more of the following items: irritable behaviour and angry outbursts, reckless or self-destructive behaviour, hypervigilance, exaggerated startle response, problems with concentration, sleep disturbance (American Psychiatric Association, 2013).

Clearly such symptoms are likely to impact on a woman's well-being and potentially interfere with mother-infant relationships. While some studies have suggested that PTSD is associated with depression, triple co-morbidities with depression and anxiety were found to be rare in a systematic review (Agius, Xuereb, Carrick-Sen, Sultana, & Rankin, 2016).

Adjustment Disorder

Emotional or behavioural symptoms developing within three months of an identifiable stressor are the key characteristic of this disorder. The symptoms must be clinically significant as evidenced by marked distress which is out of proportion for the stressor (American Psychiatric Association, 2013).

Perinatal Distress

The term 'perinatal distress' has been used to cover a broad range of constructs. At times it has been used to describe sub-clinical, but disabling, symptoms and other times interchangeably with depression, anxiety or both. A more useful definition might be to consider sources of distress that may be associated with depression or anxiety but are independent. For example, the Stress Scale of the Depression and Anxiety Scale (DASS) (Lovibond, 1995) measures a stress dimension separate from depression and anxiety. Similarly, pregnant women have been reported to be concerned about changes in appearance and physical functioning, the birth and changes in interpersonal relationships (Alderdice et al., 2013). The Prenatal Distress Questionnaire (PDQ) was designed to capture this type of 'pregnancy-specific' stress. It has been suggested that the broader construct of perinatal distress is influenced by a woman's appraisal (e.g. pessimistic ideas about the future) and coping strategies which may influence her ability to cope practically and emotionally with pregnancy and maternal-related issues (Coo, Milgrom, Kuppens, & Trinder, 2015; Milgrom & Beatrice, 2003).

Impact of Perinatal Depression and Anxiety

The biopsychosocial model of Milgrom and colleagues (Milgrom, Martin, & Negri, 1999) implicates numerous major biological, psychological and social influences contributing to the aetiology of postnatal depression. Here, we review areas of a woman's life which can be impacted negatively by perinatal depression in a substantial way in the context of a biopsychosocial model. While a fuller review of risk factors is provided by Pariante and Biaggi (Chapter 14 of this book), Figure 12.1 provides a schematic representation of some major potential influences, moderators and impacts.

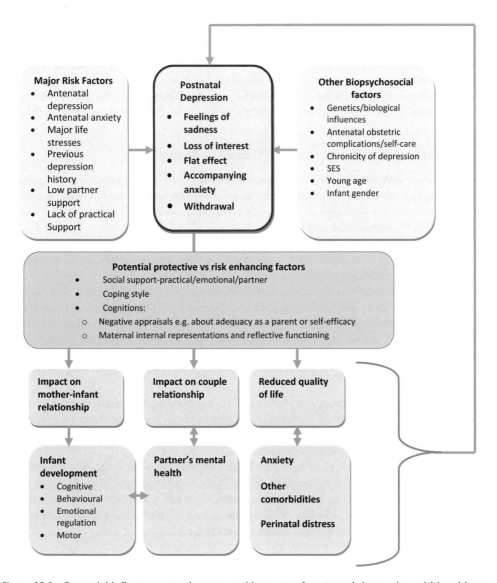

Figure 12.1   Potential influences, moderators and impacts of postnatal depression within a biopsychosocial model. Areas potentially impacted by postnatal depression are depicted. Double-headed arrows indicate where such effects can in turn re-impact on other areas (negative feedback)

Adapted from Milgrom, Martin, and Negri (1999) A Biopsychosocial Model. In: Treating Postnatal Depression- A Psychological Approach for Health Care Practitioners. Wiley, Chichester, p. 26.

Impact of Postnatal Depression on Women

Societal and cultural expectations that the transition to motherhood should be a time of un-matched joy and happiness may make the effects of a depressive or anxiety disorder even more difficult.

The symptoms of a depression will impact the subjective quality of a woman's inner experience and daily functioning (anhedonia, feelings of sadness, hopelessness, thoughts of death, psychomotor retardation or agitation, disturbed sleep). In addition, accompanying symptoms of anxiety such as constant worry will have a detrimental impact. Women's lived experiences of perinatal anxiety and depression have been the subject of numerous qualitative studies (Beck, 1992; Brockington, Macdonald, & Wainscott, 2006; Chan, Levy, Chung, & Lee, 2002; Coates et al., 2014; Highet, Stevenson, Purtell, & Coo, 2014; Mason, Rice, & Records, 2005) and, just as in the general population (Brenes, 2007; Roberts, Lenton, Keetharuth, & Brazier, 2014), postpartum depressed mood can have measurable impacts on all domains of a woman's quality of life including social activities, general health and life satisfaction (Abbasi, van den Akker, & Bewley, 2014; Alhamdan, Ajaj, Alali, & Badr, 2017; Da Costa et al., 2006; de Tychey et al., 2008; Moinmehr et al., 2016).

Potential Moderators of the Impact of Postnatal Depression

As outlined more fully in Chapter 14, in perinatal women, both during pregnancy and postpartum, negative cognitive styles, perfectionism, neuroticism, introversion, interpersonal sensitivity low self-esteem and low self-efficacy are associated with depression (Jones et al., 2010; Leigh & Milgrom, 2008; McMahon et al., 2005).

What is less well understood is how such variation in cognitive styles in different women with different personalities can mediate or moderate the impact of depression on numerous areas of a woman's life (see Figure12.1).

For example, depressed women may be further challenged in their relationship with their infant when low self-efficacy and perfectionist traits collide with the reality of the constant changes and demands associated with early parenthood. Similarly, negative appraisals and cognitive distortions such as maladaptive beliefs about motherhood are likely to impact on mother-infant relationships (Sockol, Epperson, & Barber, 2014). Pessimistic ideas about the future and certain coping strategies may also interfere with a woman's ability to cope practically and emotionally (Coo et al., 2015).

DeJong and colleagues (DeJong, Fox, & Stein, 2016) have developed a model that suggests how behavioural effects of depression on parenting are mediated via cognitive mechanisms, specifically rumination; cognitive biases and cognitive control. These variables impact on maternal processing of infant cues and subsequent parenting responses.

Social support is also known to be both a protective and risk factor for mitigating the effects of depression on the mother-infant relationship (Stein, Pearson, & Goodman, 2014). Similarly, variations in factors such as social support, cognitive style, degree of perfectionism and neuroticism can potentially moderate the influence of depression on a well-functioning couple relationship and the quality of life of the individuals involved (see Figure 12.1).

Effect on the Mother-Infant Relationship

Symptoms of sadness, flatness, loss of interest and anxiety can make it difficult for some depressed women to remain emotionally available for their infants. The many micro-behavioural exchanges between a sensitive and attuned caregiver and a developing infant are vital for healthy infant behavioural, emotional and cognitive development. Responding appropriately to infant interactional cues in a timely manner can prove difficult for depressed women who can find it difficult to engage with their infants in a reciprocal and synchronous manner way. A range of such detrimental effects on mother-child interaction have been reported (Murray et al., 2015). For example, in the early months after birth, depressed mothers have been found to make less eye contact with their infants and during interactions they are more likely to appear disengaged and emotionally flat (Field et al., 1988; Field, 2002; Murray et al., 2003; Murray, Stanley, Hooper, King, & Fiori-Cowley, 1996; Reck et al., 2004). Infants of depressed mothers in turn show increased sad affect and distress (Field, Diego, & Hernandez-Reif, 2009; Field et al., 1988).

Effects of Perinatal Depression and Anxiety on Infant and Child Development

There is now good evidence that if a mother is depressed while pregnant or in the postpartum period, her child is substantially more likely to have behavioural and emotional problems. This includes an increased risk of anxiety and attention deficit/hyperactivity in childhood (Glover, 2014, 2015; Herba, Glover, Ramchandani, & Rondon, 2016; O'Connor, Monk, & Fitelson, 2014; Talge, Neal, & Glover, 2007; Waters, Hay, Simmonds, & van Goozen, 2014). Long-lasting effects have been demonstrated; children of women with antenatal depression have an increased risk of depression (Pearson et al., 2013; Quarini et al., 2015) and anxiety disorders (Capron et al., 2015) at 18 years of age. Maternal depression during pregnancy predicts altered foetal behaviour (heart rate and motor activity), reduced scores on neonatal neurobehavioural assessments and increased fussiness in newborns (Monk, 2001; Monk et al., 2000; Monk, Spicer, & Champagne, 2012). Antenatal maternal mood is also associated with structural variation in the hippocampus, amygdala and prefrontal regions in neonates (Qiu, Anh et al., 2015; Qiu, Tuan et al., 2015). Moreover, infants born to mothers with more antenatal depressive symptoms show altered functional connectivity between brain regions (amygdala, temporal cortex), which is largely consistent with patterns observed in adults with a major depressive disorder (Qiu, Anh et al., 2015). Mechanisms that affect foetal development *in utero* (foetal programming) are likely to involve a number of biological systems and pathways ((Blakeley, Capron, Jensen, O'Donnell, & Glover, 2013; de Weerth, Buitelaar, & Mulder, 2005; Glover, 2015; O'Donnell, Glover, Barker, & O'Connor, 2014).

Maternal depression beginning or continuing into the postnatal period also impacts infant development. Several problem areas for children of depressed mothers have been consistently reported. These include emotional problems (Barker, Jaffee, Uher, & Maughan, 2011; Murray et al., 2010; Murray, Cooper, & Stein, 1991; Murray et al., 2003; O'Donnell et al., 2014; Stein et al., 2014), attention deficit hyperactivity disorder (O'Connor, Heron, Golding, Beveridge, & Glover, 2002; Van Batenburg-Eddes et al., 2013) and impaired cognitive development and academic achievement (Barker et al., 2011; Bergman et al., 2007; Huizink et al., 2003). The chronicity and severity of maternal depression symptoms is associated with the incidence of child psychiatric disorders at school age (Matijasevich et al., 2015). Higher risk of attention deficit and hyperactivity is reported (Galera et al., 2011; Mount, Crockenberg, Jo, & Wagar, 2010) along with poorer self-regulatory capacities (Feldman et al., 2009) and child anxiety (Stein et al., 2014). Enduring impact has been reported to adolescence and young adulthood (Capron et al., 2015; Murray et al., 2011; Pawlby, Hay, Sharp, Waters, & O'Keane, 2009; Pawlby et al., 2008; Pearson et al., 2016) and the sizes of these effects are clinically important.

Impact on Women's Partners and the Couple Relationship

The occurrence of perinatal psychological difficulties in men is beginning to receive increased attention in its own right (Underwood et al., 2017). Both during pregnancy and postpartum, depressive symptomatology in women has been found to be significantly correlated with that observed in their male partners (Deater-Deckard, Pickering, Dunn, & Golding, 1998). Between 5% and 10% of new/expectant fathers experience depression, anxiety and other forms of emotional distress in the perinatal period (Condon, 2004; Paulson & Bazemore, 2010; Paulson, Bazemore, Goodman, & Leiferman, 2016). Men may also develop depressive symptoms in the perinatal period independent of any problems in their partner's mood (Fletcher, Garfield, & Matthey, 2015; Fletcher et al., 2013; Garfield et al., 2014). Men appear significantly less likely to acknowledge their symptoms and to seek or engage with support (Berger, Levant, McMillan, Kelleher, & Sellers, 2005; McCarthy & Holliday, 2004). There is some evidence that the manifestation of depression in men is symptomatically different from that observed in women, typically characterised by anger, irritability and alcohol use (Cochran & Rabinowitz, 2003; Winkler, Pjrek, & Kasper, 2005). Consequently, it has been suggested that male-specific tools may be needed to accurately identify depression in fathers (Fletcher et al., 2015). Among men, just as is the case for maternal mental health, paternal depression and anxiety are sometimes associated with a heightened occurrence of emotional and behavioural difficulties in children (Dave, Sherr, Senior, & Nazareth, 2008; Gutierrez-Galve, Stein, Hanington, Heron, & Ramchandani, 2015) as well as the development of language abilities (Paulson, Keefe, & Leiferman, 2009). Lesbian and bisexual mothers (both biological and non-biological mothers) appear no less susceptible to symptoms of perinatal depression than heterosexual women (Ross, Steele, Goldfinger, & Strike, 2007).

Perhaps not surprisingly, having a depressed partner is a known risk factor for depression (Burke, 2003) and depression in one partner may be associated with, or exacerbate, mood difficulties in the other (Banker & LaCoursiere, 2014). As a consequence, a couple's relationship may be vulnerable when one partner develops depression or symptoms of emotional distress in the perinatal period (Banker & LaCoursiere, 2014; Barnes, 2006; Malus, Szyluk, Galinska-Skok, & Konarzewska, 2016; Milgrom & McCloud, 1996; Sipsma et al., 2016). Same-sex couples may face a particular set of vulnerabilities in the perinatal period (Ross & Ross, 2005; Ross et al., 2007; Trettin, Moses-Kolko, & Wisner, 2006), but the research in this area is not currently well developed.

Interventions in the Perinatal Period

Systematic reviews of the evidence (Cuijpers, Brannmark, & van Straten, 2008; Cuijpers, Smit, Bohlmeijer, Hollon, & Andersson, 2009; Dennis, 2005; Dennis & Hodnett, 2008) have confirmed that a range of treatment approaches are effective specifically for perinatal depression including cognitive behavioural therapy (CBT) (Milgrom, Negri, Gemmill, McNeil, & Martin, 2005), counselling (MacArthur et al., 2002), pharmacotherapy (Appleby et al., 1997; Milgrom, Gemmill et al., 2015a) and interpersonal psychotherapy (IPT) (O'Hara, Stuart, Gorman, & Wenzel, 2000). The largest evidence base is for CBT-based perinatal interventions (Sockol, 2015) and a wealth of evidence also supports the effectiveness of CBT interventions for depression in general (NIMH, 2003). About two in three individuals in CBT trials are no longer diagnosed with depressive disorders at follow-up (Gloaguen et al., 1998), and CBT also reduces the risk of relapse (NIMH, 2003). Milgrom and colleagues (Milgrom et al., 1999; Milgrom, Negri et al., 2005) have stressed the importance of adapting best practice treatment approaches to the particular needs of new mothers.

Cognitive Behaviour Therapy (CBT) and Other Psychological Approaches to Treatment

We have previously evaluated a 12-week group CBT programme designed specifically for postnatal depression. The manualised programme, *Getting Ahead of Postnatal Depression* (Milgrom et al., 1999), was successful in lowering depressed mood and was superior to group counselling, and at least as effective as pharmacotherapy with sertraline ((Milgrom, Gemmill et al., 2015b; Milgrom,

Negri et al., 2005). The programme development involved adapting Lewinsohn's well-validated 'coping with depression course' (Cuijpers, Muñoz, Clarke, & Lewinsohn, 2009; Lewinsohn, Antonuccio, Steinmetz, & Teri, 1984; Lewinsohn, Munoz, Youngren, & Zeiss, 1992) to more directly address the unique needs of depressed mothers with new infants. Partner sessions were introduced and the order of content was rearranged so that behavioural elements precede cognitive elements and content was re-packaged to be less demanding of time and information processing (e.g. techniques of 'relaxation on the run'). Novel components included modules on family of origin issues and securing social support.

Randomised trials have established the efficacy of this approach (Milgrom et al., 2011; Milgrom, Negri et al., 2005) and we have also successfully developed and trialled a web-based version (Danaher et al., 2013; Milgrom et al., 2016) that produced up to a four-fold increase in remission from a diagnosed episode of depression in postnatal women.

Most recently trialled and validated was an antenatal adaptation (Milgrom, Holt et al., 2015), Beating the Blues Before Birth, which proved highly effective in reducing both depression and associated anxiety in a population of pregnant women diagnosed with depression (80% with major depressive disorder).

The efficacy of a range of psychological treatment of maternal perinatal depression has support from other existing research evidence (Cuijpers, Brannmark et al., 2008; Dennis & Hodnett, 2007; Dennis, Ross, & Grigoriadis, 2007). It appears that CBT-based treatments and IPT achieve the most promising outcomes although IPT has a somewhat narrower evidence base in perinatal populations than CBT, as do non-directive counselling and psychodynamic therapy

Antidepressants

To our knowledge, there have been no published randomised controlled trials of antidepressants in the antenatal period. However, there have been 'open label' trials, as well as some controlled trials of antidepressant medications for postnatal depression. For ethical and other reasons, controlled trials in postnatal women have most often compared antidepressants to an active comparator, or combined them with a psychological treatment, rather than adopting a classic, two-group, placebo-controlled design (see the following section on combination therapy). While some open-label trials have reported positive results (Pearlstein et al., 2006), the findings of placebo-controlled trials have been more ambiguous (Yonkers et al., 2008). In weighing the overall evidence available, a recent Cochran review (Molyneaux, Howard, McGeown, Karia, & Trevillion, 2014) concludes that in perinatally depressed women, current research provides 'insufficient evidence to conclude whether, and for whom, antidepressant or psychological/psychosocial treatments are more effective, or whether some antidepressants are more effective or better tolerated than others'. However, despite these weaknesses in the specific evidence base for their perinatal use, it seems not unreasonable that the efficacy observed for antidepressant medications in the general population, including non-perinatal women, would also be expected in depressed postnatal women (O'Hara, Dennis, McCabe, & Galbally, 2015).

During pregnancy and in the postpartum period, a complicating issue is that the potential risks of exposing a foetus or breastfeeding infant need to be considered alongside the risks of untreated mental illness, or the cessation of already-commenced medication, for the woman herself (Galbally, Lewis, & Buist, 2011). Medications that are used to treat depression, or their metabolites, will enter the circulatory system and may therefore be passed to the foetus or be present in breast milk in low concentrations. Some countries (the USA, the UK and Australia) have developed national guidelines to assist with what should ideally be a collaborative decision taken together by patients and their doctors (beyondblue, 2011; NICE, 2014; O'Hara et al., 2015; Yonkers et al., 2009).

The selective serotonin reuptake inhibitors (SSRIs) are the class of antidepressants about which the most information is available. An emerging literature work suggests several potential areas of increased tetratogenicity associated with antidepressant taken during pregnancy (Galbally et al., 2011). However, the quality of evidence regarding the risks posed to infants remains somewhat limited (McDonagh et al., 2014) and there is no clear consensus on specific risks associated with most antidepressants (Robakis, Jernick, & Williams, 2017).

Information on possible long-term effects of SSRIs passed through breastfeeding is also limited. Clinical guidelines in some countries (beyondblue, 2011; Yonkers et al., 2009) advise that medication, if used, should be at the lowest effective dose, regularly reviewed and dispensed in single repeats. In the case of two or more effective alternative medications, the alternative with the shortest half-life should be chosen and, if possible, should be avoided during the first trimester of pregnancy.

Combination Therapy

There is some evidence for combining psychological and pharmacological therapies for the treatment of depression in general (Cuijpers, van Straten, Hollon, & Andersson, 2009; Cuijpers, van Straten, van Oppen, & Andersson, 2008; de Matt, Dekker, Schoevers, & de Jonghe, 2007). Efficacy may be conditional on type of antidepressant used as well as on symptom severity and chronicity. For example, where the psychological component is CBT, the additive benefit of an antidepressant appears to be relatively small.

For the treatment of postnatal depression in particular, most existing studies appear to find little or no benefit of combining SSRIs with psychological therapies (Milgrom, Gemmill et al., 2015a). For example, an early placebo-controlled study of cognitive-behaviour counselling and fluoxetine found both to be similarly beneficial (Appleby, 1997) and another study by Misri et al. (2004) reported paroxetine both alone and combined with CBT as comparable (Misri et al., 2004). Similarly, Bloch and colleagues (Bloch et al., 2012) and Milgrom and colleagues (Milgrom, Gemmill et al., 2015a) found no benefit in combining sertraline with psychological therapy. No large, high-quality randomised controlled trials have thus far reported a clear additive benefit of combining psychological and pharmacological approaches to postnatal depression. Nonetheless, at least one pragmatic trial of psychological intervention versus antidepressants provides some evidence that medication may act more rapidly which could be an advantage (Sharp et al., 2010). Large randomised controlled trials with longer follow-up periods are needed in order to understand the pros and cons of particular combinations of therapy more fully (De Crescenzo, Perelli, Fabio, Armando, & Vicari, 2014; O'Hara & McCabe, 2013).

e-Mental Health Treatments for Perinatal Depression and Anxiety

Increasingly, internet-based interventions have been used to address maternal depression and a range of psychological problems faced by women in the perinatal period (Lau, Htun, Wong, Tam, & Klainin-Yobas, 2017; Lee, Denison, Hor, & Reynolds, 2016). Beginning with the work of Danaher and colleagues (Danaher et al., 2012, 2013) and Sheeber et al. (2013), cognitive and behavioural intervention depression has been a major focus. Several feasibility and randomised studies using CBT and Behavioural Activation have shown significant effects on depressive and anxious symptoms (Danaher et al., 2013; Pugh et al., 2016). Milgrom et al. (2016) reported a four-fold increase in remission from a DSM-diagnosed depressive disorder following a six-session online CBT intervention (MumMoodBooster; Milgrom et al., 2016). O'Mahen and colleagues achieved similar reductions of symptoms with a 12-session programme of Behavioural Activation therapy (O'Mahen et al., 2013, 2015). Reaching particular perinatal cultural and demographic groups via online interventions (Latinas, socially disadvantaged communities, women suffering reproductive loss) has also shown some promise (Barrera et al., 2015; Drozd et al., 2013; Kertsing et al., 2011, 2013; Logsdon et al., 2013; Scherrer et al., 2015; Sheeber et al., 2012; Nieminen et al., 2016).

The current evidence suggests that web-based programs can overcome several of the barriers to treatment in perinatal populations, such as stigma and lack of reach of traditional services, and the emerging evidence for their efficacy is promising, if currently limited (Lee et al., 2016). Approaches including compassionate mind training are currently the subject of ongoing work (Kelman et al., 2016).

Mother-Infant Interventions

A number of studies have found that even after effectively treating symptoms of maternal depression, adverse effects on the mother-infant relationship can nonetheless persist in the longer term (Milgrom, Ericksen, McCarthy, & Gemmill, 2006; Murray et al., 2003). Interventions aimed at directly enhancing the relationship between mother and baby, in addition to the mother's depression treatment, have therefore been the subject of research (Forman et al., 2007; Nylen et al., 2010).

These interventions target areas such as parental sensitivity, parental internal working models, social supports, and maternal mental health and well-being (van IJzendoorn, Bakermans-Kranenburg, & Juffer, 2005) and shorter interventions appear particularly promising for increasing maternal sensitivity. Our own HUGS programme, for example (Milgrom et al., 1999, 2006; Milgrom & Holt, 2014), is a specialised four-week module designed to complement CBT treatment for depressed maternal mood and has shown encouraging pilot results (Milgrom et al., 2006). The four sessions include the following:

Session 1: Play and physical contact – play provides interactional opportunities, assessment of interactional strengths and deficits and modelling of alternative responses;
Session 2: Observation and understanding baby's signals – essential elements of a 'good enough' interaction are taught;
Session 3: Parental responses to infant cues – building on cognitive strategies learnt, distorted cognitions are challenged including separating past experiences from the reality of the infant;
Session 4: Consolidation of gains in a final booster session – reinforcing positive interactional behaviours and maternal cognitions about the infant.

Women's Treatment Preferences

The personal preference of a patient for a particular form of therapy affects individual adherence to both pharmacological and non-pharmacological treatment of mental health difficulties including depression (Kwan, Dimidjian, & Rizvi, 2010; Swift & Callahan, 2009). In general, 'talking' therapies are preferred by most depressed women in the perinatal period (Boath, Bradley, & Anthony, 2004; Boath, Bradley, & Henshaw, 2004). Providing women with an opportunity to take seriously difficult emotional issues in a non-judgmental space has emerged as an important facet of effective therapy (Dennis & Chung-Lee, 2006) although it is important to note that some women report a clear preference for medication (Turner et al., 2008). In weighing their possible options, depressed perinatal women have reported concerns over the possible side effects of medication passing to foetus or to breastfeeding infants, as well as a possible stigma attached to receiving pharmacological treatment for a mental health condition (Bilszta, Ericksen, Buist, & Milgrom, 2010; Dennis & Chung-Lee, 2006).

Other Therapies

Natural and complimentary therapies (e.g. herbal supplements, yoga, naturopathy, massage) are also accessed by perinatal women. However, there is, as yet, a limited evidence base for judging their effectiveness in treating depression in perinatal populations (Dennis & Dowswell, 2013).

References

Abbasi, M., van den Akker, O., & Bewley, C. (2014). Persian couples' experiences of depressive symptoms and health-related quality of life in the pre- and perinatal period. *Journal of Psychosomatic Obstetrics & Gynecology, 35*(1), 16–21.

Agius, A., Xuereb, R. B., Carrick-Sen, D., Sultana, R., & Rankin, J. (2016). The co-existence of depression, anxiety and post-traumatic stress symptoms in the perinatal period: A systematic review. *Midwifery, 36*, 70–79. doi: 10.1016/j.midw.2016.02.013

Alcorn, K. L., O'Donovan, A., Patrick, J. C., Creedy, D., & Devilly, G. J. (2010). A prospective longitudinal study of the prevalence of post-traumatic stress disorder resulting from childbirth events. *Psychological Medicine, 40*(11), 1849–1859.

Alderdice, F., McNeill, J., Gargan, P., & Perra, O. (2017). Preliminary evaluation of the Well-being in Pregnancy (WiP) questionnaire. *Journal of Psychosomatic Obstetrics and Gynaecology, 38*(2), 133–142.

Alderdice, F., Savage-McGlynn, E., Martin, C., McAuliffe, F., Hunter, A., Unterscheider, J.,… Malone, F. (2013). The prenatal distress questionnaire: An investigation of factor structure in a high risk population. *Journal of Reproductive and Infant Psychology, 31*(5), 456–464. doi: 10.1080/02646838.2013.830210

Alhamdan, N., Ajaj, A., Alali, F., & Badr, H. E. (2017). Postpartum depression and health related quality of life: A necessary assessment. *International Journal of Family & Community Medicine, 1*(11–17).

American Psychiatric Association. (2000). *Diagnostic and Statistical Manual of Mental Disorders – Text Revision* (4th ed.). Washington, DC: American Psychiatric Press.

American Psychiatric Association. (2013). *Diagnostic and Statistical Manual of Mental Disorders* (5th ed.). Arlington, VA: American Psychiatric Press.

Andersson, L., Sundström-Poromaa, I., Wulff, M., Åström, M., & Bixo, M. (2004). Implications of antenatal depression and anxiety for obstetric outcome. *Obstetrics and Gynecology, 104*(3), 467–476. doi: 10.1097/01.AOG.0000135277.04565.e9

Appleby, L., Warner, R., Whitton, A., & Faragher, B. (1997). A controlled study of fluoxetine and cognitive-behavioural counselling in the treatment of postnatal depression. *BMJ, 314*, 932.

Ayers, S. (2007). Thoughts and emotions during traumatic birth: A qualitative study. *Birth, 34*(3), 253–263.

Ayers, S., Coates, R., & Matthey, S. (2015). Identifying perinatal anxiety. In J. Milgrom & A. Gemmill (Eds.), *Identifying Perinatal Depression and Anxiety* (pp. 93–107): John Wiley & Sons, Ltd. Chichester.

Ayers, S., Jessop, D., Pike, A., Parfitt, Y., & Ford, E. (2014). The role of adult attachment style, birth intervention and support in posttraumatic stress after childbirth: A prospective study. *Journal of Affective Disorders, 155*, 295–298.

Ayers, S., & Pickering, A. D. (2001). Do women get posttraumatic stress disorder as a result of childbirth? A prospective study of incidence. *Birth, 28*(2), 111.

Banker, J. E., & LaCoursiere, D. Y. (2014). Postpartum depression: Risks, protective factors, and the couple's relationship. *Issues in Mental Health Nursing, 35*(7), 503–508.

Barker, E. D., Jaffee, S. R., Uher, R., & Maughan, B. (2011). The contribution of prenatal and postnatal maternal anxiety and depression to child maladjustment. *Depression and Anxiety, 28*(8), 696–702. doi: 10.1002/da.20856

Barnes, D. L. (2006). Postpartum depression: Its impact on couples and marital satisfaction. *Journal of Systemic Therapies, 25*(3), 25–42.

Beck, C. T. (1992). The lived experience of postpartum depression: A phenomenological study. *Nursing Research, 41*(3), 166–170.

Berger, J. M., Levant, R., McMillan, K. K., Kelleher, W., & Sellers, A. (2005). Impact of gender role conflict, traditional masculinity ideology, alexithymia, and age on men's attitudes toward psychological help seeking. *Psychology of Men & Masculinity, 6*(1), 73–78.

beyondblue. (2011). *Australian Clinical Practice Guidelines: Depression and Related Disorders in the Perinatal Period.* Melbourne, Australia: The National Depression Initiative.

Bilszta, J., Ericksen, J., Buist, A., & Milgrom, J. (2010). Women's experiences of postnatal depression - beliefs and attitudes as barriers to care. *Australian Journal of Advanced Nursing, 27*(3), 44–54.

Blakeley, P. M., Capron, L. E., Jensen, A. B., O'Donnell, K. J., & Glover, V. (2013). Maternal prenatal symptoms of depression and down regulation of placental monoamine oxidase a expression. *Journal of Psychosomatic Research, 75*(4), 341–345.

Bloch, M., Meiboom, H., Lorberblatt, M., Bluvstein, I., Aharonov, I., & Schreiber, S. (2012). The effect of sertraline add-on to brief dynamic psychotherapy for the treatment of postpartum depression: A random-ized, double-blind, placebo-controlled study. *The Journal of Clinical Psychiatry, 73*(2), 235–241.

Boath, E., Bradley, E., & Anthony, P. (2004). Users' views of two alternative approaches to the treat-ment of postnatal depression. *Journal of Reproductive and Infant Psychology, 22*(1), 13–24. doi: 10.1080/02646830310001643085

Boath, E., Bradley, E., & Henshaw, C. (2004). Women's views of antidepressants in the treatment of postnatal depression. *Journal of Psychosomatic Obstetrics & Gynecology, 25*(3–4), 221–233. doi: 10.1080/01674820400017889

Brenes, G. A. (2007). Anxiety, depression, and quality of life in primary care patients. *Primary Care Compan-ion to the Journal of Clinical Psychiatry, 9*(6), 437–443.

Brockington, I. F., Macdonald, E., & Wainscott, G. (2006). Anxiety, obsessions and morbid preoccupations in pregnancy and the puerperium. *Archives of Women's Mental Health, 9*(5), 253–263.

Brunton, R. J., Dryer, R., Saliba, A., & Kohlhoff, J. (2015). Pregnancy anxiety: A systematic review of cur-rent scales. *Journal of Affective Disorders, 176*, 24–34. doi: 10.1016/j.jad.2015.01.039

Burke, L. (2003). The impact of maternal depression of familial relationships. *International Review of Psychi-atry, 15*, 243–255.

Capron, L. E., Glover, V., Pearson, R. M., Evans, J., O'Connor, T. G., Stein, A.,… Ramchandani, P. G. (2015). Associations of maternal and paternal antenatal mood with offspring anxiety disorder at age 18 years. *Journal of Affective Disorders, 187*, 20–26.

Chan, S. W., Levy, V., Chung, T. K., & Lee, D. (2002). A qualitative study of the experiences of a group of Hong Kong Chinese women diagnosed with postnatal depression. *Journal of Advanced Nursing, 39*(6), 571–579.

Coates, R., Ayers, S., & de Visser, R. (2014). Women's experiences of postnatal distress: A qualitative study. *BMC Pregnancy Childbirth, 14*(359), 1471–2393.

Cochran, S. V., & Rabinowitz, F. E. (2003). Gender-sensitive recommendations for assessment and treat-ment of depression in men. *Professional Psychology: Research and Practice, 34*(2), 132–140.

Condon, J. (2004). The first-time fathers study: A prospective study of the mental health and wellbeing of men during the transition to parenthood. *Australian and New Zealand Journal of Psychiatry, 38*, 56–64.

Coo, S., Milgrom, J., Kuppens, P., & Trinder, J. (2015). Perinatal distress, an appraisal perspective. *Journal of Reproductive and Infant Psychology, 33*(2), 190–204. doi: 10.1080/02646838.2015.1004570

Couto, E. R., Couto, E., Vian, B., Gregorio, Z., Nomura, M. L., Zaccaria, R., & Passini, R., Jr. (2009). Quality of life, depression and anxiety among pregnant women with previous adverse pregnancy out-comes. *Sao Paulo Medical Journal, 127*(4), 185–189.

Cuijpers, P., Brannmark, J. G., & van Straten, A. (2008). Psychological treatment of postpartum depression: a meta-analysis. *Journal of Clinical Psychology, 64*(1), 103–118.

Cuijpers, P., Muñoz, R., Clarke, G., & Lewinsohn, P. (2009). Psychoeducational treatment and prevention of depression: The "coping with depression" course thirty years later. *Clinical Psychology Review, 29*(5), 449–458.

Cuijpers, P., Smit, F., Bohlmeijer, E., Hollon, S. D., & Andersson, G. (2009). Efficacy of cognitive-behavioural therapy and other psychological treatments for adult depression: meta-analytic study of pub-lication bias. *British Journal of Psychiatry, 196*, 173–178.

Cuijpers, P., van Straten, A., Hollon, S. D., & Andersson, G. (2009). The contribution of active medication to combined treatments of psychotherapy and pharmacotherapy for adult depression: A meta-analysis. *Acta Psychiatr Scand, 121*(6), 415–423.

Cuijpers, P., van Straten, A., van Oppen, P., & Andersson, G. (2008). Are psychological and pharmacologic interventions equally effective in the treatment of adult depressive disorders? A meta-analysis of compar-ative studies. *The Journal of Clinical Psychiatry, 69*(11), 1675–1685.

Da Costa, D., Dritsa, M., Rippen, N., Lowensteyn, I., & Khalife, S. (2006). Health-related quality of life in postpartum depressed women. *Archives of Women's Mental Health, 9*(2), 95–102.

Danaher, B. G., Milgrom, J., Seeley, J. R., Stuart, S., Schembri, C., Tyler, M. S.,… Lewinsohn, P. (2013). MomMoodBooster web-based intervention for postpartum depression: Feasibility trial results. *Journal of Medical Internet Research, 15*(11), e242. doi: 10.2196/jmir.2876

Danaher, B. G., Milgrom, J., Seeley, J. R., Stuart, S., Schembri, C., Tyler, M. S.,… Lewinsohn, P. (2012). Web-based intervention for postpartum depression: Formative research and design of the mummood-booster program. *JMIR Research Protocols, 1*(2), e18.

Dave, S., Sherr, L., Senior, R., & Nazareth, I. (2008). Associations between paternal depression and behaviour problems in children of 4–6 years. *European Child and Adolescent Psychiatry, 17*(5), 306–315.

Dayan, J., Creveuil, C., Marks, M. N., Conroy, S., Herlicoviez, M., Dreyfus, M.,… Tordjman, S. (2006). Prenatal depression, prenatal anxiety, and spontaneous preterm birth: A prospective cohort study among women with early and regular care. *Psychosomatic Medicine, 68*(6), 938–946.

De Crescenzo, F., Perelli, Fabio, A., Armando, M., & Vicari, S. (2014). Selective serotonin reuptake inhibitors (SSRIs) for post-partum depression (PPD): A systematic review of randomiized clinical trials. *Journal of Affective Disorders, 154*, 39–44.

de Matt, S., Dekker, J., Schoevers, R., & de Jonghe, F. (2007). Relative efficacy of psychotherapy and combined therapy in the treatment of depression: A meta-analysis. *Eurpean Psychiatry, 22*, 1–8.

de Tychey, C., Briancon, S., Lighezzolo, J., Spitz, E., Kabuth, B., de Luigi, V.,… Vincent, S. (2008). Quality of life, postnatal depression and baby gender. *Journal of Clinical Nursing, 17*(3), 312–322.

de Weerth, C., Buitelaar, J. K., & Mulder, E. J. H. (2005). Prenatal programming of behavior, physiology and cognition. *Neuroscience and Biobehavioral Reviews, 29*(2), 207–208.

Deater-Deckard, K., Pickering, K., Dunn, J. F., & Golding, J. (1998). Family structure and depressive symptoms in men preceding and following the birth of a child. The Avon longitudinal study of pregnancy and childhood study team. *American Journal of Psychiatry, 155*(6), 818–823.

DeJong, H., Fox, E., & Stein, A. (2016). Rumination and postnatal depression: A systematic review and a cognitive model. *Behaviour Research and Therapy, 82*, 38–49. doi: 10.1016/j.brat.2016.05.003

Dennis, C.-L. (2005). Psychosocial and psychological interventions for prevention of postnatal depression: Systematic review. *BMJ (Clinical research ed.), 331*(7507), 15. doi: 10.1136/bmj.331.7507.15

Dennis, C.-L., & Chung-Lee, L. (2006). Postpartum depression help-seeking barriers and maternal treatment preferences: A qualitative systematic review. *Birth (Berkeley, Calif.), 33*(4), 323–331. doi: 10.1111/j.1523-536X.2006.00130.x

Dennis, C., & Hodnett, E. (2008). Psychosocial and psychological interventions for treating postpartum depression. *Evidence-Based Mental Health, 11*(3), 79.

Dennis, C. L., & Dowswell, T. (2013). Interventions (other than pharmacological, psychosocial or psychological) for treating antenatal depression. *Cochrane Database Systematic Review, 31*(7) CD006795.

Dennis, C. L., Falah-Hassani, K., Brown, H. K., & Vigod, S. N. (2016). Identifying women at risk for postpartum anxiety: A prospective population-based study. *Acta Psychiatrica Scandinavica, 134*(6), 485–493. doi: 10.1111/acps.12648

Dennis, C. L., Falah-Hassani, K., & Shiri, R. (2017). Prevalence of antenatal and postnatal anxiety: Systematic review and meta-analysis. *British Journal of Psychiatry, 210*(5), 315–323.

Dennis, C. L., & Hodnett, E. (2007). Psychosocial and psychological interventions for treating postpartum depression. *Cochrane Database Systematic Review, 17*(4) CD006116.

Dennis, C. L., Ross, L. E., & Grigoriadis, S. (2007). Psychosocial and psychological interventions for treating antenatal dperession. *Cochrane Database of Systematic Reviews, 3*. doi: 10.1002/14615818.CD006309.pub2

Don, B. P., & Mickelson, K. D. (2012). Paternal postpartum depression: The role of maternal postpartum depression, spousal support, and relationship satisfaction. *Couple and Family Psychology: Research and Practice, 1*, 323–334.

Falah-Hassani, K., Shiri, R., & Dennis, C. L. (2017). The prevalence of antenatal and postnatal co-morbid anxiety and depression: A meta-analysis. *Psychological Medicine, 47*(12), 2041–2053.

Feldman, R., Granat, A., Pariente, C., Kanety, H., Kuint, J., Gilboa-Schechtman, E.,… Gilboa-Schechtman, E. (2009). Maternal depression and anxiety across the postpartum year and infant social engagement, fear regulation, and stress reactivity. *Journal of the American Academy of Child & Adolescent Psychiatry, 48*(9), 919–927.

Field, T., Diego, M., & Hernandez-Reif, M. (2009). Depressed mothers' infants are less responsive to faces and voices. *Infant Behavior & Development, 32*(3), 239–244.

Field, T., Healy, B., Goldstein, S., Perry, S., Bendell, D., Schanberg, S.,… Kuhn, C. (1988). Infants of depressed mothers show 'depressed' behaviour even with non-depressed adults. *Child Development, 59*, 1569–1579.

Field, T. M. (2002). Early interactions between infants and their postpartum depressed mothers. *Infant Behavior & Development, 25*(1), 25–29.

Fletcher, R., Garfield, C. F., & Matthey, S. (2015). Fathers' perinatal mental health. In J. Milgrom & A. Gemmill (Eds.), *Identifying Perinatal Depression and Anxiety: Evidence-Based Practice in Screening, Psychosocial Assessment, and Management* (pp. 165–176). Chichester, UK: Wiley.

Fletcher, R. J., Maharaj, O., Fletcher, W. C., May, C., Skeates, N., & Gruenert, S. (2013). Fathers with mental illness: Implications for clinicians and health services. *The Medical Journal of Australia, 199*(3 Suppl), S34–36.

Forman, D. R., O'Hara, M. W., Stuart, S., Gorman, L. L., Larsen, K. E., & Coy, K. C. (2007). Effective treatment for postpartum depression is not sufficient to improve the developing mother-child relationship. *Development & Psychopathology, 19*(2), 585–602.

Furuta, M., Sandall, J., Cooper, D., & Bick, D. (2016). Predictors of birth-related post-traumatic stress symptoms: Secondary analysis of a cohort study. *Archives of Women's Mental Health, 19*(6), 987–999.

Galbally, M., Lewis, A. J., & Buist, A. (2011). Developmental outcomes of children exposed to antidepressants in pregnancy. *Australian and New Zealand Journal of Psychiatry, 45*(5), 393–399. doi: 10.3109/00048674.2010.549995

Galera, C., Cote, S. M., Bouvard, M. P., Pingault, J. B., Melchior, M., Michel, G.,… Tremblay, R. E. (2011). Early risk factors for hyperactivity-impulsivity and inattention trajectories from age 17 months to 8 years. *Archives of General Psychiatry, 68*(12), 1267–1275.

Garfield, C. F., Duncan, G., Rutsohn, J., McDade, T. W., Adam, E. K., Coley, R. L., & Chase-Lansdale, P. L. (2014). A longitudinal study of paternal mental health during transition to fatherhood as young adults. *Pediatrics, 133*(5), 836–843.

Gavin, N. I., Gaynes, B. N., Lohr, K. N., Meltzer-Brody, S., Gartlehner, G., & Swinson, T. (2005). Perinatal depression: A systematic review of prevalence and incidence. *Obstetrics & Gynecology, 106*(5 Pt 1), 1071–1083.

Gloaguen, V., Cottraux, J., Cucherat, M., & Blackburn, I. M.. (1998). A meta-analysis of the effects of cognitive therapy in depressed patients.. *Journal of Affective Disorders, 28*(1), 59–72.

Glover, V. (2014). Maternal depression, anxiety and stress during pregnancy and child outcome; what needs to be done. *Best Practice & Research. Clinical Obstetrics & Gynaecology, 28*(1), 25–35. doi: 10.1016/j.bpobgyn.2013.08.017

Glover, V. (2015). Prenatal stress and its effects on the fetus and child: Possible underlying biological mechanisms. *Advanced Neurobiology, 10*, 269–283.

Gutierrez-Galve, L., Stein, A., Hanington, L., Heron, J., & Ramchandani, P. (2015). Paternal depression in the postnatal period and child development: Mediators and moderators. *Pediatrics, 135*(2), e339–e347. doi: 10.1542/peds.2014-2411

Herba, C. M., Glover, V., Ramchandani, P. G., & Rondon, M. B. (2016). Maternal depression and mental health in early childhood: An examination of underlying mechanisms in low-income and middle-income countries. *Lancet Psychiatry, 3*(10), 983–992.

Highet, N., Stevenson, A. L., Purtell, C., & Coo, S. (2014). Qualitative insights into women's personal experiences of perinatal depression and anxiety. *Women Birth, 27*(3), 179–184.

James, S. (2015). Women's experiences of symptoms of posttraumatic stress disorder (PTSD) after traumatic childbirth: A review and critical appraisal. *Archives of Women's Mental Health, 18*(6), 761–771.

Jones, L., Scott, J., Cooper, C., Forty, L., Smith, K. G., Sham, P.,… Jones, I. (2010). Cognitive style, personality and vulnerability to postnatal depression. *The British Journal of Psychiatry: the Journal of Mental Science, 196*(3), 200–205.

Kim, W. J., Lee, E., Kim, K. R., Namkoong, K., Park, E. S., & Rha, D. W. (2015). Progress of PTSD symptoms following birth: A prospective study in mothers of high-risk infants. *Journal of Perinatology, 35*(8), 575–579.

Kwan, B., Dimidjian, S., & Rizvi, S. (2010). Treatment preference, engagement, and clinical improvement in pharmacotherapy versus psychotherapy for depression. *Behaviour Research and Therapy, 48*, 799–804.

Lau, Y., Htun, T. P., Wong, S. N., Tam, W. S. W., & Klainin-Yobas, P. (2017). Therapist-supported internet-based cognitive behavior therapy for stress, anxiety, and depressive symptoms among postpartum women: A systematic review and meta-analysis. *Journal of Medical Internet Research, 19*(4), e138.

Lee, E. W., Denison, F. C., Hor, K., & Reynolds, R. M. (2016). Web-based interventions for prevention and treatment of perinatal mood disorders: A systematic review. *BMC Pregnancy and Childbirth, 16*(1). doi: 10.1186/s12884-016-0831-1

Leigh, B., & Milgrom, J. (2008). Risk factors for antenatal depression, postnatal depression and parenting stress. *BMC Psychiatry, 8*, 24. doi: 10.1186/1471-244x-8-24

Lewinsohn, P. M., Antonuccio, D. O., Steinmetz, J. L., & Teri, L. (1984). *The Coping with Depression Course: A Psycho-educational Intervention for Unipolar Depression.* Eugene: Castalsa Publishing Company.

Lewinsohn, P. M., Munoz, R. F., Youngren, M. A., & Zeiss, A. M. (1992). *Control Your Depression.* New York: Simon & Schuster.

Lovibond, S. L., PF. (1995). *Manual for the Depression Anxiety Stress Scales*. Sydney: Psychological Foundation.

MacArthur, C., Winter, H., Bick, D., Knowles, H., Lilford, R., Henderson, C.,… Gee, H. (2002). Effects of redesigned community postnatal care on women's health 4 months after birth: A cluster randomised controlled trial. *Lancet, 359*(9304), 378–385.

Malus, A., Szyluk, J., Galinska-Skok, B., & Konarzewska, B. (2016). Incidence of postpartum depression and couple relationship quality. *Psychiatria Polska, 50*(6), 1135–1146. doi: 10.12740/pp/61569

Mason, W. A., Rice, M. J., & Records, K. (2005). The lived experience of postpartum depression in a psychiatric population. *Perspectives in Psychiatric Care, 41*(2), 52–61.

Matijasevich, A., Murray, J., Cooper, P. J., Anselmi, L., Barros, A. J. D., Barros, F. C., & Santos, I. S. (2015). Trajectories of maternal depression and offspring psychopathology at 6 years: 2004 Pelotas cohort study. *Journal of Affective Disorders, 174*, 424–431. doi: 10.1016/j.jad.2014.12.012

Mauri, M., Oppo, A., Montagnani, M. S., Borri, C., Banti, S., Camilleri, V.,… Cassano, G. B. (2010). Beyond "postpartum depressions": Specific anxiety diagnoses during pregnancy predict different outcomes: Results from PND-ReScU. *Journal of Affective Disorders, 127*(1–3), 177–184. doi: 10.1016/j.jad.2010.05.015

McCarthy, J., & Holliday, E. L. (2004). Help-seeking and counseling within a traditional male gender role: An examination from a multicultural perspective. *Journal of Counseling & Development, 82*(1), 25–30. doi: 10.1002/j.1556-6678.2004.tb00282.x

McDonagh, M. S., Matthews, A., Phillipi, C., Romm, J., Peterson, K., Thakurta, S., & Guise, J. M. (2014). Depression drug treatment outcomes in pregnancy and the postpartum period: A systematic review and meta-analysis. *Obstetrics and Gynecology, 124*(3), 526–534.

McMahon, C., Barnett, B., Kowalenko, N., Tennant, C., McMahon, C., Barnett, B.,… Tennant, C. (2005). Psychological factors associated with persistent postnatal depression: Past and current relationships, defence styles and the mediating role of insecure attachment style. *Journal of Affective Disorders, 84*(1), 15–24.

Meades, R., & Ayers, S. (2011). Anxiety measures validated in perinatal populations: A systematic review. *Journal of Affective Disorders, 133*(1–2), 1–15. doi: 10.1016/j.jad.2010.10.009

Milgrom, J., & Beatrice, G. (2003). Coping with the stress of motherhood: Cognitive and defence style of women with postnatal depression. *Stress and Health, 19*, 281–287.

Milgrom, J., Danaher, B. G., Gemmill, A. W., Holt, C., Holt, C. J., Seeley, J. R.,… Ericksen, J. (2016). Internet cognitive behavioral therapy for women with postnatal depression: A randomized controlled trial of MumMoodBooster. *Journal of Medical Internet Research, 18*(3). doi: 10.2196/jmir.4993

Milgrom, J., Ericksen, J., McCarthy, R. M., & Gemmill, A. W. (2006). Stressful impact of depression on early mother-infant relations. *Stress and Health, 22*(4), 229–238.

Milgrom, J., Ericksen, J., Negri, L., & Gemmill, A. (2005). Screening for postnatal depression in routine primary care: Properties of the Edinburgh Postnatal Depression Scale in an Australian sample. *The Australian and New Zealand Journal of Psychiatry, 39*, 833–839.

Milgrom, J., Gemmill, A., Ericksen, J., Burrows, G., Buist, A., & Reece, J. (2015a). Treatment of postnatal depression with cognitive behavioural therapy, sertraline and combination therapy: A randomised controlled trial. *Australian & New Zealand Journal of Psychiatry, 49*(3), 236–245. doi: 10.1177/0004867414565474

Milgrom, J., & Gemmill, A. W. (2014). Screening for perinatal depression. *Best Practice & Research Clinical Obstetrics & Gynaecology, 28*(1), 13–23. doi: 10.1016/j.bpobgyn.2013.08.014

Milgrom, J., Gemmill, A. W., Ericksen, J., Burrows, G., Buist, A., & Reece, J. (2015b). Treatment of postnatal depression with cognitive behavioural therapy, sertraline and combination therapy: A randomised controlled trial. *Australian and New Zealand Journal of Psychiatry, 49*(3), 236–245. doi: 10.1177/0004867414565474

Milgrom, J., & Holt, C. (2014). Early intervention to protect the mother-infant relationship following postnatal depression: Study protocol for a randomised controlled trial. *Trials, 15*, 385.

Milgrom, J., Holt, C., Gemmill, A., Ericksen, J., Leigh, B., Buist, A., & Schembri, C. (2011). Treating postnatal depressive symptoms in primary care: A randomised controlled trial of GP management, with and without adjunctive counselling. *BMC Psychiatry, 11*(1), 95.

Milgrom, J., Holt, C., Holt, C. J., Ross, J., Ericksen, J., & Gemmill, A. W. (2015). Feasibility study and pilot randomised trial of an antenatal depression treatment with infant follow-up. *Archives of Women's Mental Health, 18*(5), 717–730. doi: 10.1007/s00737-015-0512-5

Milgrom, J., Martin, P. R., & Negri, L. M. (1999). *Treating Postnatal Depression. A Psychological Approach for Health Care Practitioners*. Chichester: Wiley.

Milgrom, J., & McCloud, P. (1996). Parenting stress and postnatal depression. *Stress Medicine, 12*(3), 177–186. doi: 10.1002/(sici)1099-1700(199607)12:3<177::aid-smi699>3.0.co;2-w

Milgrom, J., Negri, L. M., Gemmill, A. W., McNeil, M., & Martin, P. R. (2005). A randomized controlled trial of psychological interventions for postnatal depression. *British Journal of Clinical Psychology, 44*(4), 529–542.

Milgrom, J., Westley, D., & Gemmill, A. W. (2004). The mediating role of maternal responsiveness in some longer-term effects of postnatal depression on infant development. *Infant Behavior & Development, 27*, 443–454.

Misri, S., Reebye, P., Corral, M., Milis, L., Misri, S., Reebye, P.,... Milis, L. (2004). The use of paroxetine and cognitive-behavioral therapy in postpartum depression and anxiety: A randomized controlled trial. *Journal of Clinical Psychiatry, 65*(9), 1236–1241.

Moinmehr, S., Afsar, M., Salehizadeh, M., Kashani, P., Karamad, J., & Foroutan, M. (2016). Relationship between women's quality of life and postpartum depression. *The Caspian Sea Journal, 10*(1, Supplement 4), 161–116.

Molyneaux, E., Howard, L. M., McGeown, H. R., Karia, A. M., & Trevillion, K. (2014). Antidepressant treatment for postnatal depression. *Cochrane Database of Systematic Reviews, 9*. doi: 10.1002/14651858. CD002018.pub2

Monk, C. (2001). Stress and mood disorders during pregnancy: Implications for child development. *Psychiatric Quarterly, 72*(4), 347–357. doi: 10.1023/a:1010393316106

Monk, C., Fifer, W. P., Myers, M. M., Sloan, R. P., Trien, L., & Hurtado, A. (2000). Maternal stress responses and anxiety during pregnancy: Effects on fetal heart rate. *Developmental Psychobiology, 36*(1), 67–77. doi: 10.1002/(sici)1098-2302(200001)36:1<67::aid-dev7>3.0.co;2-c

Monk, C., Spicer, J., & Champagne, F. A.. (2012). Linking prenatal maternal adversity to developmental outcomes in infants: The role of epigenetic pathways. *Development and Psychopathology, 24*(4), 1361–1376.

Mount, K. S., Crockenberg, S. C., Jo, P. S., & Wagar, J. L. (2010). Maternal and child correlates of anxiety in 2(1/2)-year-old children. *Infant Behavior & Development, 33*(4), 567–578.

Murray, L., Arteche, A., Fearon, P., Halligan, S., Croudace, T., & Cooper, P. J. (2010). The effects of maternal postnatal depression and child sex on academic performance at age 16 years: A developmental approach. *Journal of Child Psychology and Psychiatry, 51*(10), 1150–1159. doi: 10.1111/j.1469-7610.2010.02259.x

Murray, L., Arteche, A., Fearon, P., Halligan, S., Goodyer, I., & Cooper, P. J. (2011). Maternal postnatal depression and the development of depression in offspring up to 16 years of age. *Journal of the American Academy of Child and Adolescent Psychiatry, 50*(5), 460–470.

Murray, L., Cooper, P. J., & Stein, A. (1991). Postnatal depression and infant development. *BMJ (Clinical research ed.), 302*(6783), 978–979.

Murray, L., Cooper, P. J., Wilson, A., Romaniuk, H., Wilson, A., & Romaniuk, H. (2003). Controlled trial of the short- and long-term effect of psychological treatment of post-partum depression: 2. Impact on the mother–child relationship and child outcome. *British Journal of Psychiatry, 182*, 420–427.

Murray, L., Fearon, P., & Cooper, P. J. (2015). Postnatal depression, mother–infant interactions, and child development: Prospects for screening and treatment. In J. Milgrom & A. W. Gemmill (Eds.), *Identifying Perinatal Depression and Anxiety: Evidence-based Practice in Screening, Psychosocial Assessment and Management* (pp. 139–164). Chichester: Wiley-Blackwell.

Murray, L., Stanley, C., Hooper, R., King, F., & Fiori-Cowley, A. (1996). The role of infant factors in postnatal depression and mother-infant interactions. *Developmental Medicine and Child Neurology, 38*(2), 109–119.

NICE. (2014). *Antenatal and Postnatal Mental Health: Clinical Management and Service Guidance. The British Psychological Society & The Royal College of Psychiatrists.* National Institute for Health and Care Excellence (NICE). http://guidance.nice.org.uk/cg192.www.nice.org.uk.CG45. Leicester and London

NIMH. (2003). The strategic plan for mood disorders research *[NIH Publication No. 03-5121].*

Nylen, K. J., O'Hara, M. W., Brock, R., Moel, J., Gorman, L., & Stuart, S. (2010). Predictors of the longitudinal course of postpartum depression following interpersonal psychotherapy. *Journal of Consulting and Clinical Psychology, 78*(5), 757–763.

O'Connor, T. G., Heron, J., Golding, J., Beveridge, M., & Glover, V. (2002). Maternal antenatal anxiety and children's behavioural/emotional problems at 4 years – Report from the Avon Longitudinal Study of Parents and Children. *British Journal of Psychiatry, 180*, 502–508. doi: 10.1192/bjp.180.6.502

O'Connor, T. G., Monk, C., & Fitelson, E. M. (2014). Practitioner review: Maternal mood in pregnancy and child development – implications for child psychology and psychiatry. *Journal of Child Psychology and Psychiatry, and Allied Disciplines, 55*(2), 99–111. doi: 10.1111/jcpp.12153

O'Donnell, K., Glover, V., Barker, E. D., & O'Connor, T. G. (2014). The persisting effect of maternal mood in pregnancy on childhood psychopathology. *Development and Psychopathology, 26*(2), 393–403.

O'Hara, M. W., Dennis, C.-L., McCabe, J. E., & Galbally, M. (2015). Evidence-based treatments and pathways to care. In J. Milgrom & A. Gemmill (Eds.), *Identifying Perinatal Depression and Anxiety: Evidence-Based Practice in Screening, Psychosocial Assessment, and Management* (pp. 177–192): John Wiley & Sons, Ltd. Chichester.

O'Hara, M. W., & McCabe, J. E. (2013). Postpartum depression: Current status and future directions. *Annual Review of Clinical Psychology, 9*, 379–407.

O'Hara, M. W., Stuart, S., Gorman, L., & Wenzel, A. (2000). Efficacy of interpersonal psychotherapy for postpartum depression. *Archives of General Psychiatry, 57*(11), 1039–1045.

Paulson, J. F., & Bazemore, S. D. (2010). Prenatal and postpartum depression in fathers and its association with maternal depression: A meta-analysis. *Journal of the American Medical Association, 303*(19), 1961–1969.

Paulson, J. F., Bazemore, S. D., Goodman, J. H., & Leiferman, J. A. (2016). The course and interrelationship of maternal and paternal perinatal depression. *Archives of Women's Mental Health, 19*(4), 655–663. doi: 10.1007/s00737-016-0598-4

Paulson, J. F., Keefe, H. A., & Leiferman, J. A. (2009). Early parental depression and child language development. *Journal of Child Psychology and Psychiatry, 50*(3), 254–262.

Pawlby, S., Hay, D. F., Sharp, D., Waters, C. S., & O'Keane, V. (2009). Antenatal depression predicts depression in adolescent offspring: Prospective longitudinal community-based study. *Journal of Affective Disorders, 113*(3), 236–243. doi: 10.1016/j.jad.2008.05.018

Pawlby, S., Sharp, D., Hay, D., O'Keane, V., Pawlby, S., Sharp, D.,... O'Keane, V. (2008). Postnatal depression and child outcome at 11 years: The importance of accurate diagnosis. *Journal of Affective Disorders, 107*(1–3), 241–245.

Pearlstein, T. (2008). Perinatal depression: Treatment options and dilemmas. *Journal of Psychiatry & Neuroscience, 33*(4), 302–318.

Pearlstein, T. B., Zlotnick, C., Battle, C. L., Stuart, S., O'Hara, M. W., Price, A. B.,... Howard, M. (2006). Patient choice of treatment for postpartum depression: A pilot study. *Archives of Women's Mental Health, 9*(6), 303–308. doi: 10.1007/s00737-006-0145-9

Pearson, R. M., Bornstein, M. H., Cordero, M., Scerif, G., Mahedy, L., Evans, J.,... Stein, A. (2016). Maternal perinatal mental health and offspring academic achievement at age 16: The mediating role of childhood executive function. *Journal of Child Psychology and Psychiatry and Allied Disciplines, 57*(4), 491–501. doi: 10.1111/jcpp.12483

Pearson, R. M., Evans, J., Kounali, D., Lewis, G., Heron, J., Ramchandani, P. G.,... Stein, A. (2013). Maternal depression during pregnancy and the postnatal period risks and possible mechanisms for offspring depression at age 18 years. *JAMA Psychiatry, 70*(12), 1312–1319. doi: 10.1001/jamapsychiatry.2013.2163

Qiu, A., Anh, T. T., Li, Y., Chen, H., Rifkin-Graboi, A., Broekman, B. F. P.,... Gluckman, P. D. (2015). Prenatal maternal depression alters amygdala functional connectivity in 6-month-old infants. *Translational Psychiatry, 5*(2), e508.

Qiu, A., Tuan, T., Ong, M., Li, Y., Chen, H., Rifkin-Graboi, A.,... Chong, Y. S. (2015). COMT haplotypes modulate associations of antenatal maternal anxiety and neonatal cortical morphology. *The American Journal of Psychiatry, 172*(2), 163–172.

Quarini, C., Pearson, R. M., Stein, A., Ramchandani, P. G., Lewis, G., & J., E. (2015). Are female children more vulnerable to the long-term effects of maternal depression during pregnancy? *Journal of Affective Disorders, 189*(329–335).

Rallis, S., Skouteris, H., McCabe, M. P., & Milgrom, J. (2014). A prospective examination of depression, anxiety and stress throughout pregnancy. *Women & Birth, 27*(1), 68–71.

Reck, C., Hunt, A., Fuchs, T., Weiss, R., Noon, A., Moehler, E.,... Mundt, C. (2004). Interactive regulation of affect in postpartum depressed mothers and their infants: An overview. *Psychopathology, 37*(6), 272–280.

Robakis, T., Jernick, E., & Williams, K. (2017). Recent advances in understanding maternal perinatal mood disorders. *F1000Res, 15*(6). F1000 Faculty Rev-916.

Roberts, J., Lenton, P., Keetharuth, A. D., & Brazier, J. (2014). Quality of life impact of mental health conditions in England: Results from the adult psychiatric morbidity surveys. *Health Qual Life Outcomes, 12*(6), 1477–7525.

Ross, L., & McLean, L. (2006). Anxiety disorders during pregnancy and the psotpartum period: A systematic review. *Journal of Clinical Psychiatry, 67*, 1285–1298.

Ross, L. E., & Ross, L. E. (2005). Perinatal mental health in lesbian mothers: A review of potential risk and protective factors. *Women & Health, 41*(3), 113–128.

Ross, L. E., Steele, L., Goldfinger, C., & Strike, C. (2007). Perinatal depressive symptomatology among lesbian and bisexual women. *Archives of Women's Mental Health, 10*(2), 53–59.

Sharp, D., Chew-Graham, C., Tylee, A., Lewis, G., Howard, L., Anderson, I.,... Peters, T. J. (2010). A pragnataic randomised controlled tria; to comaper antidepressants with acommunity-based psychosocial intervention for the treatment of women with postnatal depression: The RESPOND trial. *Health Technology Assessment, 14*(43), 1–181.

Sheeber, L. B., Seeley, J. R., Feil, E. G., Davis, B., Sorensen, E., Kosty, D. B., & Lewinsohn, P. M. (2012). Development and pilot evaluation of an Internet-facilitated cognitive-behavioral intervention for maternal depression. *Journal of Consulting and Clinical Psychology, 80*(5), 739–749.

Shlomi Polachek, I., Dulitzky, M., Margolis-Dorfman, L., & Simchen, M. J. (2016). A simple model for prediction postpartum PTSD in high-risk pregnancies. *Archives of Women's Mental Health, 19*(3), 483–490.

Simpson, M., & Catling, C. (2016). Understanding psychological traumatic birth experiences: A literature review. *Women Birth, 29*(3), 203–207.

Sipsma, H. L., Callands, T., Desrosiers, A., Magriples, U., Jones, K., Albritton, T., & Kershaw, T. (2016). Exploring trajectories and predictors of depressive symptoms among young couples during their transition to parenthood. *Maternal and Child Health Journal, 20*(11), 2372–2381. doi: 10.1007/s10995-016-2064-3

Sockol, L. E. (2015). A systematic review of the efficacy of cognitive behavioral therapy for treating and preventing perinatal depression. *Journal of Affective Disorders, 177*, 7–21.

Sockol, L. E., Epperson, C. N., & Barber, J. P. (2014). The relationship between maternal attitudes and symptoms of depression and anxiety among pregnant and postpartum first-time mothers. *Archives of Women's Mental Health, 17*(3), 199–212.

Staneva, A., Morawska, A., Bogossian, F., & Wittkowski, A. (2016). Pregnancy-specific distress: The role of maternal sense of coherence and antenatal mothering orientations. *Journal of Mental Health, 25*(5), 387–394. doi: 10.3109/09638237.2015.1101425

Stein, A., Pearson, R. M., & Goodman, S. H. (2014). Effects of perinatal mental disorders on the fetus and child. *The Lancet, 384*(9956), 1800–1819.

Swift, J., & Callahan, J. (2009). The impact of client treatment preferences on outcome: A meta-analysis. *Journal of Clinical Psychology, 56*(4), 368–381.

Talge, N., Neal, C., & Glover, V. (2007). Antenatal maternal stress and long-term effects on child neurodevelopment: How and why? *Journal of Child Psychology and Psychiatry, and Allied Disciplines, 48*, 245–261.

Trettin, S., Moses-Kolko, E. L., & Wisner, K. L. (2006). Lesbian perinatal depression and the heterosexism that affects knowledge about this minority population. *Archives of Women's Mental Health, 9*(2), 67–73.

Turner, K. M., Sharp, D., Folkes, L., Chew-Graham, C., Turner, K. M., Sharp, D.,… Chew-Graham, C. (2008). Women's views and experiences of antidepressants as a treatment for postnatal depression: A qualitative study. *Family Practice, 25*(6), 450–455.

Underwood, L., Waldie, K. E., Peterson, E., D'Souza, S., Verbiest, M., McDaid, F., & Morton, S. (2017). Paternal depression symptoms during pregnancy and after childbirth among participants in the growing up in New Zealand study. *JAMA Psychiatry, 74*(4), 1–10.

Van Batenburg-Eddes, T., Brion, M. J., Henrichs, J., Jaddoe, V. W. V., Hofman, A., Verhulst, F. C.,… Tiemeier, H. (2013). Parental depressive and anxiety symptoms during pregnancy and attention problems in children: A cross-cohort consistency study. *Journal of Child Psychology and Psychiatry, and Allied Disciplines, 54*(5), 591–600. doi: 10.1111/jcpp.12023

van IJzendoorn, M. H., Bakermans-Kranenburg, M. J., & Juffer, F. (2005). Why less is more: From the dodo bird verdict to evidence-based interventions on sensitivity and early attachments.. In L. J. Berlin, Y. Ziv, L. Amaya-Jackson & M. T. Greenberg (Eds.), *Enhancing Early Attachments; Theory, Research, Intervention, and Policy* (pp. 297–312). New York: The Guilford Press.

Vossbeck-Elsebusch, A. N., Freisfeld, C., & Ehring, T. (2014). Predictors of posttraumatic stress symptoms following childbirth. *BMC Psychiatry, 14*(200), 14–200.

Waters, C. S., Hay, D. F., Simmonds, J. R., & van Goozen, S. H. M. (2014). Antenatal depression and children's developmental outcomes: Potential mechanisms and treatment options. *Archives of Women's Mental Health, 23*(10), 957–971. doi: DOI 10.1007/s00787-014-0582-3

Weinberg, M. K., Tronick, E. Z., Beeghly, M., Olson, K. L., Kernan, H., & Riley, J. M. (2001). Subsyndromal depressive symptoms and major depression in postpartum women. *American Journal of Orthopsychiatry, 71*(1), 87–97.

Weis, K. L., Lederman, R. P., Walker, K. C., & Chan, W. (2017). Mentors offering maternal support reduces prenatal, pregnancy-specific anxiety in a sample of military women. *Journal of Obstetric, Gynecologic, and Neonatal Nursing, 46*(5), 669–685.

Winkler, D., Pjrek, E., & Kasper, S. (2005). Anger attacks in depression—evidence for a male depressive syndrome. *Psychotherapy and Psychosomatics, 74*(5), 303–307.

Wisner, K., Sit, D. Y., McShea, M. C., Rizzo, D. M., Zoretich, R. A., Hughes, C. L.,… Hanusa, B. H. (2013). Onset timing, thoughts of self-harm, and diagnoses in postpartum women with screen-positive depression findings. *JAMA Psychiatry, 70*, 490–498. doi: 10.1001/jamapsychiatry.2013.87

Yonkers, K. A., Lin, H., Howell, H. B., Heath, A. C., Cohen, L. S., Yonkers, K. A.,… Cohen, L. S. (2008). Pharmacologic treatment of postpartum women with new-onset major depressive disorder: A randomized controlled trial with paroxetine. *Journal of Clinical Psychiatry, 69*(4), 659–665.

Yonkers, K. A., Wisner, K. L., Stewart, D. E., Oberlander, T. F., Dell, D. L., & Stotland, N. (2009). The management of depression during pregnancy: A report from the American psychiatric association and the American college of obstetricians and gynecologists. *General Hospital Psychiatry, 31.* doi: 10.1016/j.genhosppsych.2009.04.003

Zhao, Y., Kane, I., Mao, L., Shi, S., Wang, J., Lin, Q., & Luo, J. (2016). The prevalence of antenatal depression and its related factors in chinese pregnant women who present with obstetrical complications. *Archives of Psychiatric Nursing, 30*(3), 316–321. doi: 10.1016/j.apnu.2015.11.012

Zuckerman, B., Amero, A., Bauchner, H., & Cabral, H. (1989). Depressive symptoms during pregnancy: Relationship to poor health behaviours. *American Journal of Obstetrics and Gynaecology, 160*, 1107–1111.

13

Risk Factors for Depression and Anxiety during the Perinatal Period

Alessandra Biaggi and Carmine M. Pariante

Introduction

Epidemiological research has demonstrated that the risk of major depression during lifetime is twice in women compared to men and this appears to be stable across different sociocultural backgrounds. This difference in the prevalence of depression has been shown to be greater during the woman's reproductive years (Castro e Couto et al., 2016; Sundstrom Poromaa et al., 2017).

Depression and anxiety are the most common psychiatric disorders during pregnancy and in the postpartum period (Alipour et al., 2012) and they are highly present in high-, low- and middle-income countries (Biaggi et al., 2016). In fact, up to 20% of the women will experience depression and/or anxiety at some point during pregnancy and in the postpartum period (NICE, 2015) and many of them will experience symptoms for the first time in their lives during this period. In fact, pregnancy and the postpartum period are times of increased vulnerability for the onset or the relapse of a mental illness (Smith et al., 2011). This is because pregnancy and delivery bring many physiological and psychosocial changes and both mothers and fathers are required to face high levels of stress and several new challenges during this period (Biaggi et al., 2016). As such, women during the perinatal period are at high risk of experiencing depression, often comorbid with anxiety and perceived stress. However, despite this high vulnerability associated with the perinatal period, this is also an incredible and unique window of opportunity for intervention. In fact, the majority of women will have at least some sort of contact with health professionals during pregnancy and the postpartum period. Indeed, the women's access to maternity services during this period, like no other time in their lives, would allow one to identify not only the women who are currently suffering from depression and anxiety but also those who, despite being currently asymptomatic, are at risk of becoming unwell at same point during the perinatal period. Identifying women at risk would give the opportunity to develop preventive interventions during pregnancy, with the aim to reduce the likelihood that women will develop full-blow episodes of depression with the negative and long-term consequences that these episodes have not only on the woman but also on the child and the family as an all. In addition, preventive interventions during pregnancy may be associated with less stigma compared to treatments for postpartum depression (Becker et al., 2016) and, therefore, women may be more willing to engage.

Despite the increased vulnerability that the perinatal period carries and the high prevalence of these disorders, around 80% of women are not identified as suffering from depression/anxiety and do not receive adequate treatment (Heyningen et al., 2016) or symptoms are identified only much later when they are already severe and pervasive.

There are a number of reasons why depression and anxiety are so far under-diagnosed and undertreated, particularly during the antenatal period. One of the reasons is that women may present with atypical symptoms of depression and unspecified somatic complaints (Posternak & Zimmerman, 2001) such as fatigue, loss of energy, appetite and sleep changes, rather than depressed mood. Therefore, these symptoms cannot be easily differentiated from the common pregnancy-related symptoms (Lee et al., 2007; Marchesi et al., 2009). Moreover, women who are already reluctant to share symptoms of sadness and irritability due to the expectations of maternity as a time of exclusive joy (Marcus, 2009) tend to consider emotional complaints as part of the physical and hormonal changes that occur during pregnancy (Bowen & Muhajarine, 2006).

Literature has shown multiple psychosocial, environmental and obstetric risk factors for antenatal and postnatal depression and anxiety (Biaggi et al., 2016; Norhayati et al., 2015) and it is likely that these factors may combine together to increase the risk that some women will develop depression or anxiety while others will stay well.

It is indeed of major importance to identify early on, during pregnancy, the women who are at risk of developing these disorders and those who are already symptomatic, also considering that the prevalence of antenatal depression has been shown to be similar or even higher than postnatal depression (Heron et al., 2004). Moreover, antenatal depression is a very strong risk factor for postpartum depression, with half of the episodes having their onset in the antenatal period (Coll et al., 2017). Furthermore, postnatal depression has been associated with difficulties in the mother-infant relationship, parenting stress and less optimal development in the infant (Leigh & Milgrom, 2008; Murray & Cooper, 1997).

Therefore, the aim of this chapter is to give an overview on the main psychosocial, environmental and obstetric risk factors involved in the onset of antenatal and postnatal depression and anxiety. Other potential factors such as breastfeeding and maternal sleep have also been discussed in relation to postnatal depression. However, other possible risk factors such as the health factors involved in the onset of perinatal depression have not been discussed in this review.

This chapter includes the most up-to-date findings on risk factors for antenatal and postnatal depression and anxiety. Few systematic reviews and meta-analysis have been previously published on risk factors for antenatal and postnatal depression. As such, if readers would like to obtain further information, they may refer to these reviews (Beck, 2001; Biaggi et al., 2016; Lancaster et al., 2010; Norhayati et al., 2015; Robertson et al., 2004).

Moreover, within this chapter, part of the section on risk factors for antenatal depression and anxiety builds on our recent published review (Biaggi et al., 2016).

Risk Factors for Antenatal Depression and Anxiety

Anxiety and depression are very common during pregnancy. In particular, approximately one in six women will experience anxiety symptoms and one in ten will experience depressive symptoms during the antenatal period (Kastello et al., 2016). Depression and anxiety are highly comorbid during pregnancy with women who experience antenatal anxiety being up to three times more likely to suffer from depression as well (Alvarado-Esquivel et al., 2016; Della Vedova et al., 2011; Leigh & Milgrom, 2008; Mohamad Yusuff et al., 2016; Waldie et al., 2015). Within the research into anxiety, studies have shown that "pregnancy-related anxiety" is a clinical distinct phenomenon that can be differentiated from the conventional clinical presentation of anxiety, even if it has shown to have a moderate correlation with antenatal anxiety and depression (Blackmore et al., 2016). "Pregnancy-related anxiety" refers to the preoccupation regarding the pregnancy (developing child, labour and birth, changes in maternal body, and future parenting role and concerns) and has been found to be an independent risk factor for antenatal depression in one study conducted in Tanzania where there is a high pregnancy-related mortality (Rwakarema et al., 2015). Because it has been observed that the correlated factors of "pregnancy-related anxiety" can sometimes be differentiated from those associated with the conventional symptoms of anxiety (Blackmore et al., 2016), in this chapter we will focus on understanding which are the main psychosocial, environmental and obstetric risk factors that have been associated with the common clinical presentation of antenatal depression and anxiety.

Psychiatric, Psychological and Childhood-Related Risk Factors

Women who have a previous history of mental illness, in particular of depression and anxiety at any time during their lifetime, are at greater risk of experiencing a new episode during pregnancy (Akcali Aslan et al., 2014; Balestrieri et al., 2012; Bayrampour et al., 2015; Coll et al., 2017; Dayan et al., 2010; Heyningen et al., 2016; Lydsdottir et al., 2014; Marchesi et al., 2014; Martini et al., 2015; Patton et al., 2015; Redshaw & Henderson, 2013; Rich-Edwards et al., 2006; Shakeel et al., 2015). In particular, about 50% of the women who are depressed during pregnancy experienced major depressive disorder at some point before in their lifespan (Marcus et al., 2003), while for the remaining 50%, this is their first episode of depression (Raisanen et al., 2014). As such, a previous history of depression or anxiety has been shown to be one of the strongest risk factors for antenatal depression/anxiety, and research has observed a more than ten-fold increased risk for women with lifetime major depression (Castro e Couto et al., 2016; Waldie et al., 2015).

The role of a history of personality disorder as a risk factor for anxiety and depression during pregnancy has been recently investigated for the first time in one study (Hudson et al., 2017). The authors have found that a preconception personality disorder increased the risk of developing anxiety symptoms of more than three times, also after adjusting for preconception background factors and common mental disorders. Regarding depressive symptoms, the risk was increased of just below two times, after adjusting for the above-mentioned factors. A possible explanation to this increased risk is that women with personality disorders may be more likely to be in context of financial difficulties, substance misuse and social isolation which may reduce their ability to cope with the stressors of pregnancy (Hudson et al., 2017).

A family history of psychiatric illness during the lifespan has also been shown to be a risk factor for antenatal depression (Jeong et al., 2013; Lydsdottir et al., 2014), although there is much less evidence in the literature compared to a personal history of mental illness.

Research into antenatal depression has also considered smoking, alcohol and substance consumption as possible risk factors. As such, studies have found a significant correlation between antenatal anxiety and depression and past (Lee et al., 2007) or current (Marcus et al., 2003) use of alcohol. Substance use during pregnancy has also been found to be strongly associated with antenatal depression (Fellenzer & Cibula, 2014; Holzman et al., 2006). Smoking before or during pregnancy has also been observed to be associated with antenatal depression and anxiety (Abuidhail & Abujilban, 2014; Alvarado-Esquivel et al., 2016; Bottomley & Lancaster, 2008; Bowen et al., 2009; Lydsdottir et al., 2014; Marcus et al., 2003; Raisanen et al., 2014; Rubertsson et al., 2014). Despite the evidence supporting the association between antenatal depression and smoking, alcohol and substance use, it is not always clear whether smoking or alcohol consumption increase the risk of depression or if it is depression that is associated with less healthy behaviours. In fact, it is well established that people who are depressed are more likely to smoke compared to those who are not (Waldie et al., 2015).

Research has also highlighted the important role of maternal childhood experiences of being parented and maternal attachment style towards her caregivers. In particular, it has been shown that women who had a parenting's style characterized by both low care and high control were six times more likely to experience anxiety during pregnancy and seven times more likely to develop postnatal depression (Grant et al., 2012). Similarly to the study of Grant et al., another study (Della Vedova et al., 2011) found that women who had a relationship with their mothers characterized by low affection and high control in childhood were at an increased risk of depression during pregnancy. The authors also found that a history of miscarriage in the woman's mother was an independent risk factor for antenatal depression, showing that the experience of sufferance in the mother figure could have an impact on the child and could arise again when a woman is about to become a mother (Della Vedova et al., 2011).

Likewise, a research conducted by Bifulco et al. found that women with an avoidant style of attachment (but not those with an anxious style of attachment) were more likely to develop antenatal depression (Bifulco et al., 2004). One of the possible explanations could be that for women with an avoidant attachment style, pregnancy could be perceived as intrusive because of their tendency to avoid close relationships and this may increase their risk of developing depression. On the contrary, for women with an anxious attachment style, pregnancy could satisfy their needs of closeness and reduce their fear of separation and therefore may reduce their chance of developing depression during this period (Bifulco et al., 2004).

Research has also highlighted that women who did not experience an adequate emotional support from their own mother (Jeong et al., 2013) or women who had developed ambivalent attachment styles (and who also perceive low level of support from their partners) are more likely to experience depressive symptoms during the perinatal period (Simpson et al., 2003). Similarly, another study has found parental rejection during childhood to be associated with depression during pregnancy although this was only significant in the univariate analyses and not in the multivariate analyses (Dayan et al., 2010). The results of the studies conducted to investigate the quality of the woman's experiences of being parented as a source of risk are in accordance with the clinical evidence that the woman's relationship with her parents, in particular the mother, is extremely important for her well-being during pregnancy. The absence of a caring relationship with the mother figure makes more difficult for the mother-to-be to adapt to the pregnancy and to develop a positive identity as mother. We know that a woman during pregnancy goes through a mental reorganization which helps her to prepare for motherhood and the quality of the relationship with her own parents, in particular the mother, has an important influence in this process (Ammaniti & Trentini, 2009). As such, a positive internalized experience with her own mother helps the mother-to-be to manage negative emotions more efficiently and to develop a positive relationship with her baby (Jeong et al., 2013). On the contrary, unresolved issues and memories can be reactivated during this process and can negatively impact the mother's response to the baby after the birth (Raphael-Leff, 2010). To this end, experiences of abuse during childhood have been observed to be strong risk factors for depression and anxiety during pregnancy (Brittain et al., 2015; Leigh & Milgrom, 2008; Plant et al., 2013; Robertson-Blackmore et al., 2013; Wosu et al., 2015). In particular, women who experienced sexual abuse during childhood are two times more likely to become depressed during pregnancy (Robertson-Blackmore et al., 2013). One of the mechanisms that could explain why the experience of childhood maltreatment is a strong risk factor for antenatal depression is that childhood maltreatment has been associated with a persistent activation of the two main systems involved in the stress response: the hypothalamic-pituitary-adrenal (HPA) axis and the inflammatory system (Baumeister et al., 2014; Pariante & Lightman, 2008). The hyperactivity of these two systems is also present in depression, and it is therefore considered to be part of its pathogenesis. As both systems are over-stimulated during normal pregnancy, this may make mothers more susceptible to depression in the context of previous exposure to childhood maltreatment (Danese et al., 2007; Heim et al., 2008; Pariante, 2014; Pariante & Lightman, 2008; Robertson-Blackmore et al., 2013). Psychological mechanisms, including for example the reactivation of a previous sexual trauma during pregnancy, experiences and feelings of shame and low self-esteem, are also considered to be very important (Mezey et al., 2005; Plant et al., 2013).

Adverse Life Events and Perceived Stress

Although it has been suggested that childhood abuse may have a specific negative impact on maternal mental health during pregnancy, research has shown (Biaggi et al., 2016) that experiences of abuse, sexual assault and domestic violence in any time during adult life, even beyond childhood, are some of the most powerful risk factors for depression, anxiety and post-traumatic symptoms during pregnancy (Akcali Aslan et al., 2014; Brittain et al., 2015; Castro e Couto et al., 2016; Dibaba et al., 2013; Heyningen et al., 2016; Karmaliani et al., 2009; Lydsdottir et al., 2014; Mahenge et al., 2013; Martini et al., 2015), particularly if the abusive experiences are perpetrated by intimate partners (Martin et al., 2006). Specifically, a recent study has found that women who had experienced severe psychological and sexual violence perpetrated by their intimated partners at any time in the 12 months before were respectively 3.16 times and 2.29 times more likely to experience depressive symptoms during pregnancy (Kastello et al., 2016). To this end, a systematic review on domestic violence and perinatal mental disorders (Howard et al., 2013) has shown that the women with probable depression during pregnancy and in the postnatal period were three to five times more likely to have experienced domestic violence during the adult lifetime, including the current pregnancy. These data show a strong association between antenatal depression and the probability that women may experience domestic violence. This may suggest not only that women who experience domestic violence may be more at risk of experiencing depression but also that women who are depressed may be more at risk of experiencing domestic violence (Howard et al., 2013).

It is well established in the literature that the experience of adverse events and high levels of stress can have a negative impact on an individual well-being at any time during lifetime and research has shown that about 80% of the episodes of depression in women follow the experience of stressful life events (Wright et al., 2015). Pregnancy is itself a time of stress due to the high number of changes and challenges that parents are asked to dial with. As such, the occurrence of adverse life events during this period, such as the death or the illness of a relative, a relationship breakdown, losing a job, a major financial crisis and high perceived stress, can have a particular detrimental effect on the woman's mental health and have been shown to be some of the strongest risk factors for antenatal depression and anxiety (Abujilban et al., 2014; Bayrampour et al., 2015; Bowen et al., 2009; Brittain et al., 2015; Della Vedova et al., 2011; Heyningen et al., 2016; Leigh & Milgrom, 2008; Melville et al., 2010; Ratcliff et al., 2015; Rubertsson et al., 2003; Shakeel et al., 2015; Underwood et al., 2017; Verreault et al., 2014). In particular, a recent study has found that a one-point increase in perceived stress was associated with a 1.34 increase in the probability that women may experience antenatal depression (Waldie et al., 2015) and similar results have been found regarding state anxiety (Akiki et al., 2016). However, very little research has been conducted to understand whether certain types of events, for example those who involve the interpersonal area of the woman, may be more associated with antenatal depression than others. In particular, the partner has a very important supporting role during the transition to motherhood and stressful life events within the intimate relationship may be very distressing for the woman. A study (Wright et al., 2015) has addressed this research question and found that despite stressful life events both related and not related to the partner relationship were associated with an increased risk of depression during pregnancy and in the first six months after the delivery, those related to the partner relationship carried a significantly higher risk compared to other types of events. Similarly, another study found that stress related to severe marital conflict, and stress related to the health of the foetus and to serious difficulties at work were some of the strongest risk factors for antenatal depression (Dayan et al., 2010).

Social Support and Marital Relationship

Research has shown that social support, in particular partner support, and marital satisfaction have a very strong protective role towards maternal mental health during pregnancy (Lee et al., 2007; Rich-Edwards et al., 2006; Zeng et al., 2015) and can attenuate the negative impact of adverse life events, reducing the probability that women may suffer from emotional distress when facing stressful events (Glazier et al., 2004). In particular, research has highlighted that lack of social support, in particular of partner support, is one of the most powerful risk factors for depression and anxiety during pregnancy (Agostini et al., 2015; Dibaba et al., 2013; Faisal-Cury et al., 2009; Golbasi et al., 2010; Jeong et al., 2013; Leigh & Milgrom, 2008; Marchesi et al., 2014; Nasreen et al., 2011; Ratcliff et al., 2015; Srinivasan et al., 2015; Waqas et al., 2015; Westdahl et al., 2007; Yanikkerem et al., 2013). This is not surprising giving the fact that pregnancy is already a highly stressful time for the woman. During this period, a problematic, conflictual and not supporting relationship can increase the levels of stress which may make more difficult for the mother to adjust to the changes that pregnancy and motherhood bring and, therefore, may rise the risk of depression (George et al., 2016; Giardinelli et al., 2012; Marchesi et al., 2009; Srinivasan et al., 2015; Underwood et al., 2017). To this end, a recent study (Akiki et al., 2016) has found that lack of support from the family and the partner was significantly associated with higher levels of state anxiety, while low level of support from friends was not a significant determinant, suggesting that close relationships may have a distinct role in protecting woman's mental health during this period.

Socio-Demographic and Environmental Risk Factors

Because lack of social and partner support has been associated with an increased risk of antenatal depression and anxiety, other factors such as marital status may be associated with the level of support the woman receives and, therefore, may be themselves a source of risk. To this end, although some studies have found that single women or women with partners not living in the same house are more at risk of antenatal depression (Brittain et al., 2015; Faisal-Cury et al., 2009; Figueiredo et al., 2007; Jeong et al., 2013; Manikkam & Burns, 2012; Marcus et al., 2003; Weobong et al., 2014), other studies have not found such results (Agostini et al., 2015; Dayan et al., 2010; Glazier et al., 2004; Husain et al., 2012). And interestingly, a study found that women with unsupported partners had higher levels of depression than single mothers (Bilszta et al., 2008). This may suggest that marital status cannot be considered per se as a source of risk but needs to be considered together with other important information such as the level of support that the partner provides and the woman's level of satisfaction with the relationship.

Together with marital status, many other socio-demographic factors have been considered in the literature but the results are not always consistent and further research is needed to better understand the role of these factors. Regarding age, some studies have found that young women are more at risk of depression and anxiety during pregnancy (Bodecs et al., 2013; Fellenzer & Cibula, 2014; Hartley et al., 2011; Martini et al., 2015; Rubertsson et al., 2014; Sundstrom Poromaa et al., 2017), while other studies found older women to be more at risk (Ali et al., 2012; Fisher et al., 2013; Golbasi et al., 2010; Luke et al., 2009; Nasreen et al., 2011; Yanikkerem et al., 2013). It has also been observed that adolescent mothers and very young mothers under the age of 17 are at particular high risk of depression (Figueiredo et al., 2007; Siegel & Brandon, 2014). However, many other studies have not found age to be a significant contributor for antenatal depression and anxiety (Agostini et al., 2015; Balestrieri et al., 2012; Castro e Couto et al., 2016; Dayan et al., 2010; Srinivasan et al., 2015; Wright et al., 2015).

Antenatal depression and anxiety seem to be more prevalent in women with low educational achievements (Abujilban et al., 2014; Bodecs et al., 2013; Bunevicius et al., 2009; Dayan et al.,

2010; Dmitrovic et al., 2014; Faisal-Cury & Rossi Menezes, 2007; Fellenzer & Cibula, 2014; Gavin et al., 2011; Marcus et al., 2003; Qiao et al., 2009), in women who are unemployed or housewives (Bodecs et al., 2013; Giardinelli et al., 2012; Lydsdottir et al., 2014; Marchesi et al., 2009; Marcus et al., 2003; Rubertsson et al., 2014; Rubertsson et al., 2003; Underwood et al., 2017) and in women with financial difficulties (Leigh & Milgrom, 2008; Prady et al., 2013; Weobong et al., 2014; Zeng et al., 2015). In particular, one recent study found that the prevalence of antenatal depression was inversely related to maternal education level. To this end, the study found that women with 0–4 years, 5–8 years and 9–11 years of education were respectively 5.5, 4.3 and 2.3 times more likely to present depression compared to women with 12 or more years of education (Coll et al., 2017). The authors have suggested that the magnitude of this association may be partly explained by other socio-economic factors, such as low income, often associated with lower educational level. Some research has also been conducted regarding food insecurity (Heyningen et al., 2016), which is considered a proxy measure of poverty, and has found that women experiencing food insecurity were two and half times more likely to experience an episode of major depression during pregnancy. Research has also shown that women whose partners are unemployed are more likely to experience depression during pregnancy (Akcal et al., 2014; Husain et al., 2011; Karmaliani et al., 2009).

The results of these studies show that negative outcomes are more common when multiple risk factors are present and we know that this often happens in contexts of economical and social adversity where women are exposed to multiple sources of risk.

Nevertheless, some studies have not found education, employment and financial hardships to be significant risk factors (Agostini et al., 2015; Glazier et al., 2004; Husain et al., 2012; Josefsson et al., 2002; Karmaliani et al., 2009; Lanzi et al., 2009; Ratcliff et al., 2015; Srinivasan et al., 2015; Zelkowitz et al., 2004).

Inconsistent results have also been found regarding the differences in prevalence of antenatal depression between different ethnic groups. In fact, some studies have reported higher levels of depression in women who belong to minority ethnic groups such as Black, Latina and Asian mothers compared to White mothers (Gavin et al., 2011; Melville et al., 2010; Redshaw & Henderson, 2013; Shakeel et al., 2015; Verreault et al., 2014; Waldie et al., 2015). It has been suggested that these higher levels of depression could be a consequence of the stress that these women may experience due to discrimination (Prady et al., 2013). However, research conducted in the United Kingdom has shown that Black mothers, despite belonging to a minority ethnic group and living in more deprived areas, did not show higher levels of depression during the perinatal period compared to White British mothers (Edge, 2007) and some studies did not find any difference in the levels of depressive symptoms in women belonging to minority groups (Canady et al., 2008; Castro e Couto et al., 2016; Dayan et al., 2010; Jesse et al., 2005; Marcus et al., 2003). On the contrary, a recent systematic review on the prevalence of antenatal depression among different ethnicities in the United States has found that, despite a few exceptions, the majority of studies reported higher levels of depression in Black and Hispanic mothers compared to White mothers (Mukherjee et al., 2016). It is likely that the role of ethnicity, similarly to marital status, may be more complex than what it does appear to be. As such, it is possible that the higher levels of depressive symptoms found in the minorities ethnic groups may be the results of other contextual and socio-demographic risk factors such as financial difficulties (Rich-Edwards et al., 2006) and lower educational level (Coll et al., 2017), often present in women who belong to minority ethnic groups. As such, low socio-economic factors and, in particular, income are likely to play a role behind the differences in the prevalence of antenatal depression between different ethnicities and not all the studies have accounted for income (Mukherjee et al., 2016). In fact, although some research has found that, even after controlling for education, age, parity and income, depression was still higher in Hispanic and Black mothers compared to White mothers (Stewart et al., 2007), other research has found that after adjusting for income, ethnicity was not an independent factor anymore (Rich-Edwards et al., 2006). It is also possible that although women who belong to minority groups and live in more deprived areas may be more at risk of depression, they may also have more resources such as a strong sense of community and spirituality, and these may function as protective factors and may prevent them from experiencing depressive symptoms (Jesse et al., 2005; Prady et al., 2013).

Obstetric- and Pregnancy-Related Risk Factors

Within the factors that have been considered in the onset of antenatal depression and anxiety, obstetric- and pregnancy-related factors have received a considerable attention in the literature. In particular, an unplanned and/or unwanted pregnancy has been found to be another strong risk factor for antenatal depression and anxiety, with a high number of studies consistently reporting an increased risk in these women (Akcali Aslan et al., 2014; Bayrampour et al., 2015; Brittain et al., 2015; Dibaba et al., 2013; Giardinelli et al., 2012; Jeong et al., 2013; Manikkam & Burns, 2012; Marchesi et al., 2009; Mohamad Yusuff et al., 2016; Redshaw & Henderson, 2013; Rich-Edwards et al., 2006; Underwood et al., 2017; Waqas et al., 2015; Weobong et al., 2014; Yanikkerem et al., 2013). Specifically, an unwanted pregnancy seems to be associated with an increased risk of depression particularly in the first trimester. It has been reported that women may be more at risk during this period because this is when they are coping with the new, unexpected and, perhaps, undesired event (Lee et al., 2007). Moreover, women who feel unsure/unhappy about the pregnancy have been observed to suffer from higher levels of anxiety and depression during pregnancy (Akiki et al., 2016; Heyningen et al., 2016). It has been suggested that negative feelings towards the pregnancy may make more difficult for the mother to cope with stress and, therefore, may negatively impact her mental health during this period (Akiki et al., 2016). It has also been observed that women who feel unhappy with the foetal gender (Alvarado-Esquivel et al., 2016) or women who feel the pressure of having a male infant, particularly in certain cultural backgrounds such as the Indian society (George et al., 2016), may be more likely to experience depressive symptoms.

A history of pregnancy or delivery complications, current pregnancy complications and a history of pregnancy loss or termination have also been repeatedly reported in the literature to be strong risk factors for a woman suffering from depression, anxiety and pregnancy-specific anxieties during pregnancy (Adewuya et al., 2007; Chojenta et al., 2014; Faisal-Cury et al., 2009; Fisher et al., 2013; Gong et al., 2013; Raisanen et al., 2014; Stewart et al., 2014; Weobong et al., 2014; Zeng et al., 2015) even if some studies have not reported any significant association (Bicking Kinsey et al., 2015; Fisher et al., 2010). Pregnancy and delivery complications and the unexpected loss of a pregnancy are highly traumatic events and the level of distress can easily persist or be reactivated during a new pregnancy. This level of distress and the fear for a new loss can significantly increase the risk that the woman may experience depression and/or anxiety. Specifically, the risk for the woman to experience depression is higher if the interval between pregnancies is less than six months. In fact, the Word Health Organization recommends an interval of at least six months after a pregnancy loss (Gong et al., 2013). This is because women need time to recover not only physically but also mentally from the traumatic event (WHO, 2005).

While an unwanted pregnancy and a history of pregnancy complications or pregnancy loss have been consistently found to be quite clear risk factors for antenatal depression and anxiety, the role of parity and gravidity is still controversial within the literature. Some studies have found multiparous women to be more at risk (Coll et al., 2017; Lanzi et al., 2009; Redshaw & Henderson, 2013; Yanikkerem et al., 2013), while other studies have found nulliparous or primiparous women to be more at risk (Ali et al., 2012; Fisher et al., 2013; Raisanen et al., 2014) and other studies have not found parity to be a significant contributor for antenatal depression (Abujilban et al., 2014; Akiki et al., 2016; Fisher et al., 2010; Ratcliff et al., 2015; Rubertsson et al., 2003;

Underwood et al., 2017). It has been hypothesized that the higher levels of depression found in multiparous women in some studies may possibly be explained by the increased levels of parenting stress that these women are often experiencing, which make them more vulnerable to depression. The association between parenting stress and depression in multiparous women may be particularly present in the context of low socio-economic status (Coll et al., 2017). However, primiparous women may be equally at an increased risk, due to the many new challenges that they are facing during this period. Further research is needed to better understand the role of parity in the onset of antenatal depression and, particularly, whether multiparous or primiparous/nulliparous women are more at risk. Similarly to parity, regarding gravidity, some studies have reported that women with a greater number of pregnancies are more at risk (Ajinkya et al., 2013; Records & Rice, 2007), while others have reported women at their first pregnancy to be more at risk (Karmaliani et al., 2009) and other studies have not found any association between gravidity and antenatal depression (Fisher et al., 2010; Srinivasan et al., 2015).

There is also some evidence that women who experience fear of childbirth have more than twice the risk of developing depression during pregnancy (Raisanen et al., 2014).

Personality Factors

Research into antenatal depression has also highlighted the role of personality factors in increasing the risk of depression and anxiety during pregnancy. We know from the literature in depression outside the perinatal period that negative cognitive styles, perfectionism and low self-esteem are often present in people who are depressed. Literature has shown that women with these personality factors are also more at risk of becoming depressed and anxious during pregnancy (Akiki et al., 2016; Bayrampour et al., 2015; Bunevicius et al., 2009; Ginsburg et al., 2008; Leigh & Milgrom, 2008; Mohammad et al., 2011). In fact, women with low self-esteem and self-efficacy may experience more difficulties in dealing with the stresses during pregnancy and, therefore, may be more likely to develop anxiety and depression (Lee et al., 2007).

Risk Factors for Postnatal Depression and Anxiety

Postpartum depression is the second most common complication related to childbirth after caesarean section (Gregoire, 1995), affecting approximately 13% of the women (Robertson et al., 2004; Stewart & Vigod, 2016). Postpartum depression, as antenatal depression, is often comorbid with anxiety (Falah-Hassani et al., 2016; Farr et al., 2014).

Many psychosocial and environmental risk factors have been shown to play a role in the onset of depression and anxiety in the postpartum period and many of them are common risk factors to the antenatal period.

Psychiatric, Psychological and Childhood-Related Risk Factors

A history of mental health disorders, in particular depression and anxiety, has been observed to be one of the strongest risk factors for postpartum depression and anxiety (Alfayumi-Zeadna et al., 2015; Bell et al., 2016; Cohen et al., 2002; De Venter et al., 2016; Leigh & Milgrom, 2008; Milgrom et al., 2008; O'Hara & Swain, 1996; Parker et al., 2015; Raisanen et al., 2013; Rich-Edwards et al., 2006; Robertson et al., 2004; Roomruangwong et al., 2016; Seimyr et al., 2013; Theme Filha et al., 2016). Women with a history of depression have been observed to be over six times more likely to develop symptoms of depression in the postpartum period (de Castro et al., 2015).

A family history of psychiatric disorders is associated with an increased risk of postnatal depression, although the associated risk seems not to be as high as having a personal history of mental illness. However, this information sometimes is hard to be collected as patients are not always aware of the psychiatric history of their relatives (Robertson et al., 2004).

Literature has also shown that antenatal depression and anxiety are strong predictors of postpartum depression and anxiety (Alipour et al., 2012; Bell et al., 2016; De Venter et al., 2016; Gaillard et al., 2014; Leigh & Milgrom, 2008; Milgrom et al., 2008; Mohamad Yusuff et al., 2015; Ngai & Ngu, 2015; O'Hara & Swain, 1996; Parker et al., 2015; Raisanen et al., 2013; Rich-Edwards et al., 2006; Robertson et al., 2004; Roomruangwong et al., 2016; Tachibana et al., 2015; Tham et al., 2016; Weobong et al., 2015). Women with untreated depression during pregnancy are seven times more likely to experience postnatal depression compared to women with no antenatal depression (Stewart & Vigod, 2016).

Alcohol use (Theme Filha et al., 2016) and smoking (Raisanen et al., 2013) during pregnancy have been found to be associated with an increased risk of postnatal depression.

Research has also investigated the role of maternal attachment style in relation to postnatal depression, although only a few studies have been conducted in this area. In particular, a study conducted by Bifulco et al. found that women with an anxious attachment style (but not those with an avoidant attachment style) are at an increased risk of experiencing depression in the postpartum period (Bifulco et al., 2004). One of the possible explanations could be that for women with an anxious attachment style, the birth of the baby could reduce closeness and activate fear of separation and loss and this could increase the risk of depressive symptoms. On the contrary, for women with an avoidant attachment style, the birth of the baby could recreate boundaries that have been previously threated by the pregnancy and this could reduce their risk of experiencing depressive symptoms (Bifulco et al., 2004).

Research on childhood maltreatment and postnatal depression has shown inconsistent results. In fact, although some studies have found positive associations, they have not always controlled for the influence of other possible factors in the analyses (Wosu et al., 2015). Also, some studies have not found childhood maltreatment to be associated with an increased risk of postpartum depression (Cohen et al., 2002; De Venter et al., 2016). This is in line with the research that has shown that childhood maltreatment is a risk factor for antenatal depression but not for postnatal depression (Alvarez-Segura et al., 2014; Robertson-Blackmore et al., 2013). Moreover, it is well known that childhood maltreatment is a risk factor for depression during the lifetime, which in turn has been shown to be one of the strongest predictor of perinatal depression.

Adverse Life Events and Perceived Stress

Studies have observed that women who have experienced domestic violence before pregnancy, during pregnancy or in the postnatal period are at an increased risk of developing postnatal depression (de Castro et al., 2015; Jackson et al., 2015; Turkcapar et al., 2015). For example, one study (Khalifa et al., 2016) found that history of violence was the strongest determinant for postpartum depression, increasing the risk to seven times. Another study (Shamu et al., 2016) found that women who had experienced severe violence from the intimate partner during pregnancy were at an increased risk of developing postpartum depression. In particular, although all types of severe intimate partner violence were found to be associated with postpartum depression, severe emotional violence or severe combined forms of intimate partner violence were found to be strongly associated with postpartum depression. These results highlight the importance of evaluating not only whether the woman has suffered from intimate partner violence but also violence severity (Shamu et al., 2016). Similarly, another research found that intimate partner violence intensity was significantly associated with postnatal depression symptom severity. The authors showed not only that intimate partner violence was associated with subsequent greater depression symptom severity but also that depression symptom severity was associated with a greater risk of subsequent experience of intimate partner violence (Tsai et al., 2016b). Stressful life events happened during pregnancy, in the postpartum period or in the last 12 months (Bell et al., 2016; Muscat et al., 2014; O'Hara & Swain, 1996; Robertson et al., 2004; Wright et al., 2015) as well as high perceived levels of stress experienced in the last six months (Giri et al., 2015; Parker et al., 2015; Underwood et al., 2017) have also been observed to be risk factors for depressive and anxiety symptomatology in the postpartum period.

Social Support and Marital Relationship

Social support is a very important element in the postpartum period as it helps to cope with the stressors of becoming a new mother, functioning as a strong protective factor against postpartum depressive symptoms (Rich-Edwards et al., 2006). As such, women who report to be satisfied with their marital relationship, to have had a high number of supportive people during pregnancy and to have received high levels of support from their partners during the perinatal period are less likely to develop depression in the postpartum period (Milgrom et al., 2008; Mohamad Yusuff et al., 2015; Morikawa et al., 2015). On the contrary, women who report low instrumental and emotional support, high perceived isolation and marital problems during pregnancy and in the postpartum period are at an increased risk of developing postpartum depressive symptoms (Alfayumi-Zeadna et al., 2015; Cohen et al., 2002; de Castro et al., 2015; Muscat et al., 2014; Ngai & Ngu, 2015; O'Hara & Swain, 1996; Robertson et al., 2004). To this end, studies have shown that depressive symptoms in the postpartum period are up to two-fold higher in immigrant women compared to non-immigrant women (Falah-Hassani et al., 2015; Gaillard et al., 2014). In particular, immigrant women have been observed to be at risk of developing depression if they have been living in the country for a short period of time, if they have low social support, marital problems and perceived low income (Falah-Hassani et al., 2015). Thus, research has shown that living in areas of lower own ethnic density (proportion of individuals from the individual same ethnic group) is independently associated with postpartum depression in White women (but not in women belonging to BME groups). As such, living in areas of high own ethnic density is protective against postpartum depression in White women (Du Preez et al., 2016). Having a baby can be very challenging and it is possible that living in an area with a high number of co-ethnics people (most likely other mums) may help women to feel less isolated during this time when they are predominantly at home and may increase the level of practical and emotional support they receive, which we know is a strong protective factor for maternal mental health during the perinatal period (Du Preez et al., 2016).

Single marital status has also been shown to be a risk factor for postnatal depression in a few studies (Lara et al., 2015), although others did not report any significant association (de Castro et al., 2015; Gaillard et al., 2014; Rich-Edwards et al., 2006). There is also some evidence that a short length of partner relationship may be associated with depressive symptomatology (Seimyr et al., 2013).

Socio-Demographic and Environmental Risk Factors

Young age has been found to be another risk factor for postpartum depressive symptomatology (Khalifa et al., 2016; Lara et al., 2015; Seimyr et al., 2013). In particular, one study (Khalifa et al., 2016) found that an increase in age reduced the risk of developing postnatal depression by almost 20% per year. However, other studies found opposite results and have observed an increased risk of depression in older women (Bell et al., 2016; Glavin et al., 2009), while some studies did not find age to be a significant risk factor for postpartum depression and anxiety (Alfayumi-Zeadna et al., 2015; Beck, 2001; Clout & Brown, 2015; de Castro et al., 2015; Gaillard et al., 2014; McMahon et al., 2011;

Morikawa et al., 2015; O'Hara & Swain, 1996; Roomruangwong et al., 2016), a part from teen-age mothers who are considered at an increased risk (Robertson et al., 2004). A study examined whether first-time older mothers would be at an increased risk but the study did not find any association (McMahon et al., 2015). There is some evidence in the literature that age may have a U-shaped relationship with regard to postnatal depression, with younger and older women being more at risk of experiencing depression (Garcia-Blanco et al., 2017). Although this may explain why studies have found contradictory results, the role of age still needs to be clarified in further research as there are a number of studies that did not found age to be a contributing factor.

Some studies have found low level of education, unemployment, low income and financial hardship to be associated with an increased risk of postnatal depression (Alfayumi-Zeadna et al., 2015; Lara et al., 2015; Rich-Edwards et al., 2006; Seimyr et al., 2013; Shivalli & Gururaj, 2015; Theme Filha et al., 2016; Underwood et al., 2017), while other studies have not found them to be significant contributing factors to postnatal depression and anxiety (Clout & Brown, 2015; de Castro et al., 2015; Gaillard et al., 2014; Giri et al., 2015; Khalifa et al., 2016; Leigh & Milgrom, 2008; Roomruangwong et al., 2016; Turkcapar et al., 2015).

A study conducted in South Africa found food insufficiency (a proxy measure for poverty) to be significantly associated with depressive symptom severity during the perinatal period. However, the authors also found that instrumental support had a modifier effect on symptom severity. In particular, among women who had suffered from food insufficiency, those who had lower level of instrumental support had higher level of depressive symptoms compared to women with higher levels of support who remained more resilient (Tsai et al., 2016a). This is in line with the idea that supportive interactions have a buffering effect against stressful situations and can protect individuals from negative consequences (Cobb, 1976).

Breastfeeding and Sleep

Research into breastfeeding and postnatal depression has shown inconsistent results. Some studies have shown that exclusive breastfeeding is a protective factor for postnatal depression (Khalifa et al., 2016; Mezzacappa & Katlin, 2002). However, other studies have found opposite results, showing that women who breastfeed for longer are at an increased risk of depression (Alder & Bancroft, 1988) and other studies did not find any association (Turkcapar et al., 2015). The majority of studies have not controlled for pre-existing mental health symptoms, so it is not always clear whether it is depression that predicts breastfeeding duration or it is breastfeeding that has an impact on maternal mental health (Borra et al., 2015). To this end, a systematic review on breast-feeding and depression (Dias & Figueiredo, 2015) has shown that, despite there is an unequivocal association between depressive symptoms and shorter duration of breastfeeding, the direction of the relationship is still unclear. Although most studies seem to suggest that depressive symptoms (in both the antenatal and postnatal period) precede and lead to an early cessation of breastfeeding, research has also shown that negative breastfeeding experiences (negative breastfeeding attitudes, breastfeeding difficulties, worries and pain, low breastfeeding self-efficacy) predict the development of postnatal depression. Moreover, some evidence seems to suggest that breastfeeding may function as a moderator in the relationship between antenatal and postnatal depression. In particular, starting to breastfeeding could reduce the levels of depression from the pregnancy to the postpartum period, while breastfeeding cessation could increase depressive scores from the pregnancy to the postpartum period (Dias & Figueiredo, 2015). Furthermore, according to a recent study, the effects of breastfeeding on maternal depressive symptoms are complicated and mediated by breastfeeding intentions and maternal mental health during pregnancy (Borra et al., 2015). As such, among the women who had not been depressed during pregnancy, breastfeeding decreased the risk of depression in women who had wanted to breastfeed their babies, while increased the risk in women who had not planned to breastfeed. Among women who had been depressed during pregnancy, breastfeeding had a protective role not only on women who intended to breastfeed (although the effect was smaller) but also on women who had not planned to breastfeed (Borra et al., 2015).

The results of this studies show that the relationship between breastfeeding and postnatal depression is complicated and not fully clear and that breastfeeding may have a distinct effect on different women.

Regarding infant patterns of sleep and feeding, a study has found that a more disturbed infant sleep and more frequent feeding at six weeks were associated with higher depressive symptomatology scores at 6 and 16 weeks postpartum and higher levels of stress (Sharkey et al., 2016). Similarly, another study has observed that sleeping problems and, to a less extent, feeding problems were significant predictors of depressive symptoms in the postpartum period. Moreover, women with high and rigid baby's regulation beliefs had a significant risk of experiencing depressive symptoms, when the infant pattern of sleep was problematic (Muscat et al., 2014). This confirms previous findings about the role of unmet rigid expectations in the development of depression, when expectations do not meet reality (Muscat et al., 2014). To this end, high levels of parenting stress in the postpartum period have been found to be a significant contributor for postnatal depression (Leigh & Milgrom, 2008).

Poor subjective quality of sleep during pregnancy has also been observed to be associated with postnatal depression, but not with anxiety, independently from prenatal depressive symptoms (Lawson et al., 2015; Okun, 2015; Tham et al., 2016). One of the possible pathways is that poor subjective quality of sleep during pregnancy may impact the mother's coping skills, which in turn increase the risk of depression in the postpartum period. Alternatively, poor subjective sleep during pregnancy may be associated with poor subjective postnatal sleep quality, which in turn increases the risk of depressive symptoms (Tham et al., 2016). To this end, another study (Park et al., 2013) found that a poor subjective quality of sleep in the last trimester of pregnancy and in the early postpartum period was highly associated with postpartum depressive symptom severity.

Obstetric-and Pregnancy-Related Risk Factors

Unplanned pregnancy has been found to be a risk factor for postpartum depression in some studies (Alfayumi–Zeadna et al., 2015; de Castro et al., 2015; Theme Filha et al., 2016), even if others have not reported pregnancy intention to be a significant factor (Clout & Brown, 2015; Gaillard et al., 2014; Khalifa et al., 2016; Rich–Edwards et al., 2006). Negative attitudes towards the pregnancy have been found to be associated with depressive symptomatology in some studies (Limlomwongse & Liabsuetrakul, 2006), while others have found no association (Kitamura et al., 2006). Some studies have found multiparous women to be more at risk of developing depression in the postpartum period (Theme Filha et al., 2016), while some studies have found primiparous women to be more at risk (Glavin et al., 2009; Morikawa et al., 2015; Raisanen et al., 2013; Tachibana et al., 2015) and some studies did not find any significant association between the number of previous children and postpartum depression (Clout & Brown, 2015; Gaillard et al., 2014; Giri et al., 2015; Robertson et al., 2004; Turkcapar et al., 2015). The birth of the first child is associated with greater psychological distress compared to the birth of a second or third child. However, multiparous women may be equally stressed as they need to take care of more children while trying to recover from childbirth.

Research has demonstrated that mothers of preterm and low birth-weight infants are at an increased risk of developing symptoms of depression and anxiety in the postpartum period (Barroso et al., 2015; Helle et al., 2015; Rich–Edwards et al., 2006; Voegtline & Stifter, 2010). In particular, a systematic review found that the prevalence of depression in women of premature babies was up to 40% in the early postpartum (Vigod et al., 2010). Furthermore, mothers of infants with health problems are at an increased risk of developing depressive symptomatology in the postpartum period (Alfayumi-Zeadna et al., 2015; Weobong et al., 2015).

Studies investigating the relationship between previous miscarriage, stillbirth and postnatal depression have shown inconsistent results. In fact, while there is more evidence on the impact of previous pregnancy loss on antenatal depression and anxiety, it is unclear whether depressive symptoms will improve after the birth of a healthy baby (Bicking Kinsey et al., 2015). In fact, although some studies have reported a decrease over time in the level of depressive symptoms in the postpartum period (Armstrong et al., 2009), others have reported that depressive symptoms remain constant during pregnancy and up to 33 months postpartum, suggesting that pregnancy loss may have an impact on mother's well-being also in the postpartum period (Blackmore et al., 2011). To this end, although some researchers have found a significant relationship between history of miscarriage and stillbirth and postnatal depression (Weobong et al., 2015), others have not found any significant association (Roomruangwong et al., 2016). It has been suggested that the number of pregnancy losses that the woman has experienced may possibly play an important role. As such, a study found that while having a history of a pregnancy loss was not associated with an increased risk of depression, having multiple pregnancy losses was associated with a slight elevation in depressive symptoms (Price, 2008). Some studies found pregnancy or delivery complications, stillbirth, congenital anomalies and caesarean section to be significant predictors of postnatal depression (Raisanen et al., 2013; Shivalli & Gururaj, 2015; Weobong et al., 2015), although the effect seems to be small according to a systematic review (Robertson et al., 2004). However, other studies did not find mood delivery, obstetric complications or abnormalities in the baby to be associated with an increased risk of postpartum depression and anxiety (Bell et al., 2016; Fairbrother & Woody, 2007; Roomruangwong et al., 2016; Theme Filha et al., 2016; Turkcapar et al., 2015). A study found that postpartum physical complications were significantly associated with postpartum depression but it did not find mode of delivery to be a significant predictor of postpartum depression (Gaillard et al., 2014). To this end, a review conducted with the purpose to investigate the relationship between caesarean section and postpartum depression did not find any significant association (Carter et al., 2006). Another systematic review on risk factors for postnatal depression (Robertson et al., 2004) reported that although there is a little evidence about the association between caesarean section and postnatal depression, women who had an emergency caesarean are more likely to develop postnatal depression.

While some studies have found fear of childbirth to be a strong risk factor for postnatal depression, increasing the risk to nearly three times in women without a history of depression and to five times in women with a history of depression (Raisanen et al., 2013), other studies have not found such results (Alipour et al., 2012; Fairbrother & Woody, 2007). However, a woman's perception of her birth experience as negative has been found to be associated with elevated anxiety symptoms both at two and eight months postpartum but not with depressive symptoms (Bell et al., 2016). To this end, it has been shown that women who had received a good support and care for them and their babies during labour and birth reported less level of depressive symptomology (Theme Filha et al., 2016). This is in line with the results of a previous review that showed that continuous support during childbirth was associated with multiple positive outcomes such as less instrumental and caesarean birth, shorter labours, babies less likely to have low Apgar scores and women with higher levels of satisfaction with their birth experiences (Hodnett et al., 2013).

Some studies have reported infant gender, in most of the cases female, to be a contributing factor for postnatal depression (Lee et al., 2000; Patel et al., 2002; Shivalli & Gururaj, 2015), while other studies have not found infant gender or satisfaction with the gender (Mohamad Yusuff et al., 2015; Turkcapar et al., 2015; Weobong et al., 2015) to be associated with depressive symptoms. It is likely that the role of infant gender on maternal well-being may vary according to the culture the woman belongs to.

Personality Factors

Research into personality factors has shown that personality traits and negative cognitive styles such as neuroticism, perfectionism, introversion, interpersonal sensitivity and low self-esteem have an impact on the possibility that women may develop postpartum depression and anxiety (Oddo-Sommerfeld et al., 2016; Robertson et al., 2004). One of the cognitive styles that have been found to be associated with an increased risk of postpartum depression is perfectionism (Milgrom et al., 2008). In particular, women with perfectionism often show high standards of performance, high concerns over mistakes, and experience frequent self-doubts, which can produce high levels of stress and can increase the risk of depression during the perinatal period (Gelabert et al., 2012; Maia et al., 2012; Rosan et al., 2016). Moreover, dysfunctional perfectionism and avoidant personality style have been shown to increase the risk of antenatal depression and anxiety, which in turn increase the risk of postpartum depression and anxiety. As such, these negative cognitive styles may not have a direct effect on postpartum depression; however, the combination of cognitive styles and antenatal mental illness would significantly increase the probability that women may develop postpartum depression and anxiety (Oddo-Sommerfeld et al., 2016). Passive coping strategies have also been found to be associated with depressive symptomatology both at 8 and 32 weeks postpartum. The authors also found that neuroticism had a strong effect on coping strategies, with high neuroticism being associated with more passive strategies, suggesting that neuroticism has a key role in the relationship between coping strategies and depressive symptoms in the postpartum period (Gutierrez-Zotes et al., 2015).

Neuroticism itself has been observed to be a strong risk factor for postpartum depression, with non-depressed pregnant women with high levels of neuroticism being up to six times more likely to develop postnatal depression in the first year after giving birth (Boyce et al., 1991; Iliadis et al., 2015; Verkerk et al., 2005). Low self-esteem has been observed to be another strong predictor of postpartum depression (Beck, 2001), although some researchers have found that self-esteem instability (temporal fluctuations in self-esteem in response to stressors and mood changes) may be a better predictor than the general level of self-esteem (Franck et al., 2016).

Research has also shown that women who have maladaptive beliefs about motherhood (such as "I should be more devoted to my baby") are at an increased risk of experiencing depressive symptoms during the perinatal period where their feelings do not match their expectations (Sockol et al., 2014).

It is possible that these cognitive styles may make these women particularly vulnerable when they need to cope with the many changes and unpredictable stressors of motherhood (lack of sleep, infant crying) and this may increase their risk of depression and anxiety (Iliadis et al., 2015; Milgrom et al., 2008). On the contrary, a moderate but realistic antenatal optimism regarding motherhood has been shown to be more protective against postnatal depression compared to both pessimism and high optimism (Churchill & Davis, 2010; Robakis et al., 2015). In fact, having very positive perhaps unrealistic expectations is associated with an increased risk of depressive symptoms as these expectations are likely to be disconfirmed when facing the reality of motherhood (Robakis et al., 2015).

Conclusion

Research has shown that multiple psychosocial, environmental and obstetric risk factors are involved in the aetiology of mood disorders during pregnancy and in the postpartum period (Bilszta et al., 2008). Different sources of risk have been shown to be involved in the onset of antenatal and postnatal depression and anxiety: psychological and psychiatric factors, social support, adverse life events, socio-demographic and environmental factors, obstetric factors and personality factors.

Table 13.1 Most significant risk factors for antenatal and postnatal depression and anxiety

Risk factors	Pregnancy	Postpartum
Personal history of mental illness	✓	✓
Antenatal depression/anxiety		✓
Childhood maltreatment	✓	?
History of abuse, domestic violence	✓	✓
Adverse events during adult life and high perceived stress	✓	✓
Lack of partner/social support	✓	✓
Unplanned/unwanted pregnancy	✓	?
Current/history of pregnancy complications/history of pregnancy loss	✓	?

In particular, literature has shown that some of the most significant contributors of antenatal depression and anxiety include previous history of mental illness, lack of partner or social support, history of abuse including childhood maltreatment or domestic violence, unplanned or unwanted pregnancy, stressful life events and high perceived stress, current or previous pregnancy complications or pregnancy loss (Biaggi et al., 2016; Lancaster et al., 2010). Regarding postnatal depression and anxiety, some of the most significant contributors include antenatal depression and anxiety, previous history of mental illness, poor marital relationship and low partner and social support, stressful life events and history of/current abuse (particularly in developed countries) (Norhayati et al., 2015; Robertson et al., 2004). However, many other factors such as obstetric factors, personality factors and socio-demographic factors also seem to play an important role in the onset of perinatal depression and anxiety, even if their impact seems to be lower compared to other factors. The role of many other factors such as age and parity remains controversial and more research is needed to better understand their contribution to perinatal depression (Table 13.1).

Research has also highlighted that some potential risk factors may have different effects on different women, depending on other associated factors. For example, breastfeeding could increase (or not) the risk of postnatal depression depending on the woman's intention to breastfeed and on her well-being during pregnancy (Borra et al., 2015). Therefore, a specialized and individualized support should be available to all women to prevent them from suffering from depression and anxiety during the perinatal period.

Furthermore, while some risk factors may not be modifiable, other factors may be the target of preventive interventions during pregnancy, a time when most parents have multiple contacts with health professionals and are particularly motivated to promote their babies' and families' well-being. Targeting "high-risk women", with the aim to intervene on modifiable risk factors during pregnancy, may help reducing the likelihood that women may experience depression and anxiety and, in turn, may help promoting the long-term well-being of the child and the family.

Research has shown that a cumulate presence of different risk factors significantly increases the risk that women may develop perinatal depression and anxiety. As such, a study (de Castro et al., 2015) has shown that women who presented four psychosocial risk factors (history of depression, low social support, intimate partner violence and unplanned pregnancy) had a predicted probability of 67% to develop depressive symptoms in the postpartum period. However, the authors have shown that if low social support, intimate partner violence and unplanned pregnancy would be removed, the risk of postpartum depressive symptoms could be reduced to 5.5%, even in the presence of a history of depression (de Castro et al., 2015). These results are extremely important because they show that if multidimensional screenings and preventive interventions would be available for all the women during the perinatal period, rates of depression could be reduced with the long-term positive outcomes that this would have on the child and the family. A such, multidimensional evaluations should be conducted with all pregnant women (Austin, 2014; Milgrom & Gemmill, 2014) and should be repeated more times at different time points during pregnancy as multiple evaluations can show differences in the rates of depression and anxiety, which would not be captured if only one screening was implemented (Lee et al., 2007; Marchesi et al., 2009). First, these screenings should aim to identify women currently suffering from depression and anxiety. Identifying and treating antenatal depression is imperative not only to reduce the well-known long-term negative consequences of the illness, but also to prevent postnatal depression (Stewart & Vigod, 2016). Moreover, these screenings should also be intended to collect information as more detailed as possible on the woman's psychosocial circumstances (e.g. sources of support, personal or family history of mental illness and if occurred during the perinatal period, quality of her relationships, recent life stressors, past or current experience of abuse, substance misuse), to be able to create an estimation of the level of risk during the perinatal period and, therefore, the necessity of preventive interventions (Austin, 2014; Milgrom & Gemmill, 2014; Stewart & Vigod, 2016).

Multidimensional screenings and individual psychosocial interventions may be used together as the combination of these has been shown to be effective among pregnant and postpartum women (Tsai et al., 2016b). Psychosocial interventions would be beneficial in reducing not only the woman's probability of developing perinatal depression but also other collateral risks such as the women's susceptibility to intimate partner violence, considering that studies have reported a strong bidirectional relationship between depression and domestic violence (Howard et al., 2013; Tsai et al., 2016b).

All this evidence seems to suggest that preventive programmes targeting high-risk women that start during pregnancy and continue in the postpartum period are likely to be the most cost-effective interventions for the long-term well-being of the family (O'Hara, 2009).

Unfortunately, many women are still not identified as being at risk for or currently suffering from perinatal depression and anxiety (Andersson et al., 2003; Marcus et al., 2003). It is well know that perinatal depression and anxiety, if untreated, can have long-lasting negative effects on the mother and the child. Therefore, being able to identify the women who are at high risk of developing anxiety and depression during the perinatal period is a crucial public health and clinical priority (Parker et al., 2015).

References

Abuidhail, J., & Abujilban, S. (2014). Characteristics of Jordanian depressed pregnant women: a comparison study. *J Psychiatr Ment Health Nurs, 21*(7), 573–579. doi: 10.1111/jpm.12125

Abujilban, S. K., Abuidhail, J., Al-Modallal, H., Hamaideh, S., & Mosemli, O. (2014). Predictors of antenatal depression among Jordanian pregnant women in their third trimester. *Health Care Women Int, 35*(2), 200–215. doi: 10.1080/07399332.2013.817411

Adewuya, A. O., Ola, B. A., Aloba, O. O., Dada, A. O., & Fasoto, O. O. (2007). Prevalence and correlates of depression in late pregnancy among Nigerian women. *Depress Anxiety, 24*(1), 15–21. doi: 10.1002/da.20221

Agostini, F., Neri, E., Salvatori, P., Dellabartola, S., Bozicevic, L., & Monti, F. (2015). Antenatal depressive symptoms associated with specific life events and sources of social support among Italian women. *Matern Child Health J, 19*(5), 1131–1141. doi: 10.1007/s10995-014-1613-x

Ajinkya, S., Jadhav, P. R., & Srivastava, N. N. (2013). Depression during pregnancy: prevalence and obstetric risk factors among pregnant women attending a tertiary care hospital in Navi Mumbai. *Ind Psychiatry J, 22*(1), 37–40. doi: 10.4103/0972-6748.123615

Akcal, X. A. P., Ayd, X. N. N., Yaz, X. C. X. E., Aksoy, A. N., Kirkan, T. S., & Daloglu, G. A. (2014). Prevalence of depressive disorders and related factors in women in the first trimester of their pregnancies in Erzurum, Turkey. *Int J Soc Psychiatry.* doi: 10.1177/0020764014524738

Akcali Aslan, P., Aydin, N., Yazici, E., Aksoy, A. N., Kirkan, T. S., & Daloglu, G. A. (2014). Prevalence of depressive disorders and related factors in women in the first trimester of their pregnancies in Erzurum, Turkey. *Int J Soc Psychiatry, 60*(8), 809–817. doi: 10.1177/0020764014524738

Akiki, S., Avison, W. R., Speechley, K. N., & Campbell, M. K. (2016). Determinants of maternal antenatal state-anxiety in mid-pregnancy: role of maternal feelings about the pregnancy. *J Affect Disord, 196*, 260–267. doi: 10.1016/j.jad.2016.02.016

Alder, E., & Bancroft, J. (1988). The relationship between breast feeding persistence, sexuality and mood in postpartum women. *Psychol Med, 18*(2), 389–396.

Alfayumi-Zeadna, S., Kaufman-Shriqui, V., Zeadna, A., Lauden, A., & Shoham-Vardi, I. (2015). The association between sociodemographic characteristics and postpartum depression symptoms among Arab-Bedouin women in Southern Israel. *Depress Anxiety, 32*(2), 120–128. doi: 10.1002/da.22290

Ali, N. S., Azam, I. S., Ali, B. S., Tabbusum, G., & Moin, S. S. (2012). Frequency and associated factors for anxiety and depression in pregnant women: a hospital-based cross-sectional study. *ScientificWorldJournal, 2012*, 653098. doi: 10.1100/2012/653098

Alipour, Z., Lamyian, M., & Hajizadeh, E. (2012). Anxiety and fear of childbirth as predictors of postnatal depression in nulliparous women. *Women Birth, 25*(3), e37–43. doi: 10.1016/j.wombi.2011.09.002

Alvarado-Esquivel, C., Sifuentes-Alvarez, A., & Salas-Martinez, C. (2016). Unhappiness with the Fetal Gender is associated with Depression in Adult Pregnant Women Attending Prenatal Care in a Public Hospital in Durango, Mexico. *Int J Biomed Sci, 12*(1), 36–41.

Alvarez-Segura, M., Garcia-Esteve, L., Torres, A., Plaza, A., Imaz, M. L., Hermida-Barros, L.,…Burtchen, N. (2014). Are women with a history of abuse more vulnerable to perinatal depressive symptoms? A systematic review. *Arch Womens Ment Health, 17*(5), 343–357. doi: 10.1007/s00737-014-0440-9

Ammaniti, M., & Trentini, C. (2009). How new knowledge about parenting reveals the neurobiological implications of intersubjectivity: a conceptual synthesis of recent research. *Psychoanalytic Dialogues, 19*(5), 537–555. doi: 10.1080/10481880903231951

Andersson, L., Sundstrom-Poromaa, I., Bixo, M., Wulff, M., Bondestam, K., & aStrom, M. (2003). Point prevalence of psychiatric disorders during the second trimester of pregnancy: a population-based study. *Am J Obstet Gynecol, 189*(1), 148–154.

Armstrong, D. S., Hutti, M. H., & Myers, J. (2009). The influence of prior perinatal loss on parents' psychological distress after the birth of a subsequent healthy infant. *J Obstet Gynecol Neonatal Nurs, 38*(6), 654–666. doi: 10.1111/j.1552-6909.2009.01069.x

Austin, M. P. (2014). Marce International Society position statement on psychosocial assessment and depression screening in perinatal women. *Best Pract Res Clin Obstet Gynaecol, 28*(1), 179–187. doi: 10.1016/j.bpobgyn.2013.08.016

Balestrieri, M., Isola, M., Bisoffi, G., Calo, S., Conforti, A., Driul, L.,… Bellantuono, C. (2012). Determinants of ante-partum depression: a multicenter study. *Soc Psychiatry Psychiatr Epidemiol, 47*(12), 1959–1965. doi: 10.1007/s00127-012-0511-z

Barroso, N. E., Hartley, C. M., Bagner, D. M., & Pettit, J. W. (2015). The effect of preterm birth on infant negative affect and maternal postpartum depressive symptoms: a preliminary examination in an under-represented minority sample. *Infant Behav Dev, 39*, 159–165. doi: 10.1016/j.infbeh.2015.02.011

Baumeister, D., Russell, A., Pariante, C. M., & Mondelli, V. (2014). Inflammatory biomarker profiles of mental disorders and their relation to clinical, social and lifestyle factors. *Soc Psychiatry Psychiatr Epidemiol, 49*(6), 841–849. doi: 10.1007/s00127-014-0887-z

Bayrampour, H., McDonald, S., & Tough, S. (2015). Risk factors of transient and persistent anxiety during pregnancy. *Midwifery, 31*(6), 582–589. doi: 10.1016/j.midw.2015.02.009

Beck, C. T. (2001). Predictors of postpartum depression: an update. *Nurs Res, 50*(5), 275–285.

Becker, M., Weinberger, T., Chandy, A., & Schmukler, S. (2016). Depression during pregnancy and postpartum. *Curr Psychiatry Rep, 18*(3), 32. doi: 10.1007/s11920-016-0664-7

Bell, A. F., Carter, C. S., Davis, J. M., Golding, J., Adejumo, O., Pyra, M.,… Rubin, L. H. (2016). Childbirth and symptoms of postpartum depression and anxiety: a prospective birth cohort study. *Arch Womens Ment Health, 19*(2), 219–227. doi: 10.1007/s00737-015-0555-7

Biaggi, A., Conroy, S., Pawlby, S., & Pariante, C. M. (2016). Identifying the women at risk of antenatal anxiety and depression: a systematic review. *J Affect Disord, 191*, 62–77. doi: 10.1016/j.jad.2015.11.014

Bicking Kinsey, C., Baptiste-Roberts, K., Zhu, J., & Kjerulff, K. H. (2015). Effect of previous miscarriage on depressive symptoms during subsequent pregnancy and postpartum in the first baby study. *Matern Child Health J, 19*(2), 391–400. doi: 10.1007/s10995-014-1521-0

Bifulco, A., Figueiredo, B., Guedeney, N., Gorman, L. L., Hayes, S., Muzik, M.,… Henshaw, C. A. (2004). Maternal attachment style and depression associated with childbirth: preliminary results from a European and US cross-cultural study. *Br J Psychiatry Suppl, 46*, s31–37.

Bilszta, J. L., Tang, M., Meyer, D., Milgrom, J., Ericksen, J., & Buist, A. E. (2008). Single motherhood versus poor partner relationship: outcomes for antenatal mental health. *Aust N Z J Psychiatry, 42*(1), 56–65. doi: 10.1080/00048670701732731

Blackmore, E. R., Cote-Arsenault, D., Tang, W., Glover, V., Evans, J., Golding, J., & O'Connor, T. G. (2011). Previous prenatal loss as a predictor of perinatal depression and anxiety. *Br J Psychiatry, 198*(5), 373–378. doi: 10.1192/bjp.bp.110.083105

Blackmore, E. R., Gustafsson, H., Gilchrist, M., Wyman, C., & T, G. O. C. (2016). Pregnancy-related anxiety: evidence of distinct clinical significance from a prospective longitudinal study. *J Affect Disord, 197*, 251–258. doi: 10.1016/j.jad.2016.03.008

Bodecs, T., Szilagyi, E., Cholnoky, P., Sandor, J., Gonda, X., Rihmer, Z., & Horvath, B. (2013). Prevalence and psychosocial background of anxiety and depression emerging during the first trimester of pregnancy: data from a Hungarian population-based sample. *Psychiatr Danub, 25*(4), 352–358.

Borra, C., Iacovou, M., & Sevilla, A. (2015). New evidence on breastfeeding and postpartum depression: the importance of understanding women's intentions. *Matern Child Health J, 19*(4), 897–907. doi: 10.1007/s10995-014-1591-z

Bottomley, K. L., & Lancaster, S. J. (2008). The association between depressive symptoms and smoking in pregnant adolescents. *Psychol Health Med, 13*(5), 574–582. doi: 10.1080/13548500801927121

Bowen, A., & Muhajarine, N. (2006). Prevalence of antenatal depression in women enrolled in an outreach program in Canada. *J Obstet Gynecol Neonatal Nurs, 35*(4), 491–498. doi: 10.1111/j.1552-6909.2006.00064.x

Bowen, A., Stewart, N., Baetz, M., & Muhajarine, N. (2009). Antenatal depression in socially high-risk women in Canada. *J Epidemiol Community Health, 63*(5), 414–416. doi: 10.1136/jech.2008.078832

Boyce, P., Parker, G., Barnett, B., Cooney, M., & Smith, F. (1991). Personality as a vulnerability factor to depression. *Br J Psychiatry, 159*, 106–114.

Brittain, K., Myer, L., Koen, N., Koopowitz, S., Donald, K. A., Barnett, W.,… Stein, D. J. (2015). Risk factors for antenatal depression and associations with infant birth outcomes: results from a South African birth cohort study. *Paediatr Perinat Epidemiol, 29*(6), 505–514. doi: 10.1111/ppe.12216

Bunevicius, R., Kusminskas, L., Bunevicius, A., Nadisauskiene, R. J., Jureniene, K., & Pop, V. J. (2009). Psychosocial risk factors for depression during pregnancy. *Acta Obstet Gynecol Scand, 88*(5), 599–605. doi: 10.1080/00016340902846049

Canady, R. B., Bullen, B. L., Holzman, C., Broman, C., & Tian, Y. (2008). Discrimination and symptoms of depression in pregnancy among African American and White women. *Womens Health Issues, 18*(4), 292–300. doi: 10.1016/j.whi.2008.04.003

Carter, F. A., Frampton, C. M., & Mulder, R. T. (2006). Cesarean section and postpartum depression: a review of the evidence examining the link. *Psychosom Med, 68*(2), 321–330. doi: 10.1097/01.psy.0000204787.83768.0c

Castro e Couto, T., Cardoso, M. N., Brancaglion, M. Y., Faria, G. C., Garcia, F. D., Nicolato, R.,… Correa, H. (2016). Antenatal depression: prevalence and risk factor patterns across the gestational period. *J Affect Disord, 192*, 70–75. doi: 10.1016/j.jad.2015.12.017

Chojenta, C., Harris, S., Reilly, N., Forder, P., Austin, M. P., & Loxton, D. (2014). History of pregnancy loss increases the risk of mental health problems in subsequent pregnancies but not in the postpartum. *PLoS One, 9*(4), e95038. doi: 10.1371/journal.pone.0095038

Churchill, A. C., & Davis, C. G. (2010). Realistic orientation and the transition to motherhood. *Journal of Social and Clinical Psychology, 29*(1), 39–67. doi: 10.1521/jscp.2010.29.1.39

Clout, D., & Brown, R. (2015). Sociodemographic, pregnancy, obstetric, and postnatal predictors of postpartum stress, anxiety and depression in new mothers. *J Affect Disord, 188*, 60–67. doi: 10.1016/j.jad.2015.08.054

Cobb, S. (1976). Presidential Address-1976. Social support as a moderator of life stress. *Psychosom Med, 38*(5), 300–314.

Cohen, M. M., Schei, B., Ansara, D., Gallop, R., Stuckless, N., & Stewart, D. E. (2002). A history of personal violence and postpartum depression: is there a link? *Arch Womens Ment Health, 4*(3), 83–92. doi: 10.1007/s007370200004

Coll, C. V., da Silveira, M. F., Bassani, D. G., Netsi, E., Wehrmeister, F. C., Barros, F. C., & Stein, A. (2017). Antenatal depressive symptoms among pregnant women: evidence from a Southern Brazilian population-based cohort study. *J Affect Disord, 209*, 140–146. doi: 10.1016/j.jad.2016.11.031

Danese, A., Pariante, C. M., Caspi, A., Taylor, A., & Poulton, R. (2007). Childhood maltreatment predicts adult inflammation in a life-course study. *Proceedings of the National Academy of Sciences of the United States of America, 104*(4), 1319–1324.

Dayan, J., Creveuil, C., Dreyfus, M., Herlicoviez, M., Baleyte, J. M., & O'Keane, V. (2010). Developmental model of depression applied to prenatal depression: role of present and past life events, past emotional disorders and pregnancy stress. *PLoS One, 5*(9), e12942. doi: 10.1371/journal.pone.0012942

de Castro, F., Place, J. M., Billings, D. L., Rivera, L., & Frongillo, E. A. (2015). Risk profiles associated with postnatal depressive symptoms among women in a public sector hospital in Mexico: the role of sociodemographic and psychosocial factors. *Arch Womens Ment Health, 18*(3), 463–471. doi: 10.1007/s00737-014-0472-1

De Venter, M., Smets, J., Raes, F., Wouters, K., Franck, E., Hanssens, M.,... Van Den Eede, F. (2016). Impact of childhood trauma on postpartum depression: a prospective study. *Arch Womens Ment Health, 19*(2), 337–342. doi: 10.1007/s00737-015-0550-z

Della Vedova, A. M., Ducceschi, B., Cesana, B. M., & Imbasciati, A. (2011). Maternal bonding and risk of depression in late pregnancy: a survey of Italian nulliparous women. *Journal of Reproductive and Infant Psychology, 29*(3), 208–222. doi: 10.1080/02646838.2011.592973

Dias, C. C., & Figueiredo, B. (2015). Breastfeeding and depression: a systematic review of the literature. *J Affect Disord, 171*, 142–154. doi: 10.1016/j.jad.2014.09.022

Dibaba, Y., Fantahun, M., & Hindin, M. J. (2013). The association of unwanted pregnancy and social support with depressive symptoms in pregnancy: evidence from rural Southwestern Ethiopia. *BMC Pregnancy Childbirth, 13*, 135. doi: 10.1186/1471-2393-13-135

Dmitrovic, B. K., DugaliÄ‡, M. G., Balkoski, G. N., Dmitrovic, A., & Soldatovic, I. (2014). Frequency of perinatal depression in Serbia and associated risk factors. *International Journal of Social Psychiatry, 60*(6), 528–532.

Du Preez, A., Conroy, S., Pawlby, S., Moran, P., & Pariante, C. M. (2016). Differential effects of ethnic density on the risk of postnatal depression and personality dysfunction. *Br J Psychiatry, 208*(1), 49–55. doi: 10.1192/bjp.bp.114.148874

Edge, D. (2007). Ethnicity, psychosocial risk, and perinatal depression—a comparative study among inner-city women in the United Kingdom. *J Psychosom Res, 63*(3), 291–295. doi: 10.1016/j.jpsychores.2007.02.013

Fairbrother, N., & Woody, S. R. (2007). Fear of childbirth and obstetrical events as predictors of postnatal symptoms of depression and post-traumatic stress disorder. *J Psychosom Obstet Gynaecol, 28*(4), 239–242. doi: 10.1080/01674820701495065

Faisal-Cury, A., Menezes, P., Araya, R., & Zugaib, M. (2009). Common mental disorders during pregnancy: prevalence and associated factors among low-income women in Sao Paulo, Brazil: depression and anxiety during pregnancy. *Arch Womens Ment Health, 12*(5), 335–343. doi: 10.1007/s00737-009-0081-6

Faisal-Cury, A., & Rossi Menezes, P. (2007). Prevalence of anxiety and depression during pregnancy in a private setting sample. *Arch Womens Ment Health, 10*(1), 25–32. doi: 10.1007/s00737-006-0164-6

Falah-Hassani, K., Shiri, R., & Dennis, C. L. (2016). Prevalence and risk factors for comorbid postpartum depressive symptomatology and anxiety. *J Affect Disord, 198*, 142–147. doi: 10.1016/j.jad.2016.03.010

Falah-Hassani, K., Shiri, R., Vigod, S., & Dennis, C. L. (2015). Prevalence of postpartum depression among immigrant women: a systematic review and meta-analysis. *J Psychiatr Res, 70*, 67–82. doi: 10.1016/j.jpsychires.2015.08.010

Farr, S. L., Dietz, P. M., O'Hara, M. W., Burley, K., & Ko, J. Y. (2014). Postpartum anxiety and comorbid depression in a population-based sample of women. *J Womens Health (Larchmt), 23*(2), 120–128. doi: 10.1089/jwh.2013.4438

Fellenzer, J. L., & Cibula, D. A. (2014). Intendedness of pregnancy and other predictive factors for symptoms of prenatal depression in a population-based study. *Matern Child Health J, 18*(10), 2426–2436. doi: 10.1007/s10995-014-1481-4

Figueiredo, B., Pacheco, A., & Costa, R. (2007). Depression during pregnancy and the postpartum period in adolescent and adult Portuguese mothers. *Arch Womens Ment Health, 10*(3), 103–109. doi: 10.1007/s00737-007-0178-8

Fisher, J., Tran, T., Duc Tran, T., Dwyer, T., Nguyen, T., Casey, G. J.,... Biggs, B. A. (2013). Prevalence and risk factors for symptoms of common mental disorders in early and late pregnancy in Vietnamese women: a prospective population-based study. *J Affect Disord, 146*(2), 213–219. doi: 10.1016/j.jad.2012.09.007

Fisher, J., Tran, T., La, B. T., Kriitmaa, K., Rosenthal, D., & Tran, T. (2010). Common perinatal mental disorders in northern Viet Nam: community prevalence and health care use. *Bull World Health Organ, 88*(10), 737–745. doi: 10.2471/blt.09.067066

Franck, E., Vanderhasselt, M. A., Goubert, L., Loeys, T., Temmerman, M., & De Raedt, R. (2016). The role of self-esteem instability in the development of postnatal depression: a prospective study testing a diathesis-stress account. *J Behav Ther Exp Psychiatry, 50*, 15–22. doi: 10.1016/j.jbtep.2015.04.010

Gaillard, A., Le Strat, Y., Mandelbrot, L., Keita, H., & Dubertret, C. (2014). Predictors of postpartum depression: prospective study of 264 women followed during pregnancy and postpartum. *Psychiatry Res, 215*(2), 341–346. doi: 10.1016/j.psychres.2013.10.003

Garcia-Blanco, A., Monferrer, A., Grimaldos, J., Hervas, D., Balanza-Martinez, V., Diago, V.,... Chafer-Pericas, C. (2017). A preliminary study to assess the impact of maternal age on stress-related variables in healthy nulliparous women. *Psychoneuroendocrinology, 78*, 97–104. doi: 10.1016/j.psyneuen.2017.01.018

Gavin, A. R., Melville, J. L., Rue, T., Guo, Y., Dina, K. T., & Katon, W. J. (2011). Racial differ-ences in the prevalence of antenatal depression. *Gen Hosp Psychiatry, 33*(2), 87–93. doi: 10.1016/j.genhosppsych.2010.11.012

Gelabert, E., Subira, S., Garcia-Esteve, L., Navarro, P., Plaza, A., Cuyas, E.,... Martin-Santos, R. (2012). Perfectionism dimensions in major postpartum depression. *J Affect Disord, 136*(1–2), 17–25. doi: 10.1016/j.jad.2011.08.030

George, C., Lalitha, A. R., Antony, A., Kumar, A. V., & Jacob, K. S. (2016). Antenatal depression in coastal South India: prevalence and risk factors in the community. *Int J Soc Psychiatry, 62*(2), 141–147. doi: 10.1177/0020764015607919

Giardinelli, L., Innocenti, A., Benni, L., Stefanini, M. C., Lino, G., Lunardi, C.,... Faravelli, C. (2012). Depression and anxiety in perinatal period: prevalence and risk factors in an Italian sample. *Arch Womens Ment Health, 15*(1), 21–30. doi: 10.1007/s00737-011-0249-8

Ginsburg, G. S., Baker, E. V., Mullany, B. C., Barlow, A., Goklish, N., Hastings, R.,... Walkup, J. (2008). Depressive symptoms among reservation-based pregnant American Indian adolescents. *Matern Child Health J, 12 Suppl 1*, 110–118. doi: 10.1007/s10995-008-0352-2

Giri, R. K., Khatri, R. B., Mishra, S. R., Khanal, V., Sharma, V. D., & Gartoula, R. P. (2015). Prevalence and factors associated with depressive symptoms among post-partum mothers in Nepal. *BMC Res Notes, 8*, 111. doi: 10.1186/s13104-015-1074-3

Glavin, K., Smith, L., & Sorum, R. (2009). Prevalence of postpartum depression in two municipalities in Norway. *Scand J Caring Sci, 23*(4), 705–710. doi: 10.1111/j.1471-6712.2008.00667.x

Glazier, R. H., Elgar, F. J., Goel, V., & Holzapfel, S. (2004). Stress, social support, and emotional distress in a community sample of pregnant women. *J Psychosom Obstet Gynaecol, 25*(3–4), 247–255.

Golbasi, Z., Kelleci, M., Kisacik, G., & Cetin, A. (2010). Prevalence and correlates of depres-sion in pregnancy among Turkish Women. *Matern Child Health J, 14*(4), 485–491. doi: 10.1007/s10995-009-0459-0

Gong, X., Hao, J., Tao, F., Zhang, J., Wang, H., & Xu, R. (2013). Pregnancy loss and anxiety and depression during subsequent pregnancies: data from the C-ABC study. *Eur J Obstet Gynecol Reprod Biol, 166*(1), 30–36. doi: 10.1016/j.ejogrb.2012.09.024

Grant, K. A., Bautovich, A., McMahon, C., Reilly, N., Leader, L., & Austin, M. P. (2012). Parental care and control during childhood: associations with maternal perinatal mood disturbance and parenting stress. *Arch Womens Ment Health, 15*(4), 297–305. doi: 10.1007/s00737-012-0292-0

Gregoire, A. J. (1995). Hormones and postnatal depression. *British Journal of Midwifery, 3*, 99–105.

Gutierrez-Zotes, A., Labad, J., Martin-Santos, R., Garcia-Esteve, L., Gelabert, E., Jover, M.,... Sanjuan, J. (2015). Coping strategies and postpartum depressive symptoms: a structural equation modelling ap-proach. *Eur Psychiatry, 30*(6), 701–708. doi: 10.1016/j.eurpsy.2015.06.001

Hartley, M., Tomlinson, M., Greco, E., Comulada, W. S., Stewart, J., le Roux, I.,... Rotheram-Borus, M. J. (2011). Depressed mood in pregnancy: prevalence and correlates in two Cape Town peri-urban settle-ments. *Reprod Health, 8*, 9. doi: 10.1186/1742-4755-8-9

Heim, C., Newport, D. J., Mletzko, T., Miller, A. H., & Nemeroff, C. B. (2008). The link between child-hood trauma and depression: insights from HPA axis studies in humans. *Psychoneuroendocrinology, 33*(6), 693–710. doi: 10.1016/j.psyneuen.2008.03.008

Helle, N., Barkmann, C., Bartz-Seel, J., Diehl, T., Ehrhardt, S., Hendel, A.,... Bindt, C. (2015). Very low birth-weight as a risk factor for postpartum depression four to six weeks postbirth in mothers and fathers: cross-sectional results from a controlled multicentre cohort study. *J Affect Disord, 180*, 154–161. doi: 10.1016/j.jad.2015.04.001

Heron, J., O'Connor, T. G., Evans, J., Golding, J., & Glover, V. (2004). The course of anxiety and depres-sion through pregnancy and the postpartum in a community sample. *J Affect Disord, 80*(1), 65–73. doi: 10.1016/j.jad.2003.08.004

Heyningen, T., Myer, L., Onah, M., Tomlinson, M., Field, S., & Honikman, S. (2016). Antenatal depression and adversity in urban South Africa. *J Affect Disord, 203*, 121–129. doi: 10.1016/j.jad.2016.05.052

Hodnett, E. D., Gates, S., Hofmeyr, G. J., & Sakala, C. (2013). Continuous support for women during child-birth. *Cochrane Database Syst Rev, 7*, Cd003766. doi: 10.1002/14651858.CD003766.pub5

Holzman, C., Eyster, J., Tiedje, L. B., Roman, L. A., Seagull, E., & Rahbar, M. H. (2006). A life course perspective on depressive symptoms in mid-pregnancy. *Matern Child Health J, 10*(2), 127. doi: 10.1007/s10995-005-0044-0

Howard, L. M., Oram, S., Galley, H., Trevillion, K., & Feder, G. (2013). Domestic violence and perinatal mental disorders: a systematic review and meta-analysis. *PLoS Med, 10*(5), e1001452. doi: 10.1371/jour-nal.pmed.1001452

Hudson, C., Spry, E., Borschmann, R., Becker, D., Moran, P., Olsson, C.,... Patton, G. C. (2017). Preconception personality disorder and antenatal maternal mental health: a population-based cohort study. *J Affect Disord, 209*, 169–176. doi: 10.1016/j.jad.2016.11.022

Husain, N., Cruickshank, K., Husain, M., Khan, S., Tomenson, B., & Rahman, A. (2012). Social stress and depression during pregnancy and in the postnatal period in British Pakistani mothers: a cohort study. *J Affect Disord, 140*(3), 268–276. doi: 10.1016/j.jad.2012.02.009

Husain, N., Parveen, A., Husain, M., Saeed, Q., Jafri, F., Rahman, R.,... Chaudhry, I. B. (2011). Prevalence and psychosocial correlates of perinatal depression: a cohort study from urban Pakistan. *Arch Womens Ment Health, 14*(5), 395–403. doi: 10.1007/s00737-011-0233-3

Iliadis, S. I., Koulouris, P., Gingnell, M., Sylven, S. M., Sundstrom-Poromaa, I., Ekselius, L.,... Skalkidou, A. (2015). Personality and risk for postpartum depressive symptoms. *Arch Womens Ment Health, 18*(3), 539–546. doi: 10.1007/s00737-014-0478-8

Jackson, C. L., Ciciolla, L., Crnic, K. A., Luecken, L. J., Gonzales, N. A., & Coonrod, D. V. (2015). Intimate partner violence before and during pregnancy: related demographic and psychosocial factors and postpartum depressive symptoms among Mexican American women. *J Interpers Violence, 30*(4), 659–679. doi: 10.1177/0886260514535262

Jeong, H. G., Lim, J. S., Lee, M. S., Kim, S. H., Jung, I. K., & Joe, S. H. (2013). The association of psychosocial factors and obstetric history with depression in pregnant women: focus on the role of emotional support. *Gen Hosp Psychiatry, 35*(4), 354–358. doi: 10.1016/j.genhosppsych.2013.02.009

Jesse, D. E., Walcott-McQuigg, J., Mariella, A., & Swanson, M. S. (2005). Risks and protective factors associated with symptoms of depression in low-income African American and Caucasian women during pregnancy. *J Midwifery Womens Health, 50*(5), 405–410. doi: 10.1016/j.jmwh.2005.05.001

Josefsson, A., Angelsioo, L., Berg, G., Ekstrom, C. M., Gunnervik, C., Nordin, C., & Sydsjo, G. (2002). Obstetric, somatic, and demographic risk factors for postpartum depressive symptoms. *Obstet Gynecol, 99*(2), 223–228.

Karmaliani, R., Asad, N., Bann, C. M., Moss, N., McClure, E. M., Pasha, O.,... Goldenberg, R. L. (2009). Prevalence of anxiety, depression and associated factors among pregnant women of Hyderabad, Pakistan. *Int J Soc Psychiatry, 55*(5), 414–424. doi: 10.1177/0020764008094645

Kastello, J. C., Jacobsen, K. H., Gaffney, K. F., Kodadek, M. P., Sharps, P. W., & Bullock, L. C. (2016). Predictors of depression symptoms among low-income women exposed to perinatal intimate partner violence (IPV). *Community Ment Health J, 52*(6), 683–690. doi: 10.1007/s10597-015-9977-y

Khalifa, D. S., Glavin, K., Bjertness, E., & Lien, L. (2016). Determinants of postnatal depression in Sudanese women at 3 months postpartum: a cross-sectional study. *BMJ Open, 6*(3), e009443. doi: 10.1136/bmjopen-2015-009443

Kitamura, T., Yoshida, K., Okano, T., Kinoshita, K., Hayashi, M., Toyoda, N.,... Nakano, H. (2006). Multicentre prospective study of perinatal depression in Japan: incidence and correlates of antenatal and postnatal depression. *Arch Womens Ment Health, 9*(3), 121–130. doi: 10.1007/s00737-006-0122-3

Lancaster, C. A., Gold, K. J., Flynn, H. A., Yoo, H., Marcus, S. M., & Davis, M. M. (2010). Risk factors for depressive symptoms during pregnancy: a systematic review. *Am J Obstet Gynecol, 202*(1), 5–14. doi: 10.1016/j.ajog.2009.09.007

Lanzi, R. G., Bert, S. C., & Jacobs, B. K. (2009). Depression among a sample of first-time adolescent and adult mothers. *J Child Adolesc Psychiatr Nurs, 22*(4), 194–202. doi: 10.1111/j.1744-6171.2009.00199.x

Lara, M. A., Navarrete, L., Nieto, L., Martin, J. P., Navarro, J. L., & Lara-Tapia, H. (2015). Prevalence and incidence of perinatal depression and depressive symptoms among Mexican women. *J Affect Disord, 175*, 18–24. doi: 10.1016/j.jad.2014.12.035

Lawson, A., Murphy, K. E., Sloan, E., Uleryk, E., & Dalfen, A. (2015). The relationship between sleep and postpartum mental disorders: A systematic review. *J Affect Disord, 176*, 65–77. doi: 10.1016/j.jad.2015.01.017

Lee, A. M., Lam, S. K., Sze Mun Lau, S. M., Chong, C. S., Chui, H. W., & Fong, D. Y. (2007). Prevalence, course, and risk factors for antenatal anxiety and depression. *Obstet Gynecol, 110*(5), 1102–1112. doi: 10.1097/01.aog.0000287065.59491.70

Lee, D. T., Yip, A. S., Leung, T. Y., & Chung, T. K. (2000). Identifying women at risk of postnatal depression: prospective longitudinal study. *Hong Kong Med J, 6*(4), 349–354.

Leigh, B., & Milgrom, J. (2008). Risk factors for antenatal depression, postnatal depression and parenting stress. *BMC Psychiatry, 8*, 24. doi: 10.1186/1471-244x-8-24

Limlomwongse, N., & Liabsuetrakul, T. (2006). Cohort study of depressive moods in Thai women during late pregnancy and 6-8 weeks of postpartum using the Edinburgh Postnatal Depression Scale (EPDS). *Arch Womens Ment Health, 9*(3), 131–138. doi: 10.1007/s00737-005-0115-7

Luke, S., Salihu, H. M., Alio, A. P., Mbah, A. K., Jeffers, D., Berry, E. L., & Mishkit, V. R. (2009). Risk factors for major antenatal depression among low-income African American women. *J Womens Health (Larchmt), 18*(11), 1841–1846. doi: 10.1089/jwh.2008.1261

Lydsdottir, L. B., Howard, L. M., Olafsdottir, H., Thome, M., Tyrfingsson, P., & Sigurdsson, J. F. (2014). The mental health characteristics of pregnant women with depressive symptoms identified by the Edinburgh Postnatal Depression Scale. *J Clin Psychiatry, 75*(4), 393–398. doi: 10.4088/JCP.13m08646

Mahenge, B., Likindikoki, S., Stockl, H., & Mbwambo, J. (2013). Intimate partner violence during pregnancy and associated mental health symptoms among pregnant women in Tanzania: a cross-sectional study. *Bjog, 120*(8), 940–946. doi: 10.1111/1471-0528.12185

Maia, B. R., Pereira, A. T., Marques, M., Bos, S., Soares, M. J., Valente, J.,… Macedo, A. (2012). The role of perfectionism in postpartum depression and symptomatology. *Arch Womens Ment Health, 15*(6), 459–468. doi: 10.1007/s00737-012-0310-2

Manikkam, L., & Burns, J. K. (2012). Antenatal depression and its risk factors: an urban prevalence study in KwaZulu-Natal. *S Afr Med J, 102*(12), 940–944. doi: 10.7196/samj.6009

Marchesi, C., Ampollini, P., Paraggio, C., Giaracuni, G., Ossola, P., De Panfilis, C.,… Viviani, D. (2014). Risk factors for panic disorder in pregnancy: a cohort study. *J Affect Disord, 156*, 134–138. doi: 10.1016/j.jad.2013.12.006

Marchesi, C., Bertoni, S., & Maggini, C. (2009). Major and minor depression in pregnancy. *Obstet Gynecol, 113*(6), 1292–1298. doi: 10.1097/AOG.0b013e3181a45e90

Marcus, S. M. (2009). Depression during pregnancy: rates, risks and consequences–Motherisk Update 2008. *Can J Clin Pharmacol, 16*(1), e15–22.

Marcus, S. M., Flynn, H. A., Blow, F. C., & Barry, K. L. (2003). Depressive symptoms among pregnant women screened in obstetrics settings. *J Womens Health (Larchmt), 12*(4), 373–380. doi: 10.1089/154099903765448880

Martin, S. L., Li, Y., Casanueva, C., Harris-Britt, A., Kupper, L. L., & Cloutier, S. (2006). Intimate partner violence and women's depression before and during pregnancy. *Violence Against Women, 12*(3), 221–239. doi: 10.1177/1077801205285106

Martini, J., Petzoldt, J., Einsle, F., Beesdo-Baum, K., Hofler, M., & Wittchen, H. U. (2015). Risk factors and course patterns of anxiety and depressive disorders during pregnancy and after delivery: a prospective-longitudinal study. *J Affect Disord, 175c*, 385–395. doi: 10.1016/j.jad.2015.01.012

McMahon, C. A., Boivin, J., Gibson, F. L., Fisher, J. R. W., Hammarberg, K., Wynter, K., & Saunders, D. M. (2011). Older first-time mothers and early postpartum depression: a prospective cohort study of women conceiving spontaneously or with assisted reproductive technologies. *Fertility and Sterility, 96*(5), 1218–1224. doi: 10.1016/j.fertnstert.2011.08.037

McMahon, C. A., Boivin, J., Gibson, F. L., Hammarberg, K., Wynter, K., & Fisher, J. R. (2015). Older maternal age and major depressive episodes in the first two years after birth: findings from the Parental Age and Transition to Parenthood Australia (PATPA) study. *J Affect Disord, 175*, 454–462. doi: 10.1016/j.jad.2015.01.025

Melville, J. L., Gavin, A., Guo, Y., Fan, M. Y., & Katon, W. J. (2010). Depressive disorders during pregnancy: prevalence and risk factors in a large urban sample. *Obstet Gynecol, 116*(5), 1064–1070. doi: 10.1097/AOG.0b013e3181f60b0a

Mezey, G., Bacchus, L., Bewley, S., & White, S. (2005). Domestic violence, lifetime trauma and psychological health of childbearing women. *Bjog, 112*(2), 197–204. doi: 10.1111/j.1471-0528.2004.00307.x

Mezzacappa, E. S., & Katlin, E. S. (2002). Breast-feeding is associated with reduced perceived stress and negative mood in mothers. *Health Psychol, 21*(2), 187–193.

Milgrom, J., & Gemmill, A. W. (2014). Screening for perinatal depression. *Best Pract Res Clin Obstet Gynaecol, 28*(1), 13–23. doi: 10.1016/j.bpobgyn.2013.08.014

Milgrom, J., Gemmill, A. W., Bilszta, J. L., Hayes, B., Barnett, B., Brooks, J.,… Buist, A. (2008). Antenatal risk factors for postnatal depression: a large prospective study. *J Affect Disord, 108*(1–2), 147–157. doi: 10.1016/j.jad.2007.10.014

Mohamad Yusuff, A. S., Tang, L., Binns, C. W., & Lee, A. H. (2015). Prevalence and risk factors for postnatal depression in Sabah, Malaysia: a cohort study. *Women Birth, 28*(1), 25–29. doi: 10.1016/j.wombi.2014.11.002

Mohamad Yusuff, A. S., Tang, L., Binns, C. W., & Lee, A. H. (2016). Prevalence of antenatal depressive symptoms among women in Sabah, Malaysia. *J Matern Fetal Neonatal Med, 29*(7), 1170–1174. doi: 10.3109/14767058.2015.1039506

Mohammad, K. I., Gamble, J., & Creedy, D. K. (2011). Prevalence and factors associated with the development of antenatal and postnatal depression among Jordanian women. *Midwifery, 27*(6), e238–245. doi: 10.1016/j.midw.2010.10.008

Morikawa, M., Okada, T., Ando, M., Aleksic, B., Kunimoto, S., Nakamura, Y.,... Ozaki, N. (2015). Relationship between social support during pregnancy and postpartum depressive state: a prospective cohort study. *Sci Rep, 5*, 10520. doi: 10.1038/srep10520

Mukherjee, S., Trepka, M. J., Pierre-Victor, D., Bahelah, R., & Avent, T. (2016). Racial/ethnic disparities in antenatal depression in the United States: a systematic review. *Matern Child Health J, 20*(9), 1780–1797. doi: 10.1007/s10995-016-1989-x

Murray, L., & Cooper, P. (1997). Effects of postnatal depression on infant development. *Arch Dis Child, 77*(2), 99–101.

Muscat, T., Obst, P., Cockshaw, W., & Thorpe, K. (2014). Beliefs about infant regulation, early infant behaviors and maternal postnatal depressive symptoms. *Birth, 41*(2), 206–213. doi: 10.1111/birt.12107

Nasreen, H. E., Kabir, Z. N., Forsell, Y., & Edhborg, M. (2011). Prevalence and associated factors of depressive and anxiety symptoms during pregnancy: a population based study in rural Bangladesh. *BMC Womens Health, 11*, 22. doi: 10.1186/1472-6874-11-22

Ngai, F. W., & Ngu, S. F. (2015). Predictors of maternal and paternal depressive symptoms at postpartum. *J Psychosom Res, 78*(2), 156–161. doi: 10.1016/j.jpsychores.2014.12.003

NICE. (2015). Antenatal and postnatal mental health: clinical management and service guidance. NICE clinical guideline 192.: National Institute for Health and Clinical Excellence (NICE).

Norhayati, M. N., Hazlina, N. H., Asrenee, A. R., & Emilin, W. M. (2015). Magnitude and risk factors for postpartum symptoms: a literature review. *J Affect Disord, 175*, 34–52. doi: 10.1016/j.jad.2014.12.041

O'Hara, M. W. (2009). Postpartum depression: what we know. *J Clin Psychol, 65*(12), 1258–1269. doi: 10.1002/jclp.20644

O'Hara, M. W., & Swain, A. M. (1996). Rates and risk of postpartum depression—a meta-analysis. *International Review of Psychiatry, 8*(1), 37–54. doi: 10.3109/09540269609037816

Oddo-Sommerfeld, S., Hain, S., Louwen, F., & Schermelleh-Engel, K. (2016). Longitudinal effects of dysfunctional perfectionism and avoidant personality style on postpartum mental disorders: pathways through antepartum depression and anxiety. *J Affect Disord, 191*, 280–288. doi: 10.1016/j.jad.2015.11.040

Okun, M. L. (2015). Sleep and postpartum depression. *Curr Opin Psychiatry, 28*(6), 490–496. doi: 10.1097/yco.0000000000000206

Pariante, C. M. (2014). Depression during pregnancy: molecular regulations of mothers' and children's behaviour. *Biochem Soc Trans, 42*(2), 582–586. doi: 10.1042/bst20130246

Pariante, C. M., & Lightman, S. L. (2008). The HPA axis in major depression: classical theories and new developments. *Trends Neurosci, 31*(9), 464–468. doi: 10.1016/j.tins.2008.06.006

Park, E. M., Meltzer-Brody, S., & Stickgold, R. (2013). Poor sleep maintenance and subjective sleep quality are associated with postpartum maternal depression symptom severity. *Arch Womens Ment Health, 16*(6), 539–547. doi: 10.1007/s00737-013-0356-9

Parker, G. B., Hegarty, B., Paterson, A., Hadzi-Pavlovic, D., Granville-Smith, I., & Gokiert, A. (2015). Predictors of post-natal depression are shaped distinctly by the measure of 'depression'. *J Affect Disord, 173*, 239–244. doi: 10.1016/j.jad.2014.10.066

Patel, V., Rodrigues, M., & DeSouza, N. (2002). Gender, poverty, and postnatal depression: a study of mothers in Goa, India. *Am J Psychiatry, 159*(1), 43–47. doi: 10.1176/appi.ajp.159.1.43

Patton, G. C., Romaniuk, H., Spry, E., Coffey, C., Olsson, C., Doyle, L. W.,... Brown, S. (2015). Prediction of perinatal depression from adolescence and before conception (VIHCS): 20-year prospective cohort study. *Lancet, 386*(9996), 875–883. doi: 10.1016/s0140-6736(14)62248-0

Plant, D. T., Barker, E. D., Waters, C. S., Pawlby, S., & Pariante, C. M. (2013). Intergenerational transmission of maltreatment and psychopathology: the role of antenatal depression. *Psychol Med, 43*(3), 519–528. doi: 10.1017/s0033291712001298

Posternak, M. A., & Zimmerman, M. (2001). Symptoms of atypical depression. *Psychiatry Res, 104*(2), 175–181.

Prady, S. L., Pickett, K. E., Croudace, T., Fairley, L., Bloor, K., Gilbody, S.,... Wright, J. (2013). Psychological distress during pregnancy in a multi-ethnic community: findings from the born in Bradford cohort study. *PLoS One, 8*(4), e60693. doi: 10.1371/journal.pone.0060693

Price, S. K. (2008). Stepping back to gain perspective: pregnancy loss history, depression, and parenting capacity in the Early Childhood Longitudinal Study, Birth Cohort (ECLS-B). *Death Stud, 32*(2), 97–122. doi: 10.1080/07481180701801170

Qiao, Y. X., Wang, J., Li, J., & Ablat, A. (2009). The prevalence and related risk factors of anxiety and depression symptoms among Chinese pregnant women in Shanghai. *Aust N Z J Obstet Gynaecol, 49*(2), 185–190. doi: 10.1111/j.1479-828X.2009.00966.x

Raisanen, S., Lehto, S. M., Nielsen, H. S., Gissler, M., Kramer, M. R., & Heinonen, S. (2013). Fear of child-birth predicts postpartum depression: a population-based analysis of 511 422 singleton births in Finland. *BMJ Open, 3*(11), e004047. doi: 10.1136/bmjopen-2013-004047

Raisanen, S., Lehto, S. M., Nielsen, H. S., Gissler, M., Kramer, M. R., & Heinonen, S. (2014). Risk factors for and perinatal outcomes of major depression during pregnancy: a population-based analysis during 2002-2010 in Finland. *BMJ Open, 4*(11), e004883. doi: 10.1136/bmjopen-2014-004883

Raphael-Leff, J. (2010). Mothers' and fathers' orientations: patterns of pregnancy, parenting and the bonding process *Parenthood and Mental Health* (pp. 9–22): John Wiley & Sons, Ltd.

Ratcliff, B. G., Sharapova, A., Suardi, F., & Borel, F. (2015). Factors associated with antenatal depression and obstetric complications in immigrant women in Geneva. *Midwifery, 31*(9), 871–878. doi: 10.1016/j. midw.2015.04.010

Records, K., & Rice, M. (2007). Psychosocial correlates of depression symptoms during the third trimester of pregnancy. *J Obstet Gynecol Neonatal Nurs, 36*(3), 231–242. doi: 10.1111/j.1552-6909.2007.00140.x

Redshaw, M., & Henderson, J. (2013). From antenatal to postnatal depression: associated factors and mitigating influences. *J Womens Health (Larchmt), 22*(6), 518–525. doi: 10.1089/jwh.2012.4152

Rich-Edwards, J. W., Kleinman, K., Abrams, A., Harlow, B. L., McLaughlin, T. J., Joffe, H., & Gillman, M. W. (2006). Sociodemographic predictors of antenatal and postpartum depressive symptoms among women in a medical group practice. *J Epidemiol Community Health, 60*(3), 221–227. doi: 10.1136/jech.2005.039370

Robakis, T. K., Williams, K. E., Crowe, S., Kenna, H., Gannon, J., & Rasgon, N. L. (2015). Optimistic outlook regarding maternity protects against depressive symptoms postpartum. *Arch Womens Ment Health, 18*(2), 197–208. doi: 10.1007/s00737-014-0446-3

Robertson, E., Grace, S., Wallington, T., & Stewart, D. E. (2004). Antenatal risk factors for postpartum depression: a synthesis of recent literature. *Gen Hosp Psychiatry, 26*(4), 289–295. doi: 10.1016/j. genhosppsych.2004.02.006

Robertson-Blackmore, E., Putnam, F. W., Rubinow, D. R., Matthieu, M., Hunn, J. E., Putnam, K. T.,... O'Connor, T. G. (2013). Antecedent trauma exposure and risk of depression in the perinatal period. *J Clin Psychiatry, 74*(10), e942–948. doi: 10.4088/JCP.13m08364

Roomruangwong, C., Withayavanitchai, S., & Maes, M. (2016). Antenatal and postnatal risk factors of postpartum depression symptoms in Thai women: A case-control study. *Sex Reprod Healthc, 10*, 25–31. doi: 10.1016/j.srhc.2016.03.001

Rosan, C., Finnis, S., Biaggi, A., Pawlby, S., & Pariante, C. (2016). Perfectionism as a warning sign for postnatal mental health difficulties. *Journal of Health Visiting, 4*(8), 400–406. doi: 10.12968/johv.2016.4.8.400

Rubertsson, C., Hellstrom, J., Cross, M., & Sydsjo, G. (2014). Anxiety in early pregnancy: prevalence and contributing factors. *Arch Womens Ment Health, 17*(3), 221–228. doi: 10.1007/s00737-013-0409-0

Rubertsson, C., Waldenström, U., & Wickberg, B. (2003). Depressive mood in early pregnancy: prevalence and women at risk in a national Swedish sample. *Journal of Reproductive and Infant Psychology, 21*(2), 113–123.

Rwakarema, M., Premji, S. S., Nyanza, E. C., Riziki, P., & Palacios-Derflingher, L. (2015). Antenatal depression is associated with pregnancy-related anxiety, partner relations, and wealth in women in Northern Tanzania: a cross-sectional study. *BMC Women's Health, 15*, 68. doi: 10.1186/s12905-015-0225-y

Seimyr, L., Welles-Nystrom, B., & Nissen, E. (2013). A history of mental health problems may predict maternal distress in women postpartum. *Midwifery, 29*(2), 122–131. doi: 10.1016/j.midw.2011.11.013

Shakeel, N., Eberhard-Gran, M., Sletner, L., Slinning, K., Martinsen, E. W., Holme, I., & Jenum, A. K. (2015). A prospective cohort study of depression in pregnancy, prevalence and risk factors in a multi-ethnic population. *BMC Pregnancy Childbirth, 15*, 5. doi: 10.1186/s12884-014-0420-0

Shamu, S., Zarowsky, C., Roelens, K., Temmerman, M., & Abrahams, N. (2016). High-frequency intimate partner violence during pregnancy, postnatal depression and suicidal tendencies in Harare, Zimbabwe. *Gen Hosp Psychiatry, 38*, 109–114. doi: 10.1016/j.genhosppsych.2015.10.005

Sharkey, K. M., Iko, I. N., Machan, J. T., Thompson-Westra, J., & Pearlstein, T. B. (2016). Infant sleep and feeding patterns are associated with maternal sleep, stress, and depressed mood in women with a history of major depressive disorder (MDD). *Arch Womens Ment Health, 19*(2), 209–218. doi: 10.1007/s00737-015-0557-5

Shivalli, S., & Gururaj, N. (2015). Postnatal depression among rural women in South India: do socio-demographic, obstetric and pregnancy outcome have a role to play? *PLoS One, 10*(4), e0122079. doi: 10.1371/journal.pone.0122079

Siegel, R. S., & Brandon, A. R. (2014). Adolescents, pregnancy, and mental health. *J Pediatr Adolesc Gynecol, 27*(3), 138–150. doi: 10.1016/j.jpag.2013.09.008

Simpson, J. A., Rholes, W. S., Campbell, L., Tran, S., & Wilson, C. L. (2003). Adult attachment, the transition to parenthood, and depressive symptoms. *J Pers Soc Psychol, 84*(6), 1172–1187.

Smith, M. V., Shao, L., Howell, H., Lin, H., & Yonkers, K. A. (2011). Perinatal depression and birth outcomes in a Healthy Start project. *Matern Child Health J, 15*(3), 401–409. doi: 10.1007/s10995-010-0595-6

Sockol, L. E., Epperson, C. N., & Barber, J. P. (2014). The relationship between maternal attitudes and symptoms of depression and anxiety among pregnant and postpartum first-time mothers. *Arch Womens Ment Health, 17*(3), 199–212. doi: 10.1007/s00737-014-0424-9

Srinivasan, N., Murthy, S., Singh, A. K., Upadhyay, V., Mohan, S. K., & Joshi, A. (2015). Assessment of burden of depression during pregnancy among pregnant women residing in rural setting of chennai. *J Clin Diagn Res, 9*(4), Lc08–12. doi: 10.7860/jcdr/2015/12380.5850

Stewart, A. L., Dean, M. L., Gregorich, S. E., Brawarsky, P., & Haas, J. S. (2007). Race/ethnicity, socioeconomic status and the health of pregnant women. *J Health Psychol, 12*(2), 285–300. doi: 10.1177/1359105307074259

Stewart, D. E., & Vigod, S. (2016). Postpartum Depression. *N Engl J Med, 375*(22), 2177–2186. doi: 10.1056/NEJMcp1607649

Stewart, R. C., Umar, E., Tomenson, B., & Creed, F. (2014). A cross-sectional study of antenatal depression and associated factors in Malawi. *Arch Womens Ment Health, 17*(2), 145–154. doi: 10.1007/s00737-013-0387-2

Sundstrom Poromaa, I., Comasco, E., Georgakis, M. K., & Skalkidou, A. (2017). Sex differences in depression during pregnancy and the postpartum period. *J Neurosci Res, 95*(1–2), 719–730. doi: 10.1002/jnr.23859

Tachibana, Y., Koizumi, T., Takehara, K., Kakee, N., Tsujii, H., Mori, R.,... Kubo, T. (2015). Antenatal risk factors of postpartum depression at 20 weeks gestation in a Japanese sample: psychosocial perspectives from a cohort study in Tokyo. *PLoS One, 10*(12), e0142410. doi: 10.1371/journal.pone.0142410

Tham, E. K., Tan, J., Chong, Y. S., Kwek, K., Saw, S. M., Teoh, O. H.,... Broekman, B. F. (2016). Associations between poor subjective prenatal sleep quality and postnatal depression and anxiety symptoms. *J Affect Disord, 202*, 91–94. doi: 10.1016/j.jad.2016.05.028

Theme Filha, M. M., Ayers, S., da Gama, S. G., & Leal Mdo, C. (2016). Factors associated with postpartum depressive symptomatology in Brazil: The Birth in Brazil National Research Study, 2011/2012. *J Affect Disord, 194*, 159–167. doi: 10.1016/j.jad.2016.01.020

Tsai, A. C., Tomlinson, M., Comulada, W. S., & Rotheram-Borus, M. J. (2016a). Food insufficiency, depression, and the modifying role of social support: evidence from a population-based, prospective cohort of pregnant women in peri-urban South Africa. *Soc Sci Med, 151*, 69–77. doi: 10.1016/j.socscimed.2015.12.042

Tsai, A. C., Tomlinson, M., Comulada, W. S., & Rotheram-Borus, M. J. (2016b). Intimate partner violence and depression symptom severity among South African women during pregnancy and postpartum: population-based prospective cohort study. *PLoS Med, 13*(1), e1001943. doi: 10.1371/journal.pmed.1001943

Turkcapar, A. F., Kadioglu, N., Aslan, E., Tunc, S., Zayifoglu, M., & Mollamahmutoglu, L. (2015). Sociodemographic and clinical features of postpartum depression among Turkish women: a prospective study. *BMC Pregnancy Childbirth, 15*, 108. doi: 10.1186/s12884-015-0532-1

Underwood, L., Waldie, K. E., D'Souza, S., Peterson, E. R., & Morton, S. M. (2017). A longitudinal study of pre-pregnancy and pregnancy risk factors associated with antenatal and postnatal symptoms of depression: evidence from growing up in New Zealand. *Matern Child Health J, 21*(4), 915–931. doi: 10.1007/s10995-016-2191-x

Verkerk, G. J., Denollet, J., Van Heck, G. L., Van Son, M. J., & Pop, V. J. (2005). Personality factors as determinants of depression in postpartum women: a prospective 1-year follow-up study. *Psychosom Med, 67*(4), 632–637. doi: 10.1097/01.psy.0000170832.14718.98

Verreault, N., Da Costa, D., Marchand, A., Ireland, K., Dritsa, M., & Khalife, S. (2014). Rates and risk factors associated with depressive symptoms during pregnancy and with postpartum onset. *J Psychosom Obstet Gynaecol, 35*(3), 84–91. doi: 10.3109/0167482x.2014.947953

Vigod, S. N., Villegas, L., Dennis, C. L., & Ross, L. E. (2010). Prevalence and risk factors for postpartum depression among women with preterm and low-birth-weight infants: a systematic review. *Bjog, 117*(5), 540–550. doi: 10.1111/j.1471-0528.2009.02493.x

Voegtline, K. M., & Stifter, C. A. (2010). Late-preterm birth, maternal symptomatology, and infant negativity. *Infant Behav Dev, 33*(4), 545–554. doi: 10.1016/j.infbeh.2010.07.006

Waldie, K. E., Peterson, E. R., D'Souza, S., Underwood, L., Pryor, J. E., Carr, P. A.,... Morton, S. M. (2015). Depression symptoms during pregnancy: evidence from growing up in New Zealand. *J Affect Disord, 186*, 66–73. doi: 10.1016/j.jad.2015.06.009

Waqas, A., Raza, N., Lodhi, H. W., Muhammad, Z., Jamal, M., & Rehman, A. (2015). Psychosocial factors of antenatal anxiety and depression in pakistan: is social support a mediator? *PLoS One, 10*(1), e0116510. doi: 10.1371/journal.pone.0116510

Weobong, B., Soremekun, S., Ten Asbroek, A. H., Amenga-Etego, S., Danso, S., Owusu-Agyei, S.,… Kirkwood, B. R. (2014). Prevalence and determinants of antenatal depression among pregnant women in a predominantly rural population in Ghana: the DON population-based study. *J Affect Disord, 165*, 1–7. doi: 10.1016/j.jad.2014.04.009

Weobong, B., Ten Asbroek, A. H., Soremekun, S., Danso, S., Owusu-Agyei, S., Prince, M., & Kirkwood, B. R. (2015). Determinants of postnatal depression in rural ghana: findings from the don population based cohort study. *Depress Anxiety, 32*(2), 108–119. doi: 10.1002/da.22218

Westdahl, C., Milan, S., Magriples, U., Kershaw, T. S., Rising, S. S., & Ickovics, J. R. (2007). Social support and social conflict as predictors of prenatal depression. *Obstet Gynecol, 110*(1), 134–140. doi: 10.1097/01.AOG.0000265352.61822.1b

WHO. (2005). Report of a WHO Technical Consultation on Birth Spacing.: World Health Organization, Geneva, Switzerland.

Wosu, A. C., Gelaye, B., & Williams, M. A. (2015). History of childhood sexual abuse and risk of prenatal and postpartum depression or depressive symptoms: an epidemiologic review. *Arch Womens Ment Health, 18*(5), 659–671. doi: 10.1007/s00737-015-0533-0

Wright, N., Hill, J., Pickles, A., & Sharp, H. (2015). The specific role of relationship life events in the onset of depression during pregnancy and the postpartum. *PLoS One, 10*(12), e0144131. doi: 10.1371/journal.pone.0144131

Yanikkerem, E., Ay, S., Mutlu, S., & Goker, A. (2013). Antenatal depression: prevalence and risk factors in a hospital based Turkish sample. *J Pak Med Assoc, 63*(4), 472–477.

Zelkowitz, P., Schinazi, J., Katofsky, L., Saucier, J. F., Valenzuela, M., Westreich, R., & Dayan, J. (2004). Factors associated with depression in pregnant immigrant women. *Transcult Psychiatry, 41*(4), 445–464. doi: 10.1177/1363461504047929

Zeng, Y., Cui, Y., & Li, J. (2015). Prevalence and predictors of antenatal depressive symptoms among Chinese women in their third trimester: a cross-sectional survey. *BMC Psychiatry, 15*, 66. doi: 10.1186/s12888-015-0452-7

Screening and Early Identification of Women at Risk of Perinatal Psychopathology[1]

Alessandra Bramante

Introduction

Depression represents the most widespread psychiatric illness among mental disorders, and it is estimated that it will become the second most serious cause of disability in the population by 2020. It is currently one of the primary causes of disability among women in the world between the ages of 15 and 44. In the USA, it is the principal cause of non-obstetric hospitalizations for women between the ages of 18 and 44. Depression is a mood disorder that affects one woman in four. It is hardly surprising that this condition can occur during pregnancy as well as after the birth of a child. Indeed, in contrast to previous thinking, scientific evidence has exposed how pregnancy is a stressful event for women, characterized by important physical, psychological and hormonal changes as well as changes in family roles. It is a period of high psychopathology risk.

According to the American College of Obstetricians and Gynecologists (ACOG), 14–23% of women manifest anxiety and/or depressive symptoms during pregnancy. The rate of perinatal depression changes depending on the study and the period analyzed, whether it is pregnancy or the child's first year. The percentage ranges between 7.4% and 20%, whereas during the postpartum period it can reach up to 22% (Littlewood et al., 2016). The American Academy of Pediatrics claims that every year 400,000 children are born to depressed mothers (McDonagh et al., 2014).

As mentioned earlier, depression can occur during pregnancy or postpartum. An American study conducted on 1,396 mothers evaluated six weeks after delivery found that in 40.1% of cases, the onset of depression occurred postpartum, while in 33.4% of cases depression occurred during pregnancy and in 26.5% of the cases it occurred before the pregnancy (Wisner et al., 2013).

The period following delivery is characterized by several biological, physical, social and emotional changes. During pregnancy both the woman and her family have many expectations about this period which is filled with immense joy for the imminent arrival of the baby. However, during the gestation period and immediately after, mothers may experience a wide range of overwhelming emotions including excitement, happiness and a sense of accomplishment. But the mother may also have feelings of anxiety, of frustration, of confusion, as well as of sadness and guilt.

As a result, the pregnancy requires significant personal and interpersonal adaptability, especially for first-time mothers.

The perinatal period renders women more vulnerable to several psychiatric disorders.

Traditionally, postpartum psychiatric disorders were classified in three different categories: baby blues, postpartum depression and postpartum psychosis. Today, we recognize that this categorization is outdated, and that the postpartum phenomenology spectrum is broad and characterized by a wide range of signs, ranging from transient emotional lability, irritability and crying, to pronounced agitation, hallucinations, confusion and delirium.

Although perinatal depression is now recognized as one of the most common medical complications of pregnancy, and in the first year of the baby's life, and has an identification code in the latest edition of the *International Classification of Disease* (ICD-10) and of the diagnostic and statistical manual of mental disorders (DSM-5), it is nonetheless too often underdiagnosed. It is estimated that less than 50% of perinatal depression is identified during routine clinical examinations and that only 12–30% of women will receive proper treatment (Bick & Howard, 2010).

Perinatal depression and anxiety, when unidentified and therefore untreated, may lead to serious consequences not only for women but also for the fetus, the infant and the mother-child relationship (Bick & Howard, 2010).

The most important of these two disorders during pregnancy are obstetrical complications during the delivery, pre-term birth, low birth weight, low Apgar score, miscarriage, as well as poor adherence to prenatal care, pre-eclampsia, smoking and use of drugs which may lead to suicide. The lack of treatment for perinatal depression is considered one of the primary causes of maternal death (Bick & Howard, 2010). Furthermore, longitudinal studies on children of depressed mothers have discovered an increase in problems regarding emotional difficulties during childhood, behavioral problems and reduced cognitive development. Children of depressed mothers are less active, less attentive and more overwrought than those born of mothers not burdened by the disorder (Ding et al., 2014; Henshaw & Ericksen, 2015; Littlewood et al., 2016; McDonagh et al., 2014; NICE, 2014; Parry, 2016).

The importance of women's physical and mental health should be central in maternity. Perinatal mental disorders may affect pregnancy and parenthood, are associated with a greater risk of obstetric and neonatal complications, and may also affect the mother's ability to bond well with the child. If left untreated, the depression may also negatively affect the well-being of the fetus and subsequently of the growing child (McDonagh et al., 2014; Milgrom & Gemmill, 2015; Centre of Perinatal Excellence COPE, 2017).

This underlines the extreme importance of early assessment of psychosocial risks and of screening for symptoms of depression and anxiety for all women in the perinatal period. This approach is essential to provide prompt intervention where necessary and desired.

Definition of Screening

The UK National Screening Committee (NSC) provides an accurate definition of screening as a way of identifying people who are apparently healthy but may be at higher risk of a disease or pathology. The screening provider then offers information, further tests and treatment. This is to reduce associated problems or complications (National Screening Committee, 2013).

Another definition of screening is the systematic application of a test or questions to identify individuals at risk of a specific disease. To benefit from further investigations or preventive actions aimed at people who have not requested medical attention due to this disorder (Packman e Dezateux, 1998).

Originally, the diagnosis focused on pathologies such as cancer, deafness in children and risk factors for cardiovascular diseases. More recently, psychological risks have been included. In 2002, the US Preventive Service Task Force recommended depression screening in adult services. Many colleagues and academics in North America are now using it when compiling the medical histories of their patients. Epidemiologists define the search for disease in those who already have a medical problem as "discovering the case". This definition precisely suits the use of screening instruments in pregnant and postpartum women. It consists of a complex process that includes identification, evaluation, involvement, intervention, and symptom and risk reduction, as well as achievement of functional improvement.

Anxiety and Perinatal Depression Screening

Pregnancy and childbirth are very important times in a woman's life. It is expected that these two events will bring delight and hope. But this is also a period during which women are at risk for depression. In most cases, the perinatal period – from conception until the first year of the child's life – is filled with both ups and downs. During periods of depression, the mom must be able to find and receive treatment.

Symptoms of depression may include depressed mood, a propensity to cry, alterations in eating and sleeping behavior, agitation, anxiety, irritability, weight gain or weight loss, a decrease in energy, a lack of ability to experience pleasure, a general loss of interest and feelings of guilt or hopelessness. A loss of concentration and the fear of hurting oneself or the child may also occur during a period of depression. Depressive symptoms range from mild to severe; the latter often includes thoughts of death or suicide. The impulse to run away, the idea of being unable to protect and care for the baby or worse to harm the child are particularly painful thoughts for the mother.

Recent studies have concluded that the identification of major depression with onset in the peripartum period, when diagnosed with a screening instrument, is significantly higher than the identification of major depression diagnosed with only a routine clinical evaluation.

Screening involves the use of a validated test or questionnaire, to identify subjects at risk for a specific disorder. These are not diagnostic tools but tools to detect risk factors. Screening is designed to identify depression or anxiety disorders. The screening must take place within a program that includes a staff properly trained in methodology and screening instruments. There must be clear rules for the further evaluation of the women who are identified as being at risk, during the screening.

Accurately detecting women with depressive and/or anxiety symptoms in the perinatal period allows immediate attention to mental health services as well as an adequate follow-up.

The history of screening has changed following the publication of the guidelines on mental health during the perinatal period (Beyondblue, 2011):

- Increased awareness of the prevalence of depression and anxiety during the pregnancy and postpartum periods.
- Further research on screening instrument efficacy, and their employment in evaluation programs.
- Development of a wide range of innovative screening methods, for example, the availability and use of electronic tools.

In general, screening is recommended for high-risk individuals which also includes women during pregnancy and postpartum. The reasons for recommending these periods are (Wisconsin Association for Perinatal Care, s.d.) as follows:

- The stigma associated with mental illness, which becomes more oppressive after the birth of a baby. The event is generally assumed to bring joy and happiness. Therefore, it may be more difficult for the mom to express her feelings and ask for help.
- Women may not recognize that what they are experiencing is depression. They may think that their emotions are a normal part of pregnancy and parenthood. Hence, they may misinterpret their depression symptoms.

- Irritability could be the main symptom of depression, especially among adolescents.
- It has been demonstrated that depression is common during pregnancy and postpartum. When not detected and then treated, depression during pregnancy can extend into the post-partum period.
- Depression can interfere with a woman's willingness to seek and continue prenatal care as well as interfere with her willingness to provide the environmental safety for the child. This may have negative consequences for both mother and child.
- Depression interferes with the mother's ability to bond with the fetus during pregnancy as well as with the child during the postpartum period.
- Depression can be associated with premature birth.
- In extreme cases, depression can be a risk factor for infanticide and suicide.

Initial and Significant International Initiatives

An informal screening modality initiated by health professionals for the detection of perinatal depression dates back many years in the United States. In fact, systematic work started in 1990 with the Edinburgh Postnatal Depression Scale (EPDS) test. Since 2001, the Health Resources and Services Administration – an American agency that deals with facilitating access to care for the population – has authorized screening to identify women at risk for perinatal depression.

The first Australian guidelines regarding the detection, management and treatment of perinatal mental disorders were established in 2011. The Royal Australian and New Zealand College of Obstetricians and Gynaecologists supports the Australian clinical practice guidelines Beyondblue, which were approved by the National Health and Medical Research Council (NHMRC) and recommend universal screening for prenatal and postnatal mental health. It administers the EPDS and conducts a psychosocial assessment. It is currently being implemented throughout Australia. Local health facilities which deal with maternity should negotiate ways to regularly implement this clinical practice.

Why Do Screening?

Depression occurs in all populations and in all periods of life. All women, therefore, are poten-tially at risk for depression. The prevalence of perinatal depression is about the same as in other periods of a woman's life. Depression has both biological and psychosocial bases. A previous his-tory of depression, anxiety or other mental disorders, especially during previous pregnancies or postpartum, and a psychiatric predisposition to anxiety or mood disorders are the primary risk factors in the perinatal period. Other social risk factors include certain stressors – poverty, unem-ployment, lack of support from the partner or family. Depressive disorders affect a woman's ability to relate to others, including and most importantly her baby. Screening is a simple and effective way to identify women whose symptoms may interfere with a variety of role functions. When identified early on, depression is more easily treatable.

The National Institute for Health and Care Excellence (NICE, 2014), recognizing the impor-tance of early identification of maternal perinatal psychopathology particularly through screening, issued the following recommendations:

1 Perinatal depression is a common psychopathology.
2 Perinatal depression has serious consequences for the mom, the newborn as well as the entire family.
3 Screening can identify those at risk who would otherwise go unidentified.
4 There is effective treatment for these disorders.

Furthermore, it is well known that there are many barriers that may prevent women from seeking help for psychiatric problems during pregnancy and the postpartum period. It is, therefore, a health worker's task to deal with them in the perinatal period to identify the cases at risk and organize an effective response (Milgrom e Gemmill, 2015).

Moreover, screening in the perinatal period:

1   is recommended by the US Preventive Task Force, ACOG, Association of Women's Health, Obstetric and Neonatal Nurses and American Academy of Pediatrics.
2   is mandated by law in many states.
3   offers the chance to reduce the suffering in women and reduce mortality in children.

Main Agencies That Recommend Perinatal Screening

The US Preventive Services Task Force (USPSTF) recommends screening for depression in the adult population, including pregnant and postpartum women. It should be carried out with adequate systems to ensure accurate diagnosis, effective treatment and adequate follow-up. The updating of depression screening recommendations strongly indicates the important focus now given to this issue. The USPSTF's advice is the first specific recommendation for pregnancy and postpartum.

Karina Davidson, PhD, a professor at the Columbia University Medical Center in New York City and a member of the task force, affirms that adding the subgroup of pregnant and postpartum women is an important innovation in the 2015 recommendations. She also points out that in previous iterations there was a lack of evidence for screening recommendations in both pregnant and postpartum women. Now the evidence has been provided.

The recommendations, published online on January 26, 2016 by "JAMA", indicate that general practitioners will provide screening for patients, using validated tests including the Patient Health Questionnaire (PHQ), the Hospital Anxiety and Depression Scales (HADS) in adults, the Geriatric Depression Scale (GDS) in the elderly and the EPDS in pregnant and postpartum women. The inclusion of the EPDS in the program has been long needed, understanding that the principals have not been open to a dialogue on the subject of depression, especially during pregnancy.

In an interview with Medscape Medical, Richard K. Argento (president and academic director of the Department of Obstetrics and Gynecology at the North Shore University Health System, Evanston, Illinois) stated that he was very satisfied with the work done by the task force.

The USPSTF has found convincing evidence that screening improves accurate identification of depressed adult patients, including pregnant and postpartum women. Although evidence of the benefits of these interventions is limited, the ACOG recommends that clinicians evaluate patients at least once during pregnancy for anxiety and depressive symptoms, using a standardized and validated instrument. It is necessary to guarantee a regular monitoring for mothers with current or previous psychopathology or present risk factors for perinatal psychopathology. Screening itself is not enough to improve clinical outcomes. It must be combined with adequate follow-up and treatment when indicated. Medical and obstetric staff therefore should be adequately trained (Albert et al., 2016).

The Association of Women's Health, Obstetric and Neonatal Nurses argues that all pregnant and postpartum women should be screened for depressive and anxiety disorders. Obstetric workers are in a key position to detect these disorders in women and provide them with instructions to help ensure timely and effective treatment. To successfully address mood disorders and perinatal anxiety, health facilities that care for pregnant women, new mothers and newborns should conduct proper screening and appropriate protocols. Psycho-education meetings should also be held in the perinatal period with staff training courses related to these disorders (AWHONN, 2015).

According to the American Academy of Pediatrics, the patient's pediatrician has the unique opportunity to identify maternal depression and help prevent any developmental and mental health problems for the baby and the mother. Screening can be integrated into the child's well-being visit and included in the prenatal visit. Pediatricians have the opportunity to screen mothers during the check-ups to monitor the child's growth at one month, two months and four months. This screening has been shown to have good clinical outcomes for family pediatricians who take care of newborns and their families. The intervention takes place in collaboration with other facilities including mental health centers (Siu and USPSTF, 2016).

The National Service Framework (NSF) for mental health emphasizes the importance of having locally managed protocols for detecting perinatal depression, promoting the use of screening to facilitate the early detection of women at risk. This led to the introduction of the routine clinical evaluation through the administration of short self-report questionnaires such as the EPDS (Department of Health, 2016).

How to Perform Screening?

The clinician could start by informing the patient for example that it is normal practice in this clinic to ask all pregnant women or new mothers how they are feeling emotionally. This indicates that he is interested in knowing about the woman's health from an emotional point of view. Valid screening tools are available such as short self-administered questionnaires which take approximately five to ten minutes to complete. As already mentioned, these tools are not diagnostic, but rather useful in highlighting risk and therefore alerting the clinician to the fact that the woman is experiencing high levels of stressful symptoms that may indicate an ongoing depression.

When to Perform Screening?

Most postpartum depressions occur in the first three months after the birth of the child. However, we know that depression may also begin in other periods up to the first year postpartum and even beyond. The latest studies have also uncovered high rates of depression and anxiety during pregnancy. As a result, many clinicians suggest carrying out one screening during pregnancy, followed by another during the postpartum period. The administration of the screening should take place based on the resources available and the relationships between the woman and her healthcare professionals. An obvious point of contact is the first antenatal visit. It is however recognized that the time available on the initial visit because of the number of other medical assessments that must be attended to can limit the opportunity for mental health assessment. However, postnatal assessment may be integrated into the mother's and child's pediatric regimen. A monitoring project carried out at the first appointment, the third trimester of pregnancy, six weeks after delivery and one other time postpartum would make it possible to identify most women suffering depression in the perinatal period. When screening is possible during the postpartum period, the best time seems to be at the six-week point. Furthermore, although women have only one check-up appointment after the birth of their child for the check-up, they will have frequent contact with the family pediatrician. These specialists not only see children but also mothers with all their vulnerabilities. They could therefore perform a routine screening for postpartum depression, as is recommended by the American Academy of Pediatrics. The literature states that when pediatricians see children, mothers willingly accept screening, and often report their health concerns. In particular, it seems that depressed mothers, compared to those who are not depressed, tend to describe their children as difficult, spoiled and colicky. To sum up, the international guidelines recommend the following times as most appropriate for screening: pregnancy (first visit and subsequent visits), delivery (or during hospitalization), two/three weeks postpartum, during postpartum check-ups and at baby health check-ups done by the pediatrician.

Box 14.1 Consensus-Based Recommendations (Centre of Perinatal Excellence COPE, 2017)

1   Complete the first antenatal screening during the first visit and repeat the screening at least once during pregnancy.

2   Complete the first postpartum screening 6–12 weeks after birth and repeat it at least once during the first year of child's life.

3   For a woman with an EPDS score between 10 and 12, monitor and repeat the EPDS after 4–6 weeks as the score may increase.

4   Readminister the EPDS at any time during pregnancy and in the first-year postpartum if clinically indicated.

Who Should Perform the Screening?

Screening can be performed by the clinicians and other staff at services who administer to the pregnant woman and the new mother. Those involved may include midwives, family doctors, gynecologists, nurses, pediatricians, psychologists, psychiatrists and lactation consultants, belonging to both public and private services. Whoever performs the screening must then provide a follow-up plan, as recommended by numerous international guidelines. It is essential that the screening staff be adequately trained and constantly updated about issues concerning perinatal psychopathology.

Screening Acceptability

Historically, there has been little consensus regarding the acceptability of screening as a strategy for risk identification. Today, it is clearly demonstrated that women who undergo evaluation consider it simple and acceptable (Milgrom e Gemmill, 2015). The percentage of mothers who have been involved and who accept screening, both in research and in the clinic, is as high as 85–90%.

Some studies directly examine women's point of views on perinatal screening (Milgrom e Gemmill, 2015). In Australia international researchers have reported high levels of acceptability for perinatal depression screening among health professionals (Bales et al., 2015; Bowen et al., 2012; Reay et al., 2011), in Canada (Kingston et al., 2015), in the United States (Miller, Shade & Vasireddy, 2009) and in many systematic reviews (El-Den, O'Reilly & Chen, 2015).

More vulnerable women also report high acceptability, including those with high depression scores (Gemmill, Leigh & Ericksen, 2006). This includes women of different mother tongues (Matthey et al., 2005), with a previous history of diagnosis and therapy for mental disorders (Kingston et al., 2015), or from domestic violence contexts (Matthey et al., 2005). Fewer than 4% of women refuse the routine screening suggested by professionals. These rates could be even lower since women's ability to be honest about emotional health is strongly associated with comfort perceived during assessment (Kingston et al., 2015).

Recent Canadian research has found that 99% of pregnant women who had not been screened would have been comfortable if health professionals had offered them a screening, and 97% of those who had been screened reported the same thing (Kingston et al., 2015). Demographics, the type of health professionals involved and a history of diagnosis or treatment for mental illness were not related to the fact that pregnant women found the screening acceptable or not (Kingston et al., 2015).

Australian studies have also evaluated the acceptability of screening in pregnant women. In the study conducted by Leigh and Milgrom in 2006, 407 women had been screened during pregnancy using the EPDS, then interviewed by telephone. In 100% of the cases the screening had been accepted, and 50% more women state that it had served to raise their awareness of postpartum depression. No stigma or stress related to screening was demonstrated. In another Australian research study, Matthey et al., in 2005, tested the acceptability of screening during pregnancy in a sample of 202 women. He recorded high levels (98%) of acceptability.

Other research, carried out in Australia, focused on the acceptability of screening for women postpartum. In this case, the data are more heterogeneous. Gemmill et al., in 2006, asked mothers what they thought about postpartum screening. Most of them found the circumstance "comfortable" and considered it "a good idea". Of the 472 women only 18.8% found that the screening was not useful, while for the rest of the participants it was a positive experience. In another Australian survey, the sample of 860 women who had been screened for postpartum depression gave a highly acceptable opinion. Ninety-three percent said that the EPDS was an easy tool to fill out and 83% considered it acceptable and comfortable.

In another small Australian qualitative study, women reported very different experiences. For some, screening was defined as a helpful process. For others, it was described as poorly acceptable. According to the authors, women who had a syntonic relationship with the screener who sent them for subsequent treatment were more accepting of the evaluation.

In summary, Australian studies suggest that screening is generally accepted by women during pregnancy, but results were mixed in postpartum women. In Australia, perinatal depression awareness campaigns are common. Therefore, women accept screening as part of the evaluation process during pregnancy and postpartum.

A small study conducted in the United Kingdom by Shakespeare, Blake and Garcia in 2003, on the acceptability of screening in clinical postpartum practice, reported that for 46% of women interviewed, screening was unacceptable. The primary reason was the stigma associated with mental illness in the perinatal period.

Yet, what is the point of view of health professionals? Although perinatal depression is a frequent and severe disorder, few healthcare providers include regular screening in clinical practice. A percentage from 0% to 50% is estimated. Some operators who want to implement screening often use invalid tools or informal assessments thus failing in their purpose. It has been proven that informal screening is not only ineffective but may also be dangerous. The reasons mentioned by doctors concerning the difficulty of recommending screening include lack of time, competition with other examination tasks, limited knowledge about feasibility, perception of patient's reluctance, concern about excessive treatment cost for the patient, limited feasibility, fear of legal repercussions and lack of training in perinatal depression. Qualitative studies on patients have shown that health worker anxiety in asking questions about depression is negatively interpreted by the more sensitive patients.

Barriers to Screening

Obstacles to screening include lack of time, lack of training and unavailability of mental health services. Each of these barriers can be alleviated by using innovative approaches to screening, by making more information available and by creating a network for referral. Barriers among women include stigma, significant others minimizing their emotional difficulties, the desire to manage mental health problems on their own, a preference to discuss feelings with only significant others, ignorance about which emotions are "normal" or a perception that the health professional is disinterested or lacks time (Highet et al., 2014; Kingston et al., 2015a,b).

This may be improved by the provision of timely, relevant information and education about emotional and mental health in the perinatal period (Kingston et al., 2015). A recent study revealed that only half of women who screen positive follow up with a subsequent mental health assessment (Reay et al., 2011) and that 30–85% do not accept the treatment (Bales et al., 2015). The situation can be improved through the creation of timely and appropriate referral pathways.

Facilitators of Screening and Subsequent Mental Health Care

Screening percentages can increase if health professionals are both educated regarding perinatal mental health and trained in the use of this invaluable tool. The increase in screening frequency is also associated with the use of e-screening, which shortens screening time. Women are more likely to accept mental health screening when the healthcare professional is sensitive and involved. Women are reassured that mental health care is part of routine antenatal care, that other women experience emotional problems during pregnancy and that help is available.

Being informed in advance about the impending screening also improves a woman's acceptance of the screening process. Women who are not asked about their emotional health are far less likely to seek formal mental health care during pregnancy or postpartum than those who do not receive a formal referral from a specialist (Centre of Perinatal Excellence COPE, 2017).

Specialist Referrals and Treatment

For the screening program to succeed, an efficient and carefully studied system of care should be provided, which includes the following steps: screening, assessment, diagnosis, specialist referral, treatment and follow-up.

When a woman is engaged at the screening, the clinician may tell her that her test score suggests ongoing depressive symptoms. He understands that it is difficult to accept now that she is pregnant (or has become a mother). He can emphasize that depression occurs because of a chemical imbalance, or stressful events in your life as well as by various hormonal, psychological and social factors. There are treatments that can help.

After this, the woman should be encouraged to follow non-medical interventions such as diet, exercise, rest and a review of her expectations. The level of social support must also be investigated, which means understanding not only how many supports that she has, but also her perception at the moment that support is received. It may be support from family, friends, a mutual aid group on the internet, etc. It is important to help the woman understand that support during pregnancy and postpartum is an important psychosocial intervention. The effects of depression on her relationships must then be assessed. She must be asked about family members, about sharing information with them and about including them in planning. She must bear in mind that those who live with depressed people often feel powerless. Choices of clinical treatment will then be considered: pharmacotherapy, psychotherapy (individual, group, couple, mother-child) or both. Compared to individual psychotherapy, evidence-based studies identify interpersonal psychotherapy and cognitive behavioral therapy as efficient treatments in the perinatal period. It is important that the type of treatment is decided together with the mother. The choice is based on effectiveness, severity of symptoms, costs and feasibility.

The clinician must also assess the risks and benefits of drug treatment for both the mother and the child. The psychiatrist who prescribes medication in pregnancy and breastfeeding has a duty to be informed and updated through the scientific literature. It is fundamental that the risk of potential self-harm or harm to the baby be considered.

A good approach is to ask the woman to talk about feelings of desperation and hopelessness. For example, the clinician may make it clear that sometimes mothers may feel so down and depressed that they think life is not worth living or they would be better off dead. The clinician may ask if the patient has ever had similar thoughts. If the answer is yes, it is important to investigate whether or not these thoughts were translated into a real plan and then determine the probability that this plan might be implemented. Does the woman have the means to do it? Has she chosen a time? Is there opportunity? Are there reasons for not doing this? Are there precipitant factors? If yes, it is advisable to refer her urgently to emergency services for hospitalization. Thoughts of hurting the child without having any intention to do so is common in women with postpartum depression but they must always be thoroughly investigated.

Treatment for prenatal and postpartum depression must be carried out and monitored by trained and experienced clinicians. It is important that the professional, in addition to the psychological and psychiatric aspects, is also aware of all elements connected to the perinatal period, to the expectations of a woman in this phase of her life and to the cultural implications of motherhood. Clinicians must be aware that the perinatal period may be lacking in the expected carefree feelings and feelings of joy. Rather, they may be characterized by ambivalence. Scientific studies indicate that a woman, who has been depressed in the weeks or months after the birth, will be statistically more likely to describe her pregnancy as a "very hard period", or "one of the most difficult moments in my life".

Saying to the mother, "You must be excited about your pregnancy" or "Oh, what a lovely baby! Isn't it great to be a mother?" may repress the woman's desire to describe how she is really feeling. The clinician may ask, "How are things going?" or say "I have learned over the years that being pregnant [or being a new mom] can be very demanding as well as rewarding. How are things going for you?" It is necessary to leave the door open to the possibility that the mother may feel sad, anxious, irritable, have little interest in doing things or feel little attachment to the child.

Screening Tools

In 2015, Henshaw and Ericksen explained the fundamental reasons for using scales to identify depression and anxiety in pregnancy and postpartum. Depression and perinatal anxiety are common, with a prevalence of about 13–15% of women depressed during pregnancy or after the birth of a child. The consequences of such untreated pathologies can be serious and involve not only the mother but also the child and the whole family. Although treatment is effective, these women often do not ask for help with their symptoms. Barriers such as stigma have been identified. It is thus important that these women be identified. To do so, it is necessary to ask women, and their partners, about their mental condition. This is accomplished frequently with the use of screening scales. Early identification is critical for the well-being of the mother and the child.

Professionals working with pregnant and postpartum women have a special role in identifying high-risk mothers, those who have a history of depression or psychosis, or abuse of drugs and alcohol. Included also are women with serious social problems or an unwanted pregnancy. After childbirth, health workers can attend to the questions of vulnerable mothers. In many countries, these health workers will visit the mother at home. Those involved in screening should know where, and to whom to refer women in difficulty because screening alone cannot be effective without an intervention and a support network. It is possible to use a series of screening questions or questionnaires to determine which mothers may need to be referred for further diagnostic investigation and treatment. Every professional will have particular questions to ask women to investigate their current and past psychopathological history. Observations on the mother-child relationship and how the mother relates to the child are equally important.

The international literature identifies the following test tools for screening (for the general characteristics of each see Table 14.1).

Table 14.1 Screening test for the most used perinatal anxiety and depression tests

Test	Number of questions	Administration time (minutes)	The questions concern	Cut-off	Score	Sensitivity	Specificity	Is anxiety evaluated?	Cost
Edinburgh Postpartum Depression Scale (EPDS) Self-Administered	10	<5	The last 7 days	≥10 general population ≥12 clinical population ≥13 during pregnancy	≥10 depressive symptoms ≥13 major depression ≥1 item 10 suicide risk	75–100	75–97	Questions 3, 4, 5	Free
Patient Health Questionnaire-9 (PHQ-9) Self-Administered	9	<5	The last 2 weeks	≥10	≥10 risk of depression ≥2 item 9 suicide risk	75	90	No	Free
General Health Questionnaire - 12 (GHQ-12) Self-Administered	12	<5	The last 2 weeks	≥4	≥4 depressive symptoms	71–78	73–76	No	Free
Postpartum Depression Screening Scale (PDSS)	35 complete form	5–10	The last 2 weeks	≥60	≥60 depressive symptoms ≥81 major depression ≥6 suicide risk	91–94	72–98	No	100 €
Self-Administered	7 short form	<5		≥14	≥14 major depression ≥2 item 7 suicide risk				
Whooley Questions Administered	Q1 Q2	5–10	Last months	–	–	88–100	56–74	No	Free
Matthey Generic Mood Question (MGMQ) Self-Administered	3	<5	The last 2 weeks	–	–	79	73	No	Free

Screening and early identification of women at risk of perinatal psychopathology

1 The EPDS is the only screening test currently recognized internationally, and is certainly the most frequently used tool in the world, thanks also to its characteristics of sensitivity and specificity in various cultures (Cox, Holden e Sagovsky, 1987; Mirabella et al., 2014). It is short and easy to administer and has been translated into many languages. The EPDS questionnaire, previously carefully validated for use during the postpartum period, has also been validated for pregnancy and is currently the most widely used screening tool in epidemiological studies related to depression during pregnancy and after childbirth.

To minimize false positives during pregnancy, a higher cut-off has been adopted (≥13), to ensure a sensitivity of 56%, a specification of 98% and a positive predictive value of 83% (Cox, Holden e Henshaw, 2015). Even if the EPDS produces false positives and false negatives, its performance remains by far the most reliable compared to other tests. The EPDS is not used for diagnosis but evaluates and identifies the risk of depression and anxiety in the perinatal period. It must be associated with a subsequent in-depth clinical evaluation. In any case, screening using the EPDS appears numerically useful at the population level, with the potential to significantly facilitate and increase identification.

2 The Patient Health Questionnaire-9 (PHQ-9) is a short, self-administered questionnaire developed for use in primary care (Spitzer e Williams, 2001) for depression screening. Composed of nine items that correspond to the symptoms of major depression, it is frequently used for somatic symptoms related to depression in the perinatal period. It includes questions about appetite, fatigue, sleep or other biological aspects that should be interpreted with caution during pregnancy, as the highlighted problem may reflect the physical effects of gestation, rather than those of depression.

3 The General Health Questionnaire 12 (GHQ-12) by Goldberg (1972) is another short self-administered 12-item questionnaire, focused on general well-being, usually used in screening for mental disorders. Like the PHQ-9, it also includes questions related to physical issues like appetite, fatigue, sleep and the like and, therefore, requires a cautious interpretation of symptoms during pregnancy that may itself cause such factors.

4 The Postpartum Depression Screening Scale (PDSS) developed by Beck and Gable (2000) is a self-report questionnaire consisting of 35 items. It is administered in postpartum and evaluates seven categories (sleeping/eating disturbances, anxiety/insecurity, emotional lability, mental confusion, loss of self, guilt/shame and suicidal thoughts).

5 The NICE Guidelines published in 2007 recommend asking the two Whooley questions: "During the last month, have you often been bothered by feeling down, depressed or hopeless?", "During the last month, have you often been bothered by having little interest or pleasure in doing things?" If both receive positive answers, ask a third question ("Is there something you feel you need or for which you want to be helped?"). These questions, validated in other clinical settings, have never been validated for use in the perinatal period. Therefore, specific studies on women are needed during pregnancy and postpartum to be able to conclude that a negative response to both the first two questions is enough to decide that the woman is not depressed (Henshaw, Cox e Barton, 2017; NICE, 2007).

6 The MGMQ (Matthey Generic Mood Question, or generic question on mood, Matthey et al., 2013) has few questions and takes little time to administer. This test showed a better ability to identify women who meet diagnostic criteria for an anxiety disorder and is also superior to other commonly used tools used in identifying subjects with high scores on self-report scales on mood or anxiety (Matthey et al., 2013). It reflects the questions that a woman should normally be asked in clinical practice when, in a screening context, the health worker is collecting information about her experiences and state of mind. It differs from other tools, such as the EPDS, as it investigates not only the symptoms but also the

impact that these may have on the mother and her desire to talk about them with someone. This element seems to reduce the number of false positives typical of screening tests that do not include these types of questions.

The indication for the use of EPDS and other self-administered screening tools can be found within various international guidelines that suggest the procedures for pregnant and postpartum women, such as those of Canada (BC Reproductive Mental Health Program & Perinatal Services BC, 2014), the United States of America (American College of Obstetricians and Gynecologists, 2015), Australia (Beyondblue, 2011) and the United Kingdom (NICE, 2014).

Investigating Psychosocial Factors That Have an Impact on Mental Health

In addition to the screening of depression and anxiety symptoms, psychosocial evaluation is essential to identify the circumstances (past and present) that can contribute to a woman's mental health problems and may need specific attention to protect the well-being of the mother and family. The number and type of psychosocial factors identified influence the assistance pathway, suggesting multicomponent approaches or support interventions, while the possible presence of risk factors will require a coordinated multidisciplinary approach for each woman.

Psychosocial assessment can be conducted as part of the clinical interview and/or using a specific structured and validated tool. The structured questionnaires are useful to provide, in a short time, an overview of the circumstances of a woman's life, especially when the professional is not an expert in carrying out a detailed psychosocial assessment as part of a wider clinical analysis. One of the tests recognized through scientific evidence as being useful for a psychosocial survey is the Antenatal Risk Questionnaire (ANRQ) (Center of Perinatal Excellence COPE, 2017). It is a structured questionnaire consisting of 13 questions with categorical (yes/no) and dimensional (1 to 5) responses, which generates a total psychosocial risk score (cumulative risk) as well as identifying specific risk factors that independently put the woman at greater psychosocial risk (past history of trauma, significant mental health condition, etc.). This tool has two functions. It provides a brief and structured approach to the psychosocial dimension as well as giving the professional an indication of the degree of the woman's risk of perinatal psychiatric morbidity or difficulty in adapting to the role of parenting. The ANRQ covers the relationship with partner, social support, recent stressful life events, anxiety or perfectionism, past history and treatment of depression or other mental health conditions, history of abuse as a child or as an adult, and quality of relationship with mother during the childhood. The use of this tool to identify the presence of issues bears a "strong" evidence-based recommendation in the 2017 *Australian practice guideline*.

Evaluation Scales of the Mother-Fetus and Mother-Child Relationship

Another important assessment concerns the mother-fetus and mother–child relationship. There are numerous questionnaires suitable for identifying early relationship disorders. They are self-administered tools that offer several advantages (simple methodology, quick administration) and are reliable for screening studies (Beck e Gable, 2000). At an international level, various tests have been developed to assess the maternal–fetal bond. The following are the most widely known and used (taken from Bramante e Brockington, 2016).

1   Maternal–Fetal Attachment Scale (MFAS) (Cranley, 1981). It is a Likert-type, self-administered scale comprising 24 items divided into 5 subscales: (1) "differentiation of self from the fetus", (2) "interaction with the fetus", (3) "attributing characteristics and intentions to the fetus",

(4) "giving of self", (5) "role-taking" (e.g. "I picture myself feeding the baby", 4 items). The items are scored on a 5-point scale: 1 (absolutely no), 2 (no), 3 (maybe), 4 (yes) and 5 (absolutely yes). The total score ranges between 24 and 120.

2   Prenatal Attachment Inventory (PAI) (Muller, 1996). It is a Likert and self-administered scale composed of 21 items with a factorial structure: 1 (almost never), 2 (sometimes), 3 (often) and 4 (almost always). It measures the levels of the mother's attachment to the fetus: high scores indicate a good prenatal attachment. The maximum score is 84.

3   Maternal Antenatal Attachment Scale (MAAS) (Condon e Corkindale, 1997). It is a Likert and self-administered scale composed of 19 items, divided into two subscales: quality of attachment (11 items) and time dedicated to interaction (8 items). All items are evaluated on a scale of 1 to 5 points, where 5 indicates a strong attachment; high scores reflect a positive quality attachment and an intense concern for the fetus.

4   Maternal Attachment Inventory (MAI) (Muller, 1994). This is a self-administered questionnaire consisting of 26 items, which investigate how the mother feels in relation to thoughts, feelings and situations of motherhood. The items are organized on a 4-point Likert scale ranging from 1 (almost never) to 4 (almost always). The total score ranges from 6 to 104; high scores indicate good mother–child attachment.

Numerous questionnaires have also been developed to investigate the mother-infant bond. The most widely known and known internationally are the following (taken from Bramante e Brockington, 2016).

1   Postpartum Bonding Questionnaire (PBQ) (Brockington et al., 2001). It is a self-administered questionnaire consisting of 25 items, each followed by a Likert scale with a score ranging from 0 (always) to 5 (never). Four factors are identified, reflecting (1) impaired bonding (12 items), (2) rejection and pathological anger (7 items), (3) anxiety about the infant (4 items) and (4) incipient infant abuse factors (2 items). The total score is 125; high scores indicate a serious disturbance in the mother-child relationship.

2   Maternal Postnatal Attachment Scale (MPAS) (Condon e Corkindale, 1998). The scale has 19 items each of which has 2, 4 or 5 response options. To guarantee the same weight for each application, the options have been calibrated to give a score ranging from 1 (low attachment) to 5 (high attachment). A three-factor structure is used:

> (1) the desire for proximity and interaction with the infant, (2) the lack of resentment and negative feelings toward the infant and (3) a sense of confidence and satisfaction in being a mother. The sum of the 19 items forms the total of the MPAS (minimum 19, maximum 95), where a low score indicates a problematic mother-child relationship.

3   Postpartum Maternal Attachment Scale (PMAS) (Nagata et al., 2000). This is a self-administered questionnaire composed of 19 items divided into two subscales: (1) core maternal attachment focus and (2) anxiety about the child.

4   Mother-to-Infant Bonding Scale (MIBS) (Taylor et al., 2005). This scale consists of eight statements, divided into three aspects (positive attachment, negative and confused), which describe an emotional response like "loving" or "disappointing". The scale has a four-point (1 = "not at all" to 4 = "very much") Likert scale. The total ranges between 0 and 24 points: low scores indicate a good bond while the reverse suggests a problem in the mother-child relationship. This scale can be administered from a few weeks after the birth until the fourth month postpartum.

5   Parent-to-Infant Attachment Questionnaire (PAQ) (Condon et al., 2008). A self-administered questionnaire consists of 19 items organized into three subscales: quality of attachment (QA),

absence of hostility (AH), pleasure in interaction (PI). It investigates the emotional response of the mother to her child in the first year of life. It is recommended to administer this scale between the fourth and fifth month postpartum.

It is important to remember again that although all these tools are very useful for screening they are not sufficient to make a reliable diagnosis.

Screening, Assessment or Both?

There is an important distinction to be made regarding two key terms: screening and assessment. The former refers to the use of a simple and reliable test that is administered to a group of people, usually asymptomatic, at high risk of having a disease or disorder for which effective remedies exist. However, the term "assessment" refers to a broad clinical evaluation of the subject – medical and psychological history, social and current status – including analysis of the risk and protection factors. Such an assessment can be improved with the inclusion of standardized screening tools.

The feasibility and usefulness of screening, as previously stated, depend on the existence of pathways for referral, diagnosis and effective treatment, which would enable the screening not only to lead to the identification of women at risk, but also to contribute in reducing the disease.

The debate around the two terms and the consequent processes has been addressed by the National Institute of Health and Care Excellence (NICE, 2014; 2015; 2016) in the evaluation guidelines and the management of perinatal clinical conditions. These indications suggest that screening performs two main functions: prediction and detection. Prediction is the identification of current and past risk factors that increase the likelihood of developing mental disorders or the recurrence of a previous psychiatric disorder, whereas detection is the identification of an existing psychiatric disorder.

Professional Organizations and International Initiatives

The NYS Medicaid program in New York provides a refund for screening, diagnosis and treatment of maternal depression. This is because good evidence exists that this disorder can be accurately identified using standardized screening tools and that treatment improves the prognosis for the woman and the whole family.

In Australia, psychological assessment conducted using structured questions and the use of the EPDS to identify depressive and anxiety symptoms is recommended during pregnancy and at 6–12 weeks postpartum.

In the United Kingdom, many guidelines (including those previously mentioned of NICE) are the leader in the study of perinatal mental disorders and the birthplace of the EPDS, but there is no structured screening such as that established in Australia.

However, there are numerous realities and studies for the identification and provision of care for women at risk during pregnancy and postpartum.

In Canada, Canada Medicare offers a universal health program, which includes women in the perinatal period. Two provinces (British Columbia and Saskatchewan) have developed guidelines recommending the use of the EPDS during pregnancy, and some weeks after birth (two and six months). In Ontario, there was a campaign to implement screening in the perinatal period.

Table 14.2 summarizes the current recommendations for screening for maternal depression of numerous professional organizations.

Table 14.2

Organization	Recommendations
US Preventive Services Task Force (USPSTF)	Recommends screening for depression in the general adult population, including pregnant and postpartum women. Screening should be implemented with adequate systems in place to ensure accurate diagnosis, effective treatment and appropriate follow-up.
American Congress of Obstetrician and Gynecologist Committee on Obstetric Practice (ACOG)	Recommends clinicians screen patients at least once during the perinatal period for depression and anxiety symptoms using a standardized, validated tool. Screening should be coupled with appropriate follow-up and treatment when indicated.
American Academy of Pediatrics Bright Futures and Mental Health Task Force	The primary care pediatrician, by virtue of having a longitudinal relationship with families, has a unique opportunity to identify maternal depression and help prevent untoward developmental and mental health outcomes for the infant and family. Screening can be integrated into the well-child care schedule and included in the prenatal visit. This screening has proven successful in practice in several initiatives and locations and is a best practice for PCPs caring for infants and their families. Intervention and referral are optimized by collaborative relationships with community resources and/or by co-located/integrated primary care and mental health practices.
AAP/ACOG Guidelines for Perinatal Care	Prior to delivery, patients should be informed about psychosocial issues that may arise during pregnancy and the postpartum period. A woman experiencing negative feelings about her pregnancy should receive additional support from the healthcare team. All patients should be monitored for symptoms of severe postpartum depression and offered culturally appropriate treatment or referral to community resources. Specifically, the psychosocial status of the mother and newborn should be subject to ongoing assessment after hospital discharge. Women with postpartum blues should be monitored for the onset of continuing or worsening symptoms because these women are at high risk for the onset of a more serious condition. The postpartum visit approximately 4–6 weeks after delivery should include a review of symptoms for clinically significant depression to determine whether intervention is needed.

Source: health.ny.gov

International Studies on Perinatal Screening

An important longitudinal study was conducted in the United States, between July 2010 and June 2014, with the aim of assessing the feasibility of large-scale, universal screening for depression during pregnancy and postpartum using the EPDS. Pregnant women were evaluated at 24–28 weeks of gestation and again six weeks after the birth. A cut-off EPDS score of ≥12 was chosen for referral to mental health services for a more in-depth diagnostic assessment and possible treatment. The study was conducted in two hospitals: Massachusetts General Hospital and Brigham and Women's Hospital in Boston.

Of the 8,985 women who were enrolled in the study, 8,840 (98%) were screened for depression during pregnancy and 7,780 (86%) were screened during the postpartum period. A total of 576 mothers (6.5%) scored positive for a probable depression (69% positive in pregnancy and 31% positive in postpartum). All the women identified at risk were sent to mental health services to be evaluated by a professional. Among the latter, more than three quarters were diagnosed with major depression and/or anxiety disorders. Of the mothers diagnosed, 35% received antidepressant drugs; this occurred more frequently after childbirth than during pregnancy (54% vs 28%; p <0.0001). This study demonstrates the feasibility of universal screening for depression both during pregnancy and after childbirth, using the EPDS. The practice may represent an initial skimming followed by referral to the services for further diagnostic evaluation and treatment. Although universal screening for depression is feasible, further studies are necessary regarding barriers to mental health assessment, treatment and its impact on obstetric outcomes (Parry, 2016; Venkatesh et al., 2016).

A survey carried out in the United Kingdom notes that the number of women suffering from depression during pregnancy is probably greatly underestimated. The survey, conducted by the parenting site Baby Centre, showed that about 30% of pregnant women had five or more symptoms of prenatal depression, such as anxiety, loss of interest in normal activity, unhappiness and frequent crying. A total of 1,000 mothers and pregnant women were interviewed. The research highlighted that 42% of the participants never spoke to a doctor or a midwife about their depressive symptoms. The main reasons were guilt, embarrassment or fear of being judged. A quarter of the women who had depressive symptoms had never discussed this with their partner or with a friend or relative.

Despite the widespread recognition of the problem of maternal depression and the potential benefits of screening, studies suggest that the latter is not yet standardized. A survey conducted among obstetricians and gynecologists shows that less than half of the subjects interviewed reported often or always evaluating their patients for depression or using standardized and validated analysis tools. A study carried out to assess screening rates among pediatricians found that only 8% of these investigated the presence of depressive symptoms in mothers, and none stated that they used standardized screening questionnaires. Hence, it seems that there are significant missed opportunities to identify women at risk of perinatal psychopathology.

Because half of postpartum depressions begin during pregnancy, and women with a personal or family history of depression are at increased risk, the prenatal period is the ideal time for screening and prevention. The screening process can be easily implemented using specific tools for the detection of perinatal psychopathology. As reported previously in the section *Screening tools*, a variety of tests are available, including self-administered tests and others that must be administered, where some of these have been designed for screening a general adult population and others were developed specifically for maternal depression. The procedure can be incorporated into routine prenatal and postpartum care and in health budgets.

The Costs of Perinatal Mental Health

Perinatal mental illnesses are an important public health problem that must be taken more seriously. Such diseases, if left untreated, can have a devastating impact on women, their children and their families. They represent one of the main causes of death for mothers during pregnancy and in the first year after the child's birth. Because of limitations in the data availability, cost estimates reported by The London School of Economics and Political Science (LSE) and the Centre for Mental Health are limited to three important perinatal mental health conditions: depression, anxiety and postpartum psychosis (mainly bipolar and schizophrenia disorders). Conditions such as eating disorders are, therefore, omitted. For this and other reasons, the data from the LSE and Centre for Mental Health underestimate the scale and costs of perinatal mental health problems.

The most complete and reliable estimates are those related to depression. Taken together, depression, anxiety and perinatal psychosis carry a long-term total cost of about £8.1 billion for each year of births for society in the United Kingdom. This is equivalent to a cost slightly lower than £10,000 for every birth in the country. Nearly three quarters (72%) of these costs concern the negative impact on the child, rather than on the mother. More than one fifth of the total (£1.7 billion) is paid for by the public sector, specifically the NHS and social services (£1.2 billion). The average cost for society of a case of perinatal depression is about £74,000, of which £23,000 refers to the consequences for the mother and £51,000 on those of the child. Perinatal anxiety, when it occurs alone and is not comorbid with depression, costs about £35,000 for each case, of which £21,000 for the mother and £14,000 for the child. The costs of psychosis are around £53,000 per case, but this figure is almost certainly underestimated because of the lack of evidence regarding the impact on children. Also costly is the loss of work due to the impact that the disease has on the person's functionality: Annette Bauer, head of LSE Personal Social Services Research Unit (PSSRU), underlines how the data show that maternal psychopathology strongly affects the economy and society, especially because of the negative impact it has on the child. Furthermore, in order to protect the health of the whole family in the long term, it is necessary for the interventions to begin before the birth of the child or immediately afterward, so that the potential benefits are maximized and the costs are minimized. Dr. Alain Gregoire (LSE and Centre for Mental Health, October, 2014), founder of Maternal Mental Health Alliance (MMHA) – a coalition of professionals that aims to improve the mental health and well-being of the woman and her child in the perinatal period – states that perinatal mental health problems are common and very expensive. They afflict about 20% of women during pregnancy or in the first year of a child's life and are a public health problem that impacts on both mother and child. According to Gregoire, the good news is that patients improve and heal when they are identified and receive the right treatment. Thus, it is fundamental that all women, wherever they live, receive the appropriate help they need from trained professionals and experts in the field.

Considering the data, the need to invest in prevention projects to identify early mothers at risk of perinatal psychopathology appears even more evident and critical.

Conclusions

Mental health problems during pregnancy and the postpartum period need more urgent intervention than at other times in a woman's life because of their potential consequence on children, on the physical health and care of the mother, and on her ability to function and take care of her family. However, these perinatal issues are often not recognized and, consequently, are not treated during the pregnancy and postpartum. Some women do not seek help because of the stigma, or for fear of intervention by other social services. The perinatal period may also present practical obstacles to treatment. For example, the needs associated with caring for a child can interfere with a woman's ability to attend regular therapeutic appointments. If mental health problems are not treated, women may continue, sometimes for many years, to suffer symptoms detrimental to their well-being, that of their children and other family members.

Motherhood represents a challenging job for all women and, especially, for those suffering from perinatal psychopathological disorders. For these women, it is certainly not a magical experience. Mothers enveloped in depression need to know that what they are feeling has both a name and a treatment. Their dream of motherhood must not be lost in darkness and hopelessness given that prenatal depression and postpartum depression can be treated.

A screening of mental illness in the perinatal period taking place as a routine clinical practice and easily accepted by women and health workers, despite existing barriers, is now considered a feasible and useful approach for improving perinatal mental health. Evidence now exists that early detection of women at risk of perinatal psychopathology decreases the risk of depression in women in the perinatal period and is more effective if associated with treatment and follow-up, although new studies are still needed to evaluate its effectiveness thoroughly. In any case, for clinicians working in the field perinatal screening may offer the chance to make a difference.

In conclusion, I report a summary overview, proposed by RANZCOG (Royal Australian and New Zealand College of Obstetricians and Gynaecologists, 2015), with the primary recommendations regarding the perinatal mental health problem. Each recommendation included in the list is based on the consent, opinion and experience of clinicians.

RANZCOG recommendations on perinatal mental health are as follows:

1 Mental health problems during the perinatal period are common. Routine screening should lead to identification, referral and treatment. There is evidence that early intervention produces the best outcomes for mothers and their families.

2 Perinatal mental health care should be culturally responsive and family-centered. Obstetricians are in a unique position to develop a long-term trusting relationship with their pregnant patients.

3 In line with the recognition by the College of the importance of reciprocal trust between practitioner and the patients and those who support them (cultural competency), it is imperative that an awareness of systemic inadequacies (such as poor communication, lack of continuity of care or non-collaborative models of care) remains a high priority in order to avoid these pitfalls.

4 The mental well-being of patients should be seen as important as physical health. Maternal anxiety and depression can have detrimental effects on fetal and infant development and on mother infant attachment.

5 All pregnant women should be screened for psychosocial risk factors. Screening for perinatal mood disorders, in the form of a psychosocial assessment or administration of a validated tool, such as the EPDS, should be considered part of routine antenatal and postpartum care.

6 Any treatment offered should involve collaborative decision-making with the woman and her partner including a full discussion of the potential risks and benefits.

7 The safety of mothers and infants must be considered at all times, as well as the safety of the entire family.

Note

1 Translation in English language edited by Roberta Mandolesi.

References

Albert L., Siu M.D., MSPH & US Preventive Services Task Force (USPSTF) (2016), *Screening for depression in adults: US Preventive Services Task Force recommendation statement,* JAMA, gennaio, vol. 26, n. 315(4).

American College of Obstetricians and Gynaecologists (2015), *Screening for perinatal depression: Committee Opinion N. 630,* Obstet Gynecol, vol. 125, pp. 1268–1271.

American Psychiatric Association (2014), *Manuale diagnostico e statistico dei disturbi mentali (DSM-5),* Milano, Raffaello Cortina Editore, quinta edizione.

AWHONN (2015), *Mood and anxiety disorders in pregnant and postpartum women,* AWHONN Position Statement, vol. 44(5), September/October.

Bales M., Pambrun E., Melchior M. et al. (2015), *Prenatal psychological distress and access to mental health care in the ELFE cohort,* European Psychiatry, vol. 30(2), pp. 322–328.

Bauer A., Personage M., Knapp M., Iemmi V. & Adelaja B. (2014), *The cost of perinatal mental health problems,* LSE and Centre For Maternal Mental Health, October (EPRINTS.lse.ac.uk).

BC Reproductive Mental Health Program & Perinatal Services BC (2014), *National action plan for perinatal mental health 2008–2010: full report: Best practice guidelines for mental health disorders in the perinatal period,* Perinatal Services BC.

Beck C.T. & Gable R.K. (2000), *Postpartum depression screening scale: Development and psychometric testing,* Nursing Research, vol. 49(5), pp. 272–282.

Beyondblue (2011), *Clinical practice guidelines for depression and related disorders — anxiety, bipolar disorder and puerperal psychosis — in the perinatal period: A guideline for primary care health professionals,* Melbourne, Beyondblue: The national depression initiative.

Bick D. & Howard L. (2010), *When should women be screened for postnatal depression?* Expert Review of Neurotherapeutics, vol. 10(2), pp. 151–154.

Bowen A., Bowen R., Butt P. et al. (2012), *Patterns of depression and treatment in pregnant and postpartum women,* Canadian Journal of Psychiatry, vol. 57(3), pp. 161–167.

Bramante A. & Brockington I.F. (2016), *Il disturbo della relazione mamma-bambino.* In P. Grussu & A. Bramante (a cura di), *Manuale di psicopatologia perinatale: Profili psicopatologici e modalità di intervento,* Trento, Erickson.

Brockington I.F. (2001), *A screening questionnaire for mother-infant bonding disorders,* Archive's Womens Mental Health, vol. 3, pp. 133–140.

Brockington I., Butterworth R., Glangeaud-Freudenthal N., Bramante A. et al. (2016), *An international position paper on mother-infant (perinatal) mental health, with guidelines for clinical practice,* Archive's Women's Mental Health, November 8.

Buist A., O'Mahen H. & Rooney R. (2015), *Acceptability, attitudes and overcoming stigma.* In J. Milgrom & A.W. Gemmill, *Identifying perinatal depression and anxiety,* Oxford, Wiley Blackwell.

Centre of Perinatal Excellence COPE (2017), *Effective mental health care in the perinatal period: Australian clinical practice guideline,* draft 2, June.

Condon J.T., Corkindale C. (1997), *The correlates of antenatal attachment in pregnant women,* Psychology and Psychotherapy, Theory, Research and Practice, vol. 70(4), pp. 359–372.

Condon J.T., Corkindale C. (1998), *The assessment of parent-to-infant attachment: Development of a self-report questionnaire instrument,* Journal of Reproductive and Infant Psychology, vol. 16(1).

Cox J., Holden J. & Henshaw C. (2015), *Perinatal mental health: The Edinburgh Postnatal Depression Scale (EPDS) manual,* Londra, RCPsych Publications, seconda edizione.

Cox J., Holden J. & Sagovsky R. (1987), *Detection of postnatal depression: Development of the 10-item Edinburgh Postnatal Depression Scale,* British Journal of Psychiatry, vol. 150, pp. 782–786.

Cranley M.S. (1981), *Development of a tool for the measurement of maternal attachment during pregnancy,* Nursing Research, vol. 30(5), pp. 281–284.

Department of Health (s.d.), *Screening for maternal depression recommendation,* health.ny.gov.

Department of Health (2016), *National service framework (NSF),* Regno Unito, NHS, november.

Ding X.X., Wu Y.L., Xu S.J. et al. (2014), *Maternal anxiety during pregnancy and adverse birth outcome: A systematic review and meta-analysis of prospective cohort studies,* Journal of Affective Disorders, vol. 159, pp. 103–110.

Donnelly L. et al. (2015), *One in three pregnant women suffer depressive signs,* The Telegraph, August 20.

El-Den S., O'Reilly C.L. & Chen T.F. (2015), *A systematic review on the acceptability of perinatal depression screening,* Journal of Affective Disorders, vol. 188, pp. 284–303.

Evans J., Heron J. & Francomb H. (2001), *Cohort study of depressed mood during pregnancy and after childbirth,* British Medical Journal, vol. 323, pp. 257–260.

Gemmill A.W., Leigh B., Ericksen J. et al. (2006), *A survey of the clinical acceptability of screening for postnatal depression in depressed and non-depressed women,* BMC Public Health, vol. 6, p. 211.

Goldberg D.P. (1972), *The detection of psychiatric illness by questionnaire,* Maudsley Monograph, vol. 21, Londra, Oxford University Press.

Goldin Evans M., Phillippi S. & Gee R.E. (2015), *Examining the screening practices of physicians for postpartum depression: Implications for improving health outcomes,* Women's Health Issues, vol. 25(6), pp. 703–710.

Henshaw C., Cox J. & Barton J. (2017), *Modern management of perinatal psychiatric disorders,* London, RCPsych Publications, second edition.

Henshaw C. & Ericksen J. (2015), *How to use the EPDS and maximize its usefulness in the consultation process.* In J. Milgrom & A.W. Gemmill, *Identifying perinatal depression and anxiety,* Oxford, Wiley Blackwell.

Highet N., Stevenson A.L., Purtell C., Coo S. (2014). *Qualitative insights into women's personal experiences of perinatal depression and anxiety.* Women and Birth, vol. 27, pp. 179–184.

Kim J.J., La Porte L.M., Corcoran M. et al. (2010), *Barriers to mental health treatment among obstetric patients at risk for depression,* American Journal of Obstetric and Gynaecologist, vol. 202(3), pp. 312 e1–5.

Kingston D., Austin M.P., McDonald S.W., Vermeyden L., Heaman M., Hegadoren K., Lasiuk G., Kingston J., Sword W., Jarema K., Veldhuyzen van Zanten S., McDonald S.D., Biringer A. (2015a), *Pregnant women's perceptions of harms and benefits of mental health screening*. PLoS One, vol. 10(12), pp. e0145189.

Kingston D.E., Biringer A., McDonald S.W. et al. (2015b), *Preferences for mental health screening among pregnant women: A cross-sectional study*, American Journal of Preventive Medicine, vol. 49(4), pp. e35–43.

Kozinszky Z., Dudas R.B., Devosa I. et al. (2012), *Can a brief antepartum preventive group intervention help reduce postpartum depressive symptomatology?* Psychother Psychosom, vol. 81(2), pp. 98–107.

Levit K. et al. (2008), *HCUP facts and figures, 2006: Statistics on hospital-based care in the United States*, Rockville, MD: Agency for Healthcare Research and Quality.

Littlewood E. et al. (2016), *Identification of depression in women during pregnancy and the early postnatal period using the Whooley questions and the Edinburgh Postnatal Depression Scale: Protocol for the Born and Bred in Yorkshire: Perinatal Depression Diagnostic Accuracy (BaBY PaNDA) study*, BMJ Open.

Matthey S., Valenti B., Souter K. & Ross-Hamid C. (2013), *Comparison of four self-report measures and a generic mood question to screen for anxiety during pregnancy in English-speaking women*, Journal of Affective Disorders, vol. 148, pp. 347–351.

Matthey S., White T., Phillips J. et al. (2005), *Acceptability of routine antenatal psychosocial assessments to women from English and non-English speaking backgrounds*, Archives of Women's Mental Health, vol. 8(3), pp. 171–180.

McDonagh M. et al. (2014), *Antidepressant treatment of depression during pregnancy and the postpartum period: Evidence report/technology assessment no. 216 (Prepared by the Pacific Northwest Evidence-based Practice Center under Contract No. 290-2007-10057-I)*, AHRQ Publication, vol. 14-E003-EF, Rockville, MD, Agency for Healthcare Research and Quality, July.

Milgrom J. & Gemmill A.W. (2015), *Identifying perinatal depression and anxiety*, Oxford, Wiley Blackwell.

Miller L., Shade M. & Vasireddy V. (2009), *Beyond screening: Assessment of perinatal depression in a perinatal care setting*, Archive of Women's Mental Health, vol. 12(5), pp. 329–334.

Mirabella F., Michelin P., Piacentini D., Veltro F., Barbano G., Cattaneo M., Cascavilla I., Palumbo G. & Gigantesco A. (2014), *Positività allo screening e fattori di rischio della depressione post partum in donne che hanno partecipato a corsi preparto*, Rivista di psichiatria, vol. 49(6), pp. 253–264.

Muller M.E. (1994), *A questionnaire to measure mother-to-infant attachment*, J Nurs, vol. 2(2), pp. 129–141.

Muller M.E. (1996), *Prenatal and postnatal attachment: A modest correlation*, Journal of Obstetric, Gynecologic, & Neonatal Nursing, vol. 25(2), pp. 161–166.

Murray D. & Cox J. (1990), *Screening for depression during pregnancy with the Edinburgh Depression Scale (EPDS)*, Journal of Reproductive Infant Psychology, vol. 8, pp. 99–107.

Nagata N., Nagai Y., Sobajima H., Ando T., Nishide Y., Honjo S. (2000), *Maternity blues and attachment to children in mothers of full-term normal infants*, Acta Psychiatrica Scandinavica, vol. 101, pp. 209–217.

National Screening Committee (2013), *Population screening explained*, Regno Unito, NHS.

NICE (2007), *Antenatal and postnatal mental health: Clinical management and service guidance: Clinical guideline CG45*, nice.org.uk.

NICE (2014), *Antenatal and postnatal mental health: Clinical management and service guidance: Clinical guideline CG192*, nice.org.uk.

NICE (2015), *Antenatal and postnatal mental health: The NICE guideline on clinical management and service guidance*, London, National Institute for Health and Care Excellence.

NICE (2016), *Antenatal and postnatal mental health: Quality standard*, nice.org.uk.

O'Connor E., Rossom R.C., Henninger M. et al. (2016), *Screening for depression in adults: An updated systematic evidence review for the us preventive services task force: Evidence synthesis No. 128*, AHRQ Publication, vol. 14-05208-EF-1, Rockville, MD, Agency for Healthcare Research and Quality.

O'Hara M. (2017), *Screening for perinatal depression and anxiety: How much is enough?* Wisconsin Dells, Wisconsin Association for Care, May.

Packman C. & Dezateux C. (1998), *Issues underlying the evaluation of screening programmes*, British Medical Bulletin, vol. 54, pp. 767–778.

Parry N.M. (2016), *Pregnancy: Universal depression screening effective, feasible*, Medscape.

Rai S., Pathak A. & Sharma I. (2015), *Postpartum psychiatric disorder: Early diagnosis and management*, Indian Journal of Psychiatry, vol. 57 (supplement 2), July.

Reay R., Matthey S., Ellwood D. et al. (2011), *Long-term outcomes of participants in a perinatal depression early detection program*, Journal of Affective Disorders, vol. 129(1–3), pp. 94–103.

Rubertsson C., Borjesson K., Berglund A., Josefsson A. & Sydsjo G. (2011), *The Swedish validation of Edinburgh Postnatal Depression Scale (EPDS) during pregnancy*, Nord J Psychiatry, vol. 65(6), pp. 414–418.

Seeahausen D.A., Baldwin L.M., Runkle H.P. & Clark G. (2005), *Are family physicians appropriately screening for postpartum depression?* Journal of American Board of Family Medicine, vol. 18, pp. 104–112.

Shakespeare J., Blake F. & Garcia J. (2003), *A qualitative study of the acceptability of routine screening of postnatal women using the Edinburgh Postnatal Depression Scale*, The British Journal of General Practice, vol. 53, pp. 614–619.

Siu A.L. & USPSTF (2016), *Screening for depression in adults US Preventive Services Task Force recommendation statement*, JAMA, vol. 26(315), n. 4.

Spitzer R.L. & Williams J.B. (2001), *The PHQ-9: Validity of a brief depression severity measure*, Journal of General Internal Medicine, vol. 16, pp. 606–663.

State wide Obstetric Support Unit (2007), *Perinatal depression and anxiety disorders.*

Tandon S.D., Cluxton-Keller F., Leis J., Le H.N. & Perry D.F. (2012), *A comparison of three screening tools to identify perinatal depression among low-income African American women*, Journal of Affective Disorders, vol. 136(1–2), pp. 155–162.

Taylor A., Atkins R., Kumar R., Asams D., Glover V. (2005), *A new mother-to-infant bonding scale: Links with early maternal mood*, Archives of Women's Mental Health, vol. 8(1), pp. 45–51.

The Royal Australian and New Zealand College of Obstetricians and Gynaecologists (2015), *Perinatal anxiety and depression*, March.

Venkatesh K.K., Nadel H., Blewett D. et al. (2016), *Implementation of universal screening for depression during pregnancy: Feasibility and impact on obstetric care*, American Journal of Obstetrics and Gynaecology, vol. 215(4), pp. 517, e1–8.

Vigod S.N. et al. (2016), *Depression in pregnancy*, BMJ, vol. 352, p. i1547, march.

Wisconsin Association for Perinatal Care (s.d.), *Position statement: Screening for prenatal and postpartum depression*, www.perinatalweb.org.

Wisner K.L. et al. (2013), *Onset timing, thoughts of self-harm, and diagnoses in postpartum women with screen-positive depression findings*, JAMA Psychiatry, vol. 70(5), pp. 490–498.

Wisner K.L. et al. (2015), *International approaches to perinatal mental health screening as a public health priority*. In J. Milgrom & A.W. Gemmill, *Identifying perinatal depression and anxiety*, Oxford, Wiley Blackwell, pp. 193–209.

World Health Organization (2008), *The global burden of disease: 2004 Update*, Ginevra, WHO Press.

World Health Organization (2016), *International statistical classification of diseases and related health problems: 10th revision (ICD-10)*, Ginevra, WHO Press.

Postpartum Psychosis, Bipolar Disorders, and Mother-Baby Unit

Florence Gressier, Ingrid Lacaze de Cordova, Elisabeth Glatigny, Nine M.-C. Glangeaud-Freudenthal, and Anne-Laure Sutter-Dallay

The perinatal period is accompanied not only by somatic and hormonal changes but also by psychological, family and social ones. It is a period at risk of occurrence or decompensation of psychiatric disorders, especially mood disorders.

Postpartum Psychosis and Bipolar Disorder during Perinatal Period

Postpartum psychosis is characterized by a rich and noisy symptomatology, with possible dramatic long-term consequences for mother, child and family. It is important to know the clinical specificities and risk factors in order to allow preventive, early and/or adapted joint mother-baby care.

Its incidence is estimated at 1–2/1,000 births (Kendell et al., 1987), with an incidence of first life-time onset varying between 0.25/1,000 and 0.6/1,000 births (Bergink et al., 2016).

Although described already in the antiquity, the place of postpartum psychosis within the classifications is still debated. In DSM-5, this disorder is classified within "psychiatric disorders (major depressive episode, manic or mixed depressive disorder, bipolar I or II, short psychotic disorder) beginning in the peripartum (during pregnancy or in the first 4 weeks of postpartum)". In ICD-10, it is with "severe mental and behavioral disorders associated with the puerperium, not elsewhere classified for episodes with onset within six weeks of delivery" (F53.1). In France, it is individualized and described as acute delirious psychosis (Dayan, 2007). Anyway, it is important to differentiate chronic psychotic illness, especially schizophrenia, from acute onset of postpartum psychosis.

Clinical Presentation

Acute delusional psychoses, mania or mixed states, major depression and schizophreniform states have been described with common elements (Kamperman et al., 2017). Symptoms are always polymorphic, with sudden onset and rapid deterioration, and usually begin within the first two weeks after delivery, sometimes even within the first 48–72 hours of the postpartum period (Heron et al., 2008). For about half of the women, this episode is their first one (Valdimarsdóttir et al., 2009). However, recent data are in favor of very early postpartum or even late pregnancy; prodromal symptoms are sleep disorders, irritability, mood lability, perplexity, detachment and confusion, as well as disturbances in the mother-baby relationship that can be confounded with a severe baby blues (Heron et al., 2008).

Mood disorders are always present, often as manic symptoms, with great mood lability and fluctuations of symptom intensity and especially with severe mood swings. Added to those symptoms, women may present with major oscillation of vigilance, confusion and high level of anxiety (Jones et al., 2014).

Psychotic delusional ideas are usually centered on birth and child (denial of maternity, feeling non-existence of the child, conviction of substitution or death of the child, mystical filiation, etc.). Mechanisms are multiple and may include hallucinations (auditory, visual, olfactory, cenesthetic).

Risk Factors

Considering risk factors, psychiatric past history is major one. A personal past history of postpartum psychosis would expose a 30–50% risk of a new episode in a subsequent pregnancy. For pregnant women, with preexisting bipolar disorders, there is a major increased risk (about 30%) of a relapse during postpartum.

Women who stopped their mood-stabilizing treatment, specifically those under lithium treatment, are more likely to have a relapse than those who have pursued their treatment (70% vs. 24%) (Viguera et al., 2007).

Family history would also be a significant risk factor. For example, women with bipolar disorder, having a first-degree relative with a past history of postpartum psychosis, would have up to 74% more risk of a new episode.

The only consistent association with obstetrical characteristics is with primiparity. However, the causal explanation remains unclear. First pregnancy, delivery and motherhood might induce greater psychological stress, and higher hormonal, biological and immunological changes than subsequent pregnancies (Jones et al., 2014). Hormonal changes, obstetric complications (low birth weight, perinatal death, delivery hemorrhage, preeclampsia, emergency caesarean section) and lack of sleep may also contribute to the onset of the disorder (Jones et al., 2014; Sit et al., 2006). With regard to socio-demographic factors, an age of more than 35 years and the status of single mother could generate a higher risk of postpartum psychosis. There seems to be no difference of risk related to socio-educational level or ethnicity. Finally, considering the risk linked to hormonal changes, one hypothesis of mechanism would be an increase in sensitivity of dopaminergic receptors to sexual steroids' rate changes, as well as an alteration in the regulation of the immune system. This hypothesis is reinforced by revised modifications in the expression of micro-RNAs, regulators of gene expression. From a genetic point of view, the serotonin transporter gene (the 5-HTTLPR and 5-HTTVNTR polymorphisms) could be an interesting track (Kumar et al., 2007). Finally, genome-wide studies have suggested the involvement of chromosomes 16p13 and 8q24 (Weigelt et al., 2013).

Considering bipolar disorder, pregnancy has been reported with having lower rates of relapse compared to other psychiatric disorders (Munk-Olsen et al., 2006, 2009); nevertheless, Viguera et al. (2007) described high rates (85%) of relapse during pregnancy, particularly in women who had interrupted their treatment. Relapse during the postpartum period is more frequent than during pregnancy – 52% vs. 23% (Viguera et al., 2011) – and relapse mainly during early postpartum period is a specially "at-risk" period for those women with 2.7 more episodes compared to women with other psychiatric disorders (Munk-Olsen, 2009). In summary, women with preexisting bipolar disorder (type 1 or 2) have at least 20% risk of suffering from a severe recurrence following delivery and even around 50% risk of experiencing any mood episode during the postpartum period including non-psychotic major depression (Jones et al., 2014; Wesseloo et al., 2016).

For what concerns **first onset of affective disorders** during the perinatal period, an affective episode, requiring inpatient treatment during the perinatal period, is recognized as a marker of a bipolar vulnerability (Judd et al., 2003). Some recent research is showing that milder postpartum affective or anxious disorders may also be a marker of underlying bipolarity (Liu et al., 2017). Consequently, the prescriptions of antidepressants in women presenting with perinatal mood or anxious disorders absolutely need a deep clinical exploration looking at any symptoms of mixed or manic episode.

Diagnostic Assessment

Postpartum psychosis is a psychiatric emergency and requires rapid assessment. Do not forget that postpartum psychosis is associated with highly elevated risk of suicide and infanticide. It is important to first exclude organic causes for acute psychosis. The main differential diagnoses are cerebral thrombophlebitis, placental retention and infectious causes of mental confusion. Thus, a thorough physical examination must be conducted urgently, including gynecological and neurological examination. It is necessary to carry out a biological check-up to eliminate a metabolic or nutritional cause, as well as cerebral angio-tomodensitometry or magnetic resonance imaging in order to rule out cerebral thrombophlebitis.

In the acute phase, the symptomatology leads to a hospitalization in an adult psychiatric department, most of the time, in particular to prevent a risk of suicide and/or infanticide. Constrained hospitalization may be required. Support in a mother-baby unit can be proposed more often in a second step, when the dangerousness of the symptomatology is over (Glangeaud-Freudenthal et al., 2014).

Treatment

Treatment should be rapidly implemented and should be guided by clinical symptoms, by personal and family psychiatric past history, as well as by previous response to psychotropic treatments, if any. No formal guidelines are currently available. Bergink et al. (2015) presented treatment response and remission outcomes at nine months postpartum using a four-step algorithm in patients with first-onset psychosis or mania in the postpartum period: a structured treatment algorithm with the sequential addition of benzodiazepines, antipsychotics and lithium may result in high rates of remission in patients with first-onset postpartum psychosis and lithium maintenance may be most beneficial for relapse prevention.

A sedative and anxiolytic treatment is usually necessary. An antipsychotic drug (risperidone, olanzapine, quetiapine, aripiprazole, amisulpride) is often the first-line treatment. Dose is adjusted according to the clinic. Breastfeeding is contraindicated on account of the clinical condition of the mother, associated with dangerousness for the child health (compartmental dangerousness but also lack of maternal adjustment to infant's needs for a satisfactory breastfeeding), and the need for infant weaning of antipsychotic or mood stabilizer, as drugs passed through the milk.

A mood stabilizer treatment, preferably lithium, may be used according to the clinical observation and/or the present personal or family past history of bipolar disorder. If depressive symptoms are present, antidepressant therapy may sometimes be prescribed after a satisfying mood regulation has been implemented but always with caution, given the link between bipolar disorder and postpartum psychosis and thus the risk of manic turn or rapid cycling. Although monotherapy is preferable, combination therapy is often indispensable.

Electroconvulsive therapy can also be the therapeutic chosen tool, allowing a more rapid improvement in symptoms (Gressier et al., 2015). It is indicated when: the symptomatology is particularly severe, there is a major risk of suicide or infanticide, a resistance to treatment and/or intolerance to psychotropic drugs.

Psychotherapy is essential and concerns not only the woman, the mother-child relationship, but also the father and the family. The mother-baby bond must thus be sustained as soon as possible with "mediated" encounters, considering the maternal mental state and the infant characteristics, as it is described in detail later on in this chapter.

After hospitalization discharge, care should be continued at an outpatient service, with a multidisciplinary follow-up, and support to mother–child relationship and child development.

There may be concern for child safety and need of referral to social services or a judge, sometimes with the use of a provisional placement order of the child (Glangeaud-Freudenthal et al., 2013).

Evolution

Evolution is usually spontaneous within a few months. In 30% of cases, it is a single episode; 60% will progress to a mood disorder and rarely to schizophrenia. Recidivism during a new pregnancy is present in about 30% of cases. Prevention and early detection screening, for women at high risk for postpartum psychosis, should be performed during early prenatal care. Women with bipolar disorder or a personal or family past history of postpartum psychosis should be monitored closely.

Women with bipolar disorder or a previous postpartum psychosis are at high risk of relapse during the postpartum period. In the case of previous postpartum psychosis, the strategy of starting prophylaxis during pregnancy or after delivery is unclear. The strategy might differ depending on whether previous episodes have occurred outside of the perinatal period (Bergink et al., 2012). Women with a history of previous illness restricted to the postpartum period are at high risk during the postpartum period but less during pregnancy, whereas in women with a history of bipolar episodes, pregnancy is also a period of high risk (Jones et al., 2014).

Potential Risks and Benefits of Psychotropic Medication

In these situations, the potential risks and benefits of psychotropic medication options should be considered (Sutter-Dallay et al., 2015). For memory, several studies have shown that lithium salts during pregnancy of women with bipolar disorders can efficiently prevent postpartum relapses. A systematic review and meta-analysis of lithium toxicity concluded that the evidence that exposure to lithium is teratogenic is weak (McKnight et al., 2012) and the risk may have been overestimated. Nevertheless, recent data suggest that exposure to lithium in utero seems to correlate with an increase in the frequency of cardiac defects (Bergink & Kushner, 2014; Diav–Citrin et al., 2014), but no more significantly after excluding anomalies that spontaneously resolved postpartum (Diav-Citrin et al., 2014). It seems impossible to assert or refute the specificity of the influence of lithium on the occurrence of Ebstein's disease (Diav-Citrin et al., 2014; Giles and Bannigan, 2006). Therefore, it is recommended that all women receiving lithium during pregnancy should undergo fetal echocardiography and level 2 ultrasound examination (Bergink and Kushner, 2014).

The use of other therapies during the perinatal period is less documented. Thus, carbamazepine may also be used in second-line therapy. One study reported a benefit of olanzapine. Valproate did not show any benefit in the prevention of postpartum psychosis and should no longer be prescribed in women of childbearing age (NICE guidelines, 2014). The use of estrogen is controversial, while progesterone would not bring any benefit (Doucet et al., 2011; Jones et al., 2014).

Prevention Strategies

Antenatal services should identify women at high risk during the perinatal period. They must identify the specificities of postpartum psychosis compared to those of postpartum depression and be able to direct the woman toward adequate psychiatric care. Prodromal symptoms have to be detected early. Education of women is primordial and the onset of symptoms should lead to a prompt consultation. Prevention strategies should be implemented in a multidisciplinary management. A perinatal care plan for women with current or past severe mental illness has to be implemented. Women should be closely monitored throughout all the pregnancy and the post-partum period.

Joint Mother-Baby Care Units (MBUs)

Brockington et al. (2017) gave a description of the specificity of perinatal psychiatric care and some guidelines on MBUs, stressing the importance of having a specific training when dealing with mother-baby joint care and the need of some guidelines which are described in their paper.

Glangeaud-Freudenthal et al. (2014) reviewed the characteristics of mother-baby inpatient psychiatric units located in different countries and present some pieces of research coming from MBU research teams. Those authors show the diversity of such institutions and stress that some regions are still without access to this type of care for mother and child, even in countries having such institutions.

Sutter-Dallay et al. (2016) had collected contribution from experts in different countries to present recent knowledge on "Joint Care for Parents and Infants in Perinatal Psychiatric". After some chapters on the history of this joint care and perinatal psychiatry, several chapters are dealing with parental illnesses, parenting skills and infant development. Different types of care are described: parent-infant psychotherapy, care based on home visit and intervention, at inpatient night-and-day MBUs or at day MBUs. Finally, perinatal care management is discussed, as well as systematic psychosocial assessment and screening (benefits, challenges and implementation) all through the perinatal period. Multidisciplinary networking for perinatal mental health, as it is practiced in France, is important as it allows having a more "person focus" care and also a continuity from pregnancy (and even from pre-conceptional time) till late postpartum. Finally, the editors of this book concluded on the importance of putting forward efficient prevention and care during this very sensitive perinatal period.

The Francophone Marcé Society has been gathering since many years data on MBUs and is updating frequently the list of such units in France, Belgium and the Netherland detailed at its website (www.marce-francophone.fr/unites-mere-enfant-umb.html).

This society had edited in 2009 a book on different types of care given at those MBUs Poinso and Glangeaud, 2009).

Presently, the Francophone societies linked to the Marcé Society and the World Association for Infant Mental Health (WAIMH) have set up together a working multidisciplinary group that aims to improving joint mother-child care during the perinatal period. Such joint care may be ambulatory care, whole-day inpatient care or night-and-day inpatient MBUs. The target of this working group is also to focus on improving research and training for such care, and to discuss how to improve visibility of joint care toward perinatal mental health deciders, especially concerning importance of parent infant joint perinatal mental health care. The visibility of day-care services is especially low and needs more support from health deciders in France. This working group also wishes to support the development of perinatal mental health care and prevention for early mother-infant attachment disorders and to improve child development. The first step would be to identify an exact mapping of all different perinatal mental health type of care and services in France, starting with an update of the ambulatory care for which we do not have information as good as information about inpatient MBUs.

Recently, Langan Martin et al. (2016) have presented a retrospective study on admission to psychiatric hospital for mental illnesses two years' pre-childbirth and post-childbirth in Scotland to assess mother and child outcomes. They emphasized that further research is needed to assess benefits or adverse effects of perinatal joint care on development of children with mothers having a mental illness.

Although we very often speak only of mother-baby care and mother's mental health, we should speak of parents and infant care and parents' health. It is now well known that fathers have an important role to play in children development and we should pay attention to fathers as caregivers and for their own mental health during the perinatal period. Some units have changed their names from "Mother-baby Unit" to "Parents-Baby Unit". The Francophone Marcé Society has edited recently a book on fathers during the perinatal period, with experts' contributions from different disciplinary background (Glangeaud-Freudenthal and Gressier, 2017).

Is There a Place for a Psychologist In MBUs?

The place for a psychologist in an inpatient MBU is probably a challenge. There is often only one consulting psychologist at a MBU: on one side, psychologists are without the benefit from peer' support to face the doubt of their legitimacy within the dyad care at an MBU; but on the other side, they are more protected from negative predictive maternal pathology evolution and closer to reach the singularity of each maternal psychopathology encountered, which should be more beneficial for mother and child relationship care.

Working at an MBU as a psychologist, involves integrating the intrapsychic dimension of the mother and of the baby "in development", and the fundamental dimension of the intersubjectivity of mother-baby relationship.

Plurality of Practices

Now, we will focus more on the psychologist's contribution to these MBUs.

At a round table, during an MBU biennial Francophone conference in 2011, we had the opportunity to discuss the diversity of our practices which are influenced by different parameters such as psychologist's status (part-time or full-time job); leader's discipline (child psychiatry or adult psychiatry); proximity to an MBU of a maternity or a neonatology intensive care unit with a liaison service involving a psychologist; and psychologist position as an external consultant, or within a unit project with a well-defined psychologist's mission. Moreover, the clinical and institutional activities of psychologists may differ according to their professional approach and expertise, but still appear relatively homogeneous with psychological assessment, psychotherapeutic care, institutional work, training and research.

Psychological Assessment

Psychological assessments, as they are usually practiced with adult or child in general, find their place within an MBU care plan.

The psychopathological functioning screening performed by psychologists remains relevant, based on projective tests such as the Rorschach and TAT (Murray et al., 1954), the Minnesota Multiphasic Personality Inventory (MMPI-2) and the Neo-Pi 3 (Costa and Mc Crae, 1992). Several screening tools for depressive or anxious symptomatology (very common symptoms during the perinatal period) can be used: Montgomery and Åsberg Depression Rating Scale (MADRS) (Montgomery and Åsberg, 1979), Beck Depression Scale (Beck et al., 1961), Hamilton Depressive Rating Scale (HDRS) (Hamilton, 1960), State-Trait Anxiety Inventory (STAI) (Spielberger et al., 1983).

However, there are screening tools more specific to the perinatal period. Among depression scales, the Edinburgh Postnatal Depression Scale (EPDS) is an internationally recognized psychometric scale to screen postpartum depression (Cox et al., 1987). It can help the clinician to screen for symptoms but also to evaluate mental health improvement during the therapy.

One of the specificities of mother-baby units is a joint management of each member of the dyad and also of mother-child interaction. Frequently observed interaction disorders question the mother attachment type. This attachment can be more or less explored in detail depending on available tools for the psychologist. The most comprehensive assessment is the Adult Attachment Interview (AAI) (Main, 1985), which is a semi-structured interview on the type of relationships an adult had with her/his own parents during childhood. This interview aims to estimate the influence of past relationship on present ones, as well as kind of attachment, especially as a mother to her child. This knowledge of the maternal attachment functioning may help for a better therapeutic care and for the choice of psychotherapeutical treatment. It may be interesting to understand the attachment process also for very young children, using the strange situation interview (Ainsworth et al., 1978) designed to evaluate the process of attachment and exploratory behavior of a child put in an unfamiliar and stressful context. Even though assessments of maternal and child attachment are not systematic, they are specific tools efficient for learning more about the dyadic functioning.

In the MBU of Bordeaux, we use mother-child interaction scales such as Bobigny's scale (Bur et al., 1989) for early detection of mother and child interactions' disorders. Such scales contribute to a more accurate clinical observation and give an objectifying evaluation (Glatigny-Dallay et al., 2005) although done in the complex context of mother-child bonding disorders and when counter-transference may be problematic.

Videotaping interactions between mother and child is also an essential good method in our practice. Observational instruments could be implemented (CIB, Feldman, 1998; CARE Index, Crittenden, 1979, 2004). In the Bordeaux unit, we use the Global Rating Scale for Mother-Infant Interactions (Murray et al., 1996), for which we were trained, to score sequences of interactions on: maternal attitude toward the baby, as well as baby's behavior. Looking at the videos shed light on some misunderstood dyads' attitudes by giving more detailed information on interaction in the dyad. Those videos can also be used for guiding and supporting maternal behavior improvement while watching them with mothers and discussing their feedback.

Use of Esther Bick's mother-infant observation method is often mentioned during meetings on MBU care. However, a specific long training is required for this method and limits its application at MBUs. Nevertheless, this type of observation is crucial for raising awareness of professionals to focus on the baby and on his/her everyday environment at home and also for training of fine observation of mother-child relationships.

A clinical observation can be implemented by assessment of a baby's psychomotor development scale such as the Brazelton Scale (1995), the Bayley Scale (2006), the Brunet-Lezine Child Development Scale (1951/1997) and the Alarm Distress Baby Scale (ADBB) (Guedeney and Fermanian, 2001).

Assessments used by psychologists are not specific to them but contribute to a multidisciplinary assessment of child development. Psychologists used them during a psychological assessment for better understanding of the dynamics of the maternal and the dyad functioning as well as an indication for the need of a psychotherapy.

The Psychotherapeutic Approach

All psychotherapeutical approaches can be considered. However, some of them are more specific to the perinatal period. Because of admission at the same time of both mother and child to an MBU, the care management in such units raises the interest of having a dyadic therapy or even a group therapy.

The training of psychologists gives them expertise to set up therapeutical groups that they may lead, attend in or even supervise. There are different psychotherapeutical approaches: individual, mother and baby, family (parents, baby and siblings ones, sometimes also with grandparents).

Moreover, depending on severity and type of maternal symptomatology, a mother-baby therapy is possible during a hospitalization using psychodynamic (Lebovici and Stoleru, 2003) or interactionist approaches. Similarly, having a family therapy will be an opportunity to redefine places of each member in the family and also the links between each of them, by taking into account couple relationship, marital adjustment and intra-familial relationships.

An individual follow-up of mothers is an opportunity to build bridges with the past history and to leave the present history to create a new future during this "sensitive postpartum period" as named by Debray and Belot (2008). The perinatal period reactivates traumatic childhood past history and also couples functioning and social support network difficulties. For those perinatal period difficulties, interpersonal psychotherapy is specially adapted (Stuart and Robertson, 2017), and aims to improve communication and interpersonal functioning, with an emphasis on social support network. This psychotherapy is recognized by the WHO to be efficient in treatment of depression and has many indications in the perinatal period mental health care (Glatigny Dallay et al., 2017).

Institutional Work

The therapeutic framework of MBUs needs an important multidisciplinary perinatal network including hospital services and extra-hospital services in a region (maternal and child protection services, adult psychiatric units, child psychiatric units, maternity units, pediatric services, consultations, etc.).

Such regional networking is essential and should be flexible but structured to be able deliver a good care although facing maternal difficulties and mother-child relationship disturbances increased by maternal pathology. Psychologists are a bit less exposed than the caregivers MBU team to massive projections and stress that may occur being in an everyday contact with mothers' and babies' disorders. Indeed, maternal difficulties and their impact on the development of the child can generate identification either to the suffering baby or to the traumatic past history of the mother as a child and her present difficulties. Psychologists are, therefore, often asked by team members to regulate their invading experiences and to support parasitic reflective activity.

During the elaboration of an individual care project, a joint nurse and psychologist care may be decided to provide a specific care during some everyday activities like a bath (especially with mothers suffering from psychosis). The contribution of a psychologist at different meetings (clinical, institutional, synthesis with the outside's partners) is necessary. Psychologists provide a third external position during discussions on women's difficulties and their effects on the caregiver team and on the misunderstood mother-child relationship improvement.

Severe symptomatology of some women may focus all the team attention and therefore make them blind to other important aspects of maternal difficulties that they should be aware of for efficient care. Psychologists may help to get out of this maternal symptomatology focus.

For all those reasons, the presence of psychologists in an MBU allows a help in team supervision in a regulated manner by a professional outside the care team, and also allows members of the care team expressing personal feeling and their understanding of the problems.

This description of the institutional function of psychologists working in a mother-baby unit is far from exhaustive. Each unit has its own specific project that defines the role of each member of the team and aims at providing continuous therapeutical care in which the psychologist's role is relevant, and plural.

Training and Research

In a multidisciplinary UMB team, psychologists contribute, like each member of the team, to improve day-to-day care for mothers and children. For that, their professional expertise must be updated by acquiring new knowledge, attending to meetings and getting new professional training (seminar, supervision, bibliographical review). This need for importance of continuous training is also for members of caregiver team and psychologists will support this need. Psychologists can participate to MBUs as reflexive agitators. They may pass on knowledge and contribute to the updating of knowledge.

MBUs offer a fundamental clinical research space in which the psychologist may contribute. The research carried out in MBUs and clinical and observational experience of teams lead to their specific expertise both in prevention of bonding disorders and their treatment and in child very early development difficulties. Sharing this knowledge with perinatal and early childhood professionals is an integral part of mother-baby unit missions.

The activity of a psychologist in MBUs is rich and may include individual, group and institutional therapies, and all the theoretical sensibilities have their place there. Apart from evaluative expertise (psychomotor and emotional development of babies) that seems to be objective, psychologists' position, a bit outside of a care team, allows a more objective point of view on maternal difficulties and mother-child relationship disturbances. This enables psychologists to analyze the institution functioning and to give support to the team.

Psychologists in such units contribute to the multidisciplinary aspect of the team with a need for reciprocal respect of the place of each one and should lead to induce constructive discussion to help professional and families.

Box 15.1 Main Points of Chapter

- Puerperal psychosis has a special place within perinatal psychiatric pathologies.
- Despite a non-specific nosographic framework, current data show the link between postpartum psychosis and bipolar disorder.
- Prevention and early intervention have to be implemented.
- Multidisciplinary management is needed with particular attention to the mother-baby relationship.

References

Ainsworth, M. D. S., Blehar, M. C., Waters, E., & Wall, S. (1978) *Patterns of Attachment: A Psychological Study of the Strange Situation*. Hillsdale, NJ: Erlbaum.

Bayley, N. (2006) *Bayley Scales of Infant Development Manual*. 3. Antonio, TX: The Psychological Corporation.

Beck, A. T., Ward, C. H., Mendelson, M., Mock, J., & Erbaugh, J. (1961) *An Inventory for Measuring Depression*, 4, 561–571.

Bergink, V., Bouvy, P. F., Vervoort, J. S., Koorengevel, K. M., Steegers, E. A., Kushner, S. A. (2012) Prevention of postpartum psychosis and mania in women at high risk. *The American Journal of Psychiatry*, 169, 609–615.

Bergink, V., Burgerhout, K. M., Koorengevel, K. M., et al. (2015) Treatment of psychosis and mania in the postpartum period. *The American Journal of Psychiatry*, 172, 15–23.

Bergink, V., Rasgon, N., & Wisner, K. L. (2016) Postpartum psychosis: Madness, mania, and melancholia in motherhood. *The American Journal of Psychiatry*, 173(12), 1179–1188.

Bergink, V., & Kushner, S. A. (2014) Lithium during pregnancy. *The American Journal of Psychiatry*, 171(7), 712–715.

Bick, E. (1964) Notes on infant observation in psycho-analytic training. *International Journal of Psycho-Analysis*, 45, 558–566.

Brazelton, T. B., & Nugent, J. K. (1995) *Neonatal Behavioral Assessment Scale*, third edition, *Clinics in Developmental Medicine*, No. 137, London: Mackeith Press.

Brockington, I., Butterworth, R., & Glangeaud-Freudenthal, N. M.-C. (2017) An international position paper on mother-infant (perinatal) mental health, with guidelines for clinical practice. *Archives of Women's Mental Health*, 20, 113–120.

Brunet, O., & Lezine, I. (1951) Le développement psychologique de la première enfance, PUF, Paris, Nouvelle version révisée (D. Josse): *Echelle de développement psychomoteur de la première enfance*, E.A.P, 1997.

Bur, V., Gozlan, Z., Lamour, M., Letronnier, P., & Rosenfeld, J. (1989) Présentation de grilles d'évaluation des interactions précoces à l'intention des consultations pédiatriques. In Lebovici, S., Mazet, P., & Visier, J. P. éd. *L'évaluation des interactions précoces entre le bébé et ses partenaires*. Paris, Eshel, Médecine et hygiène, 427–462.

Costa, P. T., & McCrae, R. R. (1992) *Revised NEO Personality Inventory (NEO-PI-R) and NEO Five-Factor Inventory (NEO-FFI) manual*. Odessa, FL: Psychological Assessment Resources.

Cox, J. L., Holden, J. M., & Sagovsky, R. (1987) Detection of postnatal depression: Development of the 10-item Edinburgh postnatal depression scale. *British Journal of Psychiatry*, 150, 782–786.

Crittenden, CARE Index, (1979, 2004).

Dayan, J. (2007) Clinique et épidémiologie des troubles anxieux et dépressifs de la grossesse et du postpartum. Revue et synthèse. *The Journal de Gynécologie Obstétrique et Biologie de la Reproduction*, 36, 549–561.

Debray, R., & Belot, R. A. (2008) *La psychosomatique du bébé*. Paris: PUF.

Diav-Citrin, O., Shechtman, S., Tahover, E., Finkel-Pekarsky, V., Arnon, J., Kennedy, D., Erebara, A., Einarson, A., & Ornoy, A. (2014) Pregnancy outcome following in utero exposure to lithium: A prospective, comparative, observational study. *The American Journal of Psychiatry*, 171(7), 785–794.

Doucet, S., Jones, I., Letourneau, N., Dennis, C. L., & Blackmore, E. R. (2011) Interventions for the prevention and treatment of postpartum psychosis: A systematic review. *Archives of Women's Mental Health*, 14, 89–98.

Feldman, CIB, (1998).

Giles, J. J., & Bannigan, J. G. (2006) Teratogenic and developmental effects of lithium. *Current Pharmaceutical Design*, 12(12), 1531–1541.

Glangeaud-Freudenthal, N. M., Howard, L. M., & Sutter-Dallay, A. L. (2014) Treatment – mother-infant inpatient units. *Best Practice & Research: Clinical Obstetrics & Gynaecology*, 28, 147–157.

Glangeaud-Freudenthal, N. M.-C., & Gressier F. (eds) (2017) Les pères en périnatalité. *Cahier de la Société Marcé Francophone*. Collection La vie de l'enfant chez érès, 260p. ISBN, 274925471X.

Glangeaud-Freudenthal, N. M.-C, Sutter-Dallay, A.-L., Thieulin, A.-C., Dagens-Lafont, V., Zimmermann, M.-A., Debourg, A., Amzallag, C., Cazas, O., Cammas, R., Klopfert, M.-E., Rainelli, C., Tielemans, P., Mertens, C., Maron, M., Nezelof, S., & Poinso, F. (2013) Predictors of infant foster care in cases of maternal psychiatric disorders. *Social Psychiatry and Psychiatric Epidemiology*, 48(4), 553–561.

Glatigny-Dallay, E., Lacaze, I., Loustau, N., Paulais, J.-Y., & Sutter, A.-L. (2005) Evaluation des interactions précoces. *Annales Médico Psychologiques*, 163, 540.

Glatigny-Dallay, E., & Omay, O. (2017) Psychothérapie Interpersonnelle en périnatalité. In sous la direction de Bayle B. *Aide-Mémoire Psychiatrie et Psychopathologie Périnatales*, Dunod, 397–401.

Gressier, F., Rotenberg, S., Cazas, O., & Hardy, P. (2015) Postpartum electroconvulsive therapy: A systematic review and case report. *General Hospital Psychiatry*, 37, 310–314.

Guedeney, A., & Fermanian, J. (2001) A validity and reliability study of assessment and screening for sustained withdrawal reaction in infancy: The Alarm Distress Baby Scale (ADBB). *Infant Mental Health Journal*, 22(5), 559–575.

Hamilton, M. (1960) A rating scale for depression. *Journal of Neurology, Neurosurgery and Psychiatry*, 23, 56–62. (PMID 14399272).

Heron, J., McGuinness, M., Blackmore, E. R., Craddock, N., & Jones, I. (2008) Early postpartum symptoms in puerperal psychosis. *BJOG*, 115, 348–353.

Jones, I., Chandra, P. S., Dazzan, P., & Howard, L. M. (2014) Bipolar disorder, affective psychosis, and schizophrenia in pregnancy and the post-partum period. *Lancet*, 384, 1789–1799.

Judd, L. L., Akiskal, H. S., Schettler, P. J., Coryell, W., Maser, J., Rice, J. A., Solomon, D. A., & Keller, M. B. (2003) The comparative clinical phenotype and long term longitudinal episode course of bipolar I and II: A clinical spectrum or distinct disorders? *Journal of Affective Disorders*, 73(1–2), 19–32.

Kamperman, A. M., Wesseloo, R., Robertson Blackmore, E., & Bergink, V. (2017) Phenotypical characteristics of postpartum psychosis: A clinical cohort study. *Bipolar Disorder*, 19(6), 450–457.

Kendell, R. E., Chalmers, J. C., & Platz, C. (1987) Epidemiology of puerperal psychoses. *British Journal of Psychiatry*, 150, 662–673.

Kumar, H. B., Purushottam, M., Kubendran, S., et al. (2007) Serotonergic candidate genes and puerperal psychosis: An association study. *Psychiatric Genetics*, 17, 253–260.

297

Langan Martin, J., McLean, G., Cantwell, R., & Smith, D. J. (2016) Admission to psychiatric hospital in the early and late postpartum periods: Scottish national linkage study. *BMJ Open*, 6: e008758. doi:10.1136/bmjopen-2015-008758.

Lebovici, S., & Stoleru, S. (2003) *Le nourrisson, sa mère et le psychanalyste*, Paris, Bayard, 384 p.

Liu, X., Agerbo, E., Li, J., Meltzer-Brody, S., Bergink, V., & Munk-Olsen, T. (2017) Depression and anxiety in the postpartum period and risk of bipolar disorder: A Danish Nationwide register-based cohort study. *The Journal of Clinical Psychiatry*, 78(5), e469–e476.

Main, M., & Goldwyn, R. (1985/1991). Adult attachment scoring and classification system. Unpublished manuscript, University of California, Berkeley.

McKnight, R. F., Adida, M., Budge, K., Stockton, S., Goodwin, G. M., & Geddes, J. R. (2012) Lithium toxicity profile: A systematic review and meta-analysis. *Lancet*, 379(9817), 721–728. doi: 10.1016/S0140-6736(11)61516-X

Montgomery, S. A., & Asberg, M. (1979) A new depression scale designed to be sensitive to change. *British Journal of Psychiatry*, 134(4), 382–389. PMID444788. doi:10.1192/bjp.134.4.382 721-28.

Munk-Olsen, T., Laursen, T. M., Mendelson, T., Pedersen, C. B., Mors, O., & Mortensen, P. B. (2009) Risks and predictors of readmission for a mental disorder during the postpartum period. *The Archives of General Psychiatry*, 66, 189–195.

Munk-Olsen, T., Laursen, T. M., Pedersen, C. B., Mors, O., & Mortensen, P. B. (2006) New parents and mental disorders: A population-based register study. *JAMA*, 296, 2582–2589.

Murray, H., et al. (1953, 1954) Exploration de la personnalité t.1, Le système de la personnalité: étude.clinique et expérimentale de cinquante sujets d'âge correspondant à celui des études universitaires; t.2 Les techniques d'investigation, PUF.

Murray, H., et al. (1996) Global Rating Scale for Mothers-Infant Interactions.

NICE guidelines Antenatal and postnatal mental health (2014) CG192, recommendations 1.2.3 and 1.4.27.

Poinso, F., & Glangeaud-Freudenthal, N. M.-C. (eds) (2009) *Orages à l'aube de la vie: Liens précoces, pathologies puerpérales et développement des nourrissons dans les unités parents-bébé. Cahier Marcé n°4* Paris, édition érès, Collection *La vie de l'enfant*, ISBN: 978-2-7492-1122-0.

Sit, D., Rothschild, A. J., & Wisner, K. L. (2006) A review of postpartum psychosis. *Journal Womens Health* (Larchmt), 15, 352–368.

Spielberger, C. D., Gorssuch, R. L., Lushene, P. R., Vagg, P. R., & Jacobs, G. A. (1983) *Manual for the State-Trait Anxiety Inventory*. Consulting Psychologists Press.

Stuart, S., & Robertson, M. (2012) Interpersonal Psychotherapy 2E A *Clinician's Guide*.

Sutter-Dallay, A.-L., Bales, M., Pambrun, E., Glangeaud-Freudenthal, N. M.-C., Wisner, K. L., & Verdoux, H. (2015) Impact of prenatal exposure to psychotropic drugs on neonatal outcome in infants of mothers with serious psychiatric illnesses. *Journal of Clinical Psychiatry*, 76(4), 967–973.

Sutter-Dallay, A.-L., Glangeaud-Freudenthal, N. M.-C., Guedeney, A., & Riecher-Rössler, A. (Eds) (2016) *Joint Perinatal Psychiatric Care for Parents and Infants*. Springer. ISBN 9783319215570 •9783319215563. doi:10.1007/978-3-319-21557-0

Valdimarsdóttir, U., Hultman, C. M., Harlow, B., Cnattingius, S., & Sparén, P. (2009) Psychotic illness in first-time mothers with no previous psychiatric hospitalizations: A population-based study, *PLoS Med*. 6(2), e13. doi: 10.1371/journal.pmed.1000013

Viguera, A. C., Tondo, L., Koukopoulos, A. E., Reginaldi, D., Lepri, B., & Baldessarini, R. J. (2011) Episodes of mood disorders in 2252 pregnancies and postpartum periods. *The American Journal of Psychiatry*, 168, 1179–1185.

Viguera, A. C., Whitfield, T., Baldessarini, R. J., et al. (2007) Risk of recurrence in women with bipolar disorder during pregnancy: Prospective study of mood stabilizer discontinuation. *The American Journal of Psychiatry*, 164, 1817–1824.

Weigelt, K., Bergink, V., Burgerhout, K. M., Pescatori, M., Wijkhuijs, A., & Drexhage, H. A. (2013) Down-regulation of inflammation-protective microRNAs 146a and 212 in monocytes of patients with postpartum psychosis. *Brain, Behavior, and Immunity*, 29, 147–155.

Wesseloo, R., Kamperman, A. M., Munk-Olsen, T., Pop, V. J., Kushner, S. A., & Bergink, V. (2016) Risk of postpartum relapse in bipolar disorder and postpartum psychosis: A systematic review and meta-analysis. *The American Journal of Psychiatry*, 173(2), 117–127.

Afterword

Perinatal mental health and perinatal psychiatry have achieved an international Public Health prominence that was unexpected 30 years ago when the EPDS was first published and the Parent and Baby Day Unit inaugurated in Stoke-on-Trent. This would not have happened without simultaneous input from nursing, psychology, and psychiatry.

This book with many thoughtful chapters has well documented new evidence bases in the field of clinical psychology that have underpinned the conspicuous current global and national developments in perinatal mental health. It has also rightly illustrated the huge contributions from clinical psychology to this burgeoning field and the increased scope for psychological therapies. Women's Health, the context and dynamics of parent-infant bonding, the vocal advocacy groups such as the Global Mental health Alliance, and the vibrancy of the International Marcé Society have each played important roles in advancing knowledge and improving services.

The interactive, dyadic nature of attending to health problems at this time, the need to incorporate knowledge of the biology of reproduction and of abnormal mental states requires a team that includes detailed expertise in ALL components of this relationship-based biopsychosocial approach are core components of perinatal mental health services. Yet I believe that perinatal psychology and perianal psychiatry have also a wider remit than that restricted to the childbearing early years alone. We hold a key that can unlock a more integrative relationship-based approach to mental health care for 'all ages' – and for medical practice as a whole. Is it possible that psychiatrists have pulled back from this field and left it to others? I hope not – because if this were to happen the mortality statistics from child birth will not be so readily reduced. There is a need for specialist perinatal psychiatrists – a need at last recognised in the UK where existing consultants are funded for additional training in perinatal psychiatry to lead four new mother-baby units and develop community services. This field also requires that both psychiatrists and clinical psychologists are trained to know what they do not know, and then listen to the voices from distraught parents and to the signals from their infants. Pre-conceptual counselling, the full understanding of the characteristics of the perinatal mental disorders, and the use and misuse of medication as well as of the EPDS are other essential tasks.

Perinatal psychology and psychiatry together thus hold a key that can facilitate a return to a more integrative relationship-based health service – a 'mixed methods' health service – and so help rescue medicine from a narrow scientism and a managerial reductionism.

This afterword is not an epilogue. It does not summarise conclusions or close off discussion but exhorts readers and contributors to think 'outside the box'. Much of the early research in this field (including that by Brice Pitt and Channi Kumar and those studies from Africa and Scotland which underpinned the EPDS) was carried out because of experience of perinatal mood disorder, and because of the energy and compassion of community workers. They were 'blue skies' research projects largely driven by clinical need and not by the whims of funding bodies. Small-scale research can sometimes help to move mountains.

This field continues to require clinicians and researchers, including anthropologists, who see below the resurface, who use metaphors to touch the depth and open discourse, and who see medicine and health care as a scientific art as well as an artistic science.

John Cox
Professor Emeritus
Keele University
United Kingdom

Index

Note: **Bold** page numbers refer to tables; *italic* page numbers refer to figures and page numbers followed by "n" denote endnotes.

interpersonal psychotherapy (IPT) 33; following
 miscarriage 119–120
intracytoplasmic sperm injection (ICSI) 62
intrauterine insemination (IUI) 62
in vitro fertilization (IVF) 62
involuntary childlessness: long-term effects of
 66–67
Ismail, K. 106

Jaffe, Janet 71
JAMA 32, 270
James, S. 134
Janssen, H. 106
Jaoul, M. 113
Johnson, J. E. 86, 112, 114, 119
joint mother-baby care units (MBUs) 292–296;
 institutional work 295; place for psychologists
 in 293; plurality of practices 293; psychological
 assessment 293–294; psychotherapeutical
 approaches 294–295; training and research
 295–296
Jolley, S. N. 107
Jongman, G. 108
Journal of Perinatology 177

Karmali, Z. A. 111
Kendler, K. S. 36
Kilby, M. 108
Kim-Godwin, Y. S. 193
Kingsbury, M. 17
Kingston, D. 10, 160, 191
Kirchmeier, R. 108
Kiselica, M. S. 113
Klein, M. 212
Klier, C. M. 108
Klinefelter syndrome 84
Korenromp, M. J. 85
Kounin, J. 132
Kroska, E. B. 12
Krowchuk, H. 119
Kruger, L. M. 117

Lahti, M. 28
Langan Martin 292
Langford, R. W. 119
Lapp, L. K. 142
Larsson, P. G. 117, 119
Lee, C. 104, 119
Leff, Raphael 213–214
Legrand, H. 118
Legros, J. P. 115
Leigh, B. 273
Leppert, P. C. 118
life event assessments 9
Lima, M. L. 111
Lloyd, B. 156, 157
Loizzo, K. 143
Lok, I. 119

London School of Economics and Political Science
 (LSE) 282–283
LSE Personal Social Services Research Unit
 (PSSRU) 283
Lubbe, T. 212
Lygo, V. 119

McCoy, T. P. 119
McCreight, B. S. 112
McDermott, S. 84
McEwen, B. S. 20
McKenzie-McHarg, K. 142
MacKinnon, N. 17
major depressive disorder (MDD) 120, 219
Mansfield, C. 84, 86
March of Dimes' NICU Family Support
 Program 179
March of Dimes website 179, 182
Markin, R. D. 122
Marteau, T.M. 84
Massachusetts Child Psychiatry Access Program for
 Moms (MCPAP for Moms) 34–35
Maternal Antenatal Attachment Scale (MAAS) 279
Maternal Attachment Inventory (MAI) 279
maternal cortisol 15
maternal depression: link between breastfeeding
 and 200–201
Maternal-Fetal Attachment Scale (MFAS) 278–279
Maternal Mental Health Alliance (MMHA) 283
Maternal Postnatal Attachment Scale (MPAS) 279
Maternal Postpartum Quality of Life (MAPP-QOL)
 tool 195
maternal prenatal depression 30
Mater University Study of Pregnancy 15
Matthey, S. 273
Matthey Generic Mood Question, or generic
 question on mood (MGMQ) 277–278
mediators of stress 12
medical personnels 88
Medical Termination of Pregnancy (MTP) 115
Meleis, A.I. 157
men: miscarriage and pregnancy loss and 112–113;
 psychological impact of ART on 65
mental health: investigating psychosocial
 factors having impact on 278; perinatal
 psychopathology and 278
mental health professionals 88–90; counseling
 after diagnosis 74; counseling after successful
 treatment 76; counseling after unsuccessful
 treatment 76; counseling during ART 74–75;
 counseling in transition to psychotherapy/
 psychiatric treatment 76–77; counseling
 on alternative medical support 75–76; first
 interview 73–74; interventions for 73–77
Mercer, R. 143, 160
micro-RNAs 18, 19, 289
Milgrom, J. 223, 228, 273
Miller, M. L. 155

For Product Safety Concerns and Information please contact our
EU representative GPSR@taylorandfrancis.com Taylor & Francis
Verlag GmbH, Kaufingerstraße 24, 80331 München, Germany